DECODING MAGRITTE

for
Sandro

Silvano Levy

DECODING MAGRITTE

Sansom & Company

First published in 2015 by Sansom & Co
A publishing imprint of Redcliffe Press Ltd.,
First edition
First impression

81g Pembroke Road, Bristol BS8 3EA
www.sansomandcompany.co.uk
info@sansomandcompany.co.uk

ISBN: 978-1-906593-95-7

British Library Cataloguing-in-Publication Data
A catalogue record for this book is available from the British Library.

Designed by Simon Bishop
Printed in the Czech Republic via Akcent Media

Cover image: René Magritte *L'Espion* (1927-8)

Contents

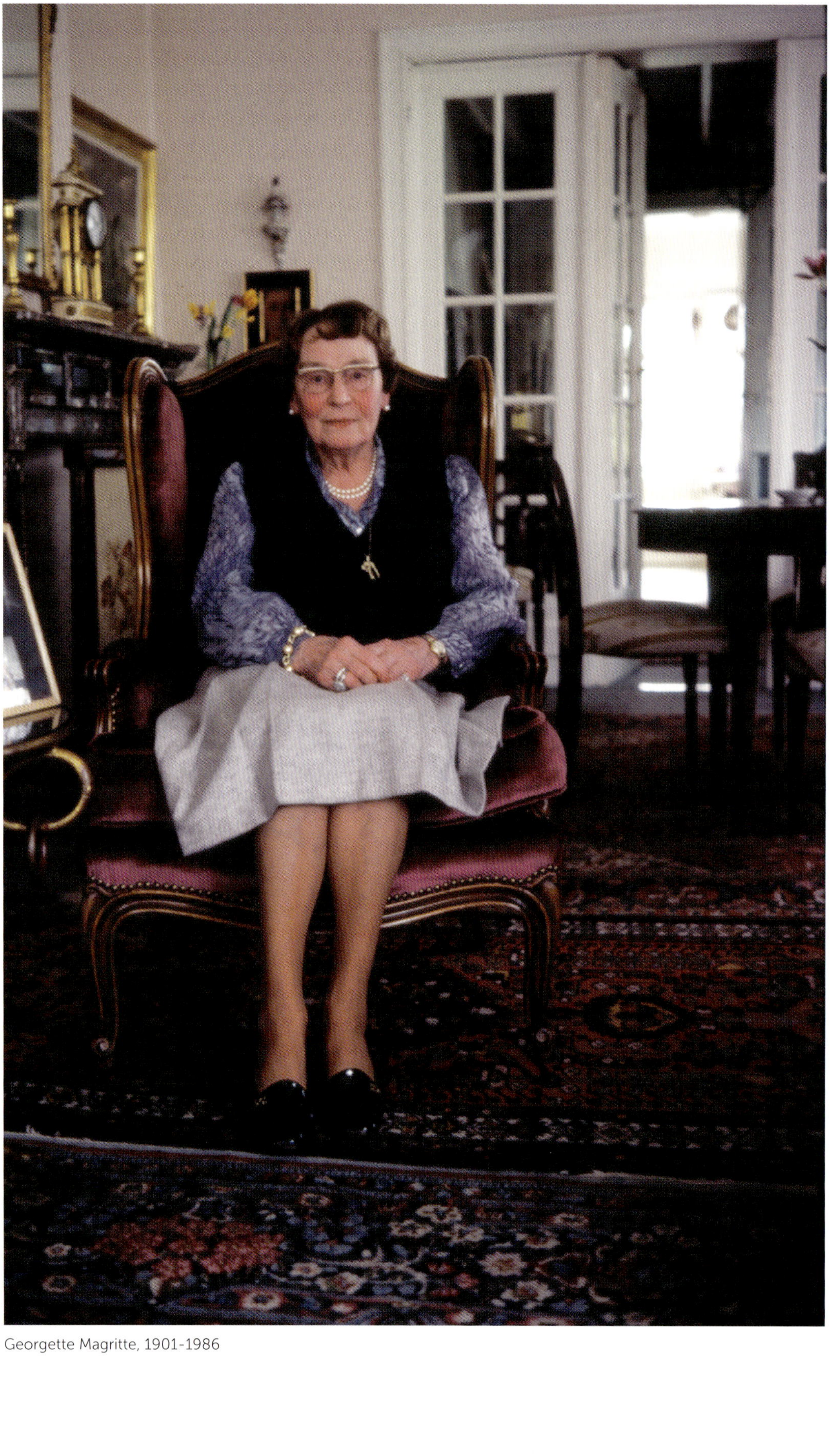

Georgette Magritte, 1901-1986

Acknowledgements

A great debt of gratitude is owed to Georgette Magritte, who unfailingly responded to my letters and repeatedly welcomed me into her home. She generously gave her time to answer questions and offer personal insights into her late husband's general outlook, mores and approaches to painting. Particularly memorable was her spontaneous piano performance in the sitting room of 97 rue des Mimosas, in response to my reminding her that René had been in the habit of asking her to play Satie's *Gymnopédies*. Her memory and inspiration lie behind this book.

I am equally appreciative for the hospitality and hours of revealing discussion that were kindly afforded by Louis Scutenaire, Irène Hamoir, Marcel Mariën, George Melly and M. and Mme DeKnop, whose first-hand testimonies of René Magritte were indispensable to the ideas developed in the pages that follow.

Central to the trajectory pursued in this book was the guidance of Roger Cardinal, from whose expertise I benefitted greatly. Michel Remy gave advice concerning translations, for which I am most appreciative. Encouragement and assistance were also kindly given by Conroy Maddox, Toni del Renzio, Desmond Morris, Randolph Quirk, Margaret Davies, Wendy Gibson, Andre Bollen, Andrew Murray, Dawn Ades, Diana Melly, Julie Lawson, David Walker, Gisèle Ollinger-Zinque, Marc Quaghebeur, Neil Matheson, Gerry White of the National Art Library in London, Luc Wanlin of the Archives et Musée de la Littérature in Brussels, Ann Simpson, Kirstie Meehan of the Scottish National Gallery of Modern Art Library, Archive and Special Books Collection, Katherine Jones and Hazel Levy.

I am grateful for the support of the British Academy.

BRITISH ACADEMY
for the humanities and social sciences

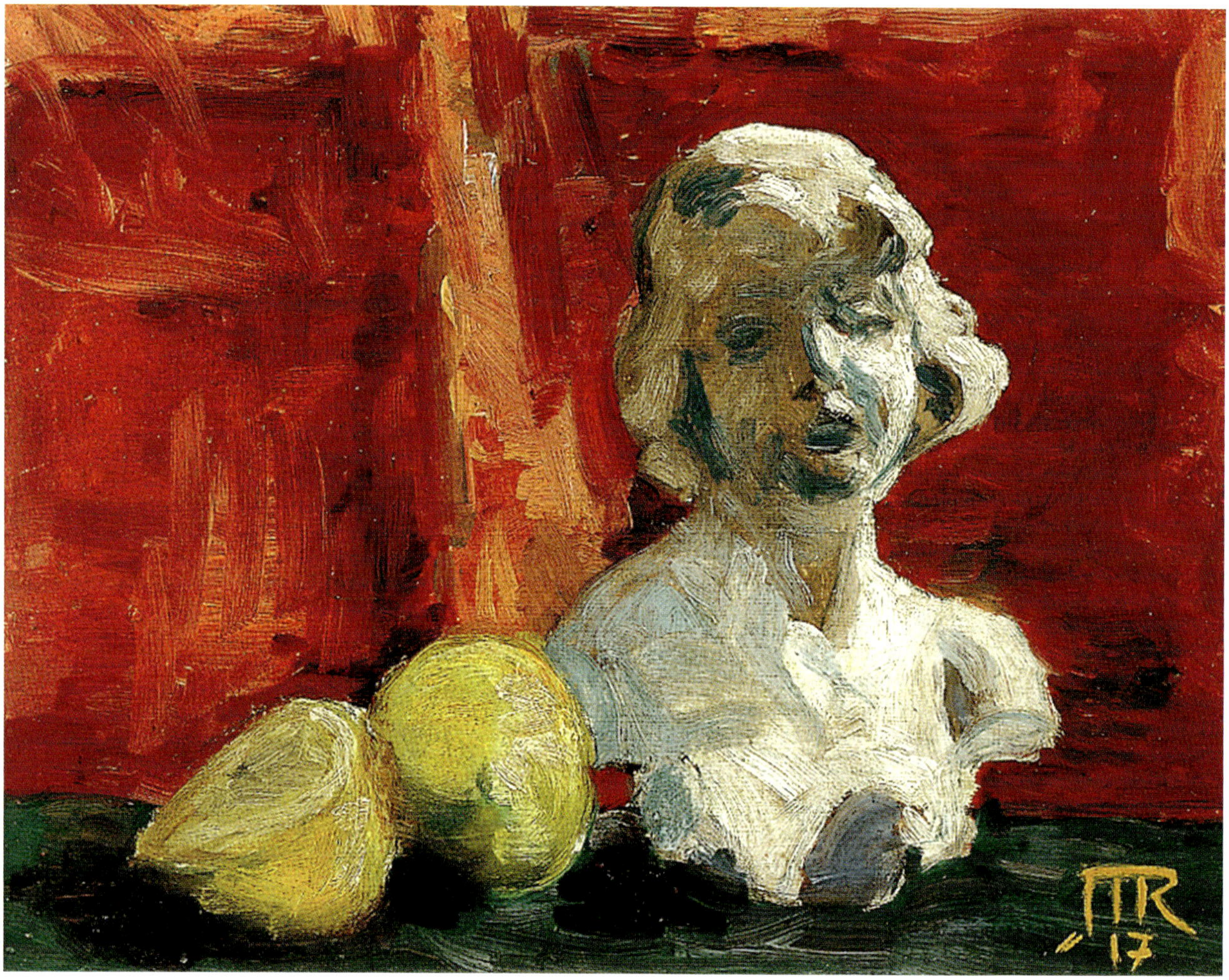

Buste en plâtre et fruits (1917)

To Decode or not to Decode

René Magritte would have been the first to condemn an attempt to decode his work. The very idea that his paintings could be accounted for in terms of a systematic conceptual mechanism, however hidden or sophisticated, would have been abhorrent to him. Indeed, he was always at pains to de-route any probing in this direction and whenever he was asked to explain his visual conundrums, he simply responded with further riddles. His favourite catch-words were 'the mysterious', 'the hidden', 'the marvellous' and 'the imagined'. He even wrote treatises around these nebulous notions that left the reader none the wiser. One of his closest surrealist collaborators, Louis Scutenaire, had to acknowledge that he couldn't make head or tail of them. Magritte incessantly and deliberately span webs of intrigue that bewildered an already perplexed audience of aficionados. This, however, was not without reason.

Bitter experience had convinced him that the best policy was to ward off his avid interpreters. What he knew only too well was that, time after time, his paintings had borne the brunt of crass explanations.[1] 'Most of the time people try to destroy the images that I paint by professing to "interpret" them.'[2] Above all, Magritte could not tolerate the reduction of his work to a banal symbolism. He was once incensed when, during a formal occasion, an ambassador set about interpreting one of his paintings as being a reflection of the political and economic situation in Israel.[3] Not surprisingly, it was not long before Magritte came to regard art criticism in general as an absurd waste of time:

> Foolishness consists in believing you understand what you really don't. You can see this clearly in those more or less endless discourses on art, which are made as academic and boring as possible.[4]

Whilst distrusting elucidation posited by his commentators, Magritte himself did make numerous statements in exhibition catalogues, lectures and manifestos, which maintained that there was, in fact, a coherent philosophical basis to his production. On rare occasions he even acknowledged that competent and edifying commentaries on his work had been produced.[5] What is clear from Magritte's comments is that he felt that analysis could be a valid exercise and even one that reinforced the intention of his work, but only, as he insisted, within specific parameters. For him, the only acceptable type of analysis was one that showed his paintings to be the consequence of unbridled intellect:

> I consider accounts that present my paintings as having been conceived as material signs of the liberty of thought to be valid.[6]

This book is just such an attempt. It maps out the complex intellectual route that Magritte pursued, his 'period of research', as he put it, that began in the early 1920s and lasted some ten years, during which he tirelessly interrogated painting and sought to extricate it from the conventions and rules that limited it.[7] With a view to uncovering the Magrittian *system*, the focus will be turned on the *deep* structures of the works, their inner configuration, which will, ultimately, emerge as functions of an algorithm of the pictorial construct. The paintings themselves will therefore be approached in terms of *surface* manifestations, capable of being unravelled into the components of their core workings, capable, that is to say, of being *decoded*.

✣ ✣ ✣

Putting a date to the beginning of Magritte's experimental phase, during which his code was elaborated, is not straightforward. Magritte himself confuses the issue by stating that this ten-year period started both in '1916' and also 'after having followed the courses at l'Académie des Beaux-Arts', which, according to E.L.T. Mesens and André Blavier, was no earlier than 1920.[8] Whilst Patrick Waldberg suggests that it was 'in 1919' that the chance discovery of some modernist trends in painting 'acted like a jolt upon Magritte and oriented him towards *new investigations*',[9] David Sylvester establishes that Magritte's Academy enrolment, which had been interrupted by National Service, definitively ended in 1920.[10] Of limited relevance is the division into periods, made by Louis Scutenaire and adopted by José Vovelle, which advances an initial demarcation of '1925' and is based on style, an aspect of Magritte's work which only became consistent by the mid twenties.[11] Scutenaire writes of 'an unusual style, rudimentary forms, earth colours'.[12] Of more significance are Magritte's fundamental motivations, which crystallized from the earliest works precisely at a time when his 'style' was far from being established.

Additionally, to say that Magritte was motivated by a desire to 'liberate' painting is problematic in its own right. Of course, artistic freedom had existed since the late nineteenth century and by the 1870s the academic techniques demanded by formal art had been abandoned by the Impressionists. Instead of following the traditional ideas of composition and drawing, which were based on line and solid colouring, artists like Monet, Sisley and Pissaro applied paint in tiny dabs and omitted the firm outline. Equally, in the 1880s, the Synthetists, Gauguin, Bernard and van Gogh, had completely rejected the aim of naturalistic representation and produced works whose relation to external reality was routinely tenuous. Against this background, the sense in which Magritte may be said to strive for liberation necessarily goes beyond the simple notion of rejecting the techniques of painting or its representational aspirations. 'Not for an instant', Scutenaire assures us, 'did Magritte concern himself with attacking painting.'[13] Indeed, the meticulous *trompe-l'œil* technique, which Magritte maintained for most of his career, demonstrates that he endorsed and practised many of its canons. Contrary to Sarah Whitfield's view that 'he wanted to break with art', Magritte remained positively entrenched within the ambit of the pictorial.[14]

Yet, whilst retaining the pictorial elements which representational convention prescribes, Magritte did diverge from formal art inasmuch as he rejected the *systematization* that traditional painting places on those elements. What Magritte did was extract the figures and settings which established art endorses from the schema of art as a whole and reorganize them in accordance with his own designs. As Louis Scutenaire puts forward, Magritte did not so much attack painting as 'bring it to heel, making it submit to the torrent of images that sprang from his internal fire'.[15] It would be more accurate to say that Magritte sought freedom *in* painting rather than freedom *from* it.

If Magritte was to have this free rein over the products of figuration, he was clearly faced with the task of divorcing them from the formal rules with which they had been associated and which, for centuries, had governed their utilization. His basic mission was to isolate the various constituents, which together made up the complex of painting. He needed to render them discrete through a decontextualization that would result in their autonomy within the pictorial structure. In other words, Magritte's 'liberation' of painting amounted to no less than the elimination of the monopoly that academic pictorial systematization had exercised over the raw material of figurative representation since the Renaissance. Even though Magritte may never have consciously articulated this particular aim, such an underlying preoccupation is implicit throughout his early work. He clearly conducted a suite of 'experiments' that progressively distanced the elements of painting from their orthodox functions and systematically diminished and subdivided the very means of depiction. As, for Magritte, the painting was 'a constructed object', he demonstrably considered it capable of being dismantled, deconstructed.[16] Indeed, he was to 'take apart' not only form, but also space; under his brush, objects became incomplete and segmented, while pictorial space was broken up into separate, self-contradictory zones. Effectively, Magritte freed the unit parts of formal art from the *order*, as well as from the *form*, that formal art had placed on them. As John Berger remarks, 'there is such a thing as a reduction, not to absurdity, but to freedom'.[17] Magritte's work centres on just such a reduction.

Inevitably, a denudation of the devices of representation must eventually verge on what may be considered to be the 'frontier' of painting. In their persistent erosion of the rules of painting, Magritte's works were destined to lead to the extremities of the system itself, to what cannot be considered as the realm of painting. Indeed, by the end of his experimental period Magritte found that his

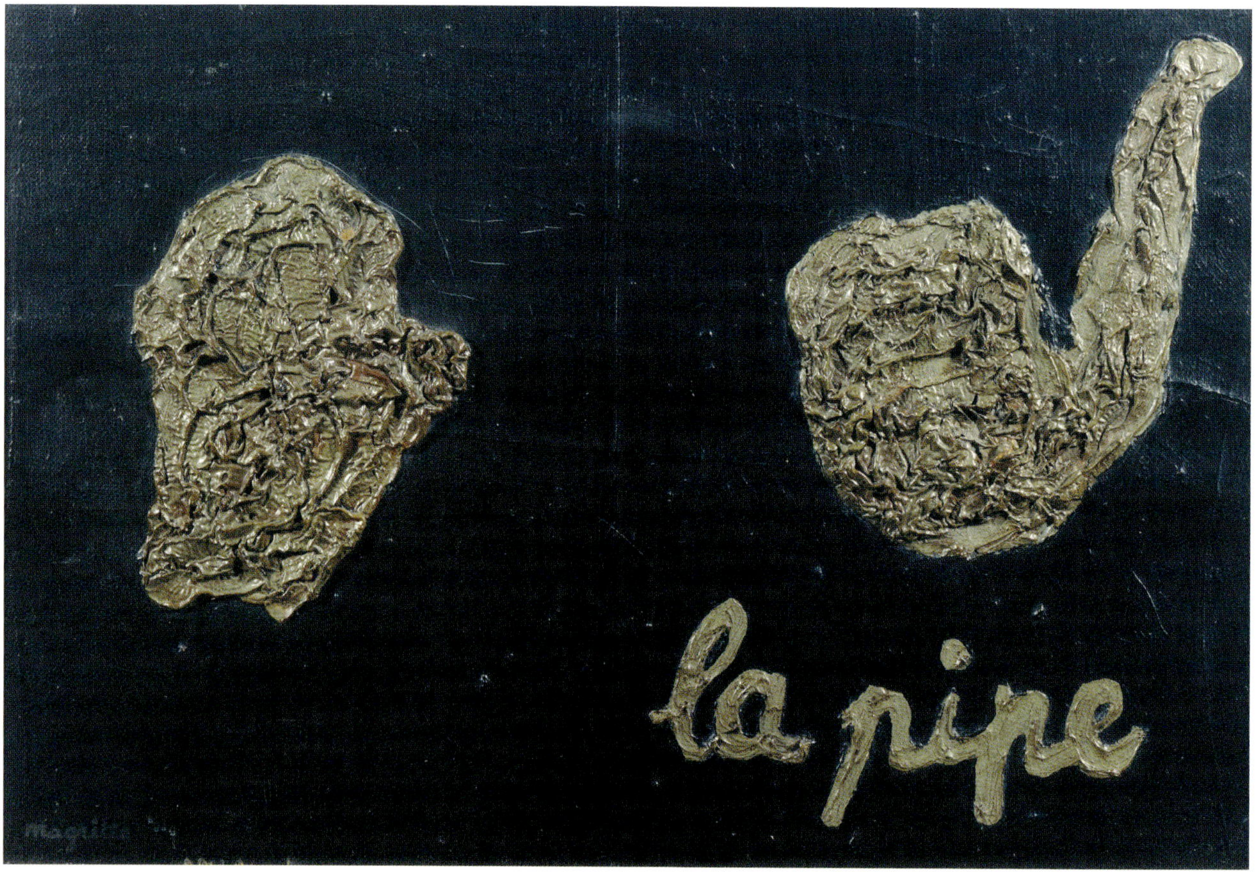

La Pipe (1923)

line of enquiry had taken him *beyond* painting. It had transgressed the pictorial to such a degree that his work of the late 1920s could be said to appertain not so much to 'painting', as to a wholly divergent system of signification, that of language. At that juncture, when Magritte could be said neither to be wholly writing nor wholly painting, the imperatives and constraints of neither system held sway. Whilst still engaging with the painter's ritual of putting paint onto canvas, he moved his work beyond the orbit of the pictorial schema with a vocabulary that became increasingly extrinsic to the rules of representation.

This conceptual step, however, honed over some ten years and centring on a systematic critique of the academic pictorial construct, was taken in progressive stages that were neither conscious nor methodical on the part of Magritte. Indeed, his route was more often than not inconsistent and non-sequential. In many instances, the paintings treat problems posed by consecutive 'stages of painting' in a meandering way. Typically, a work with a particular focus would be followed by another with a divergent theme, which may have already been investigated or not yet fully elaborated. As Suzi Gablik observes,

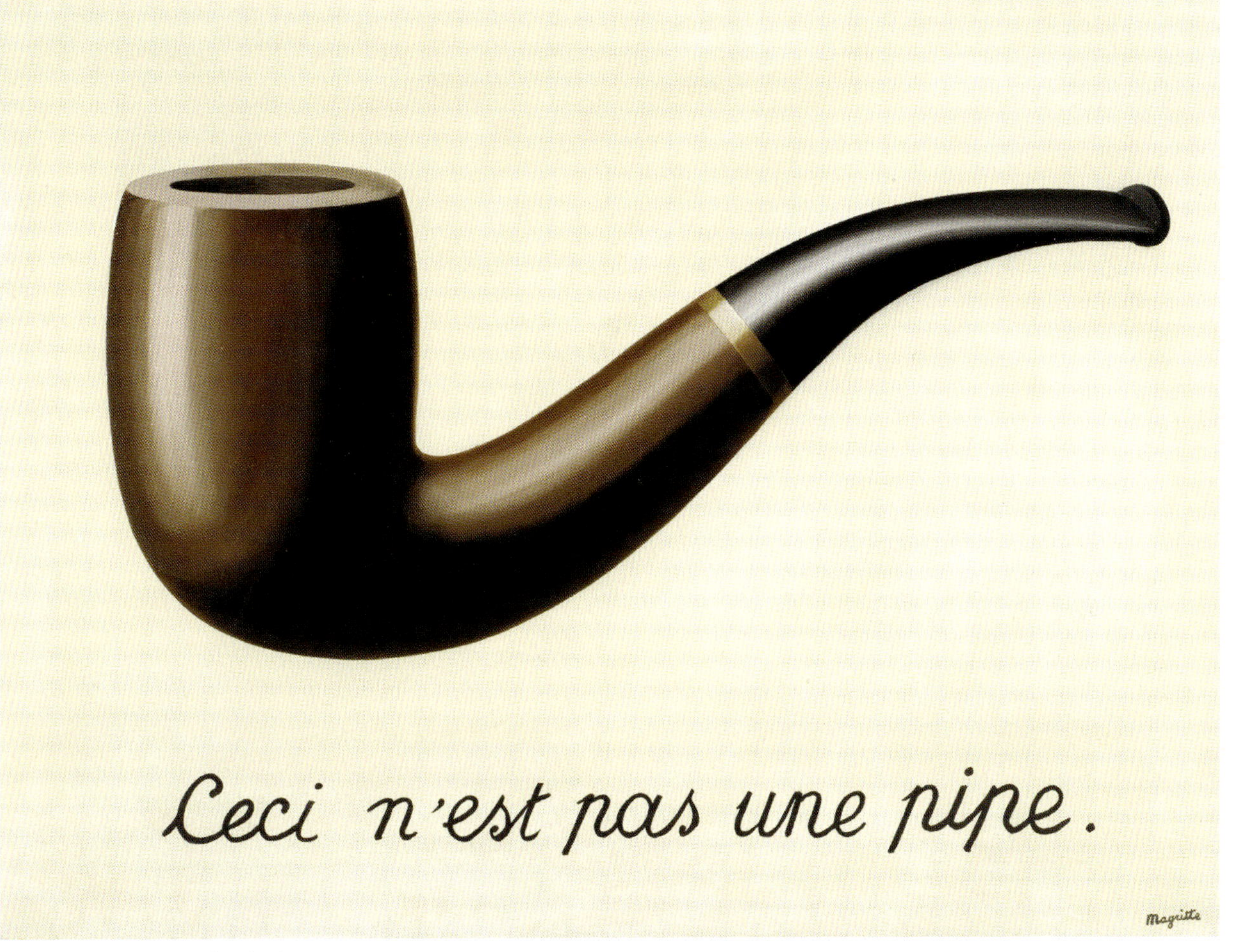

La Trahison des images (1928-9)

Magritte 'tended to work back and forth through a small range of variants at different times, elaborating on certain key ideas'.[18] For this reason, any critique of Magritte's work would only be de-routed by more than a cursory regard for chronology, being far better served by an approach that, as Suzi Gablik advocates, proceeds 'taxonomically rather than chronologically' and appreciates that 'each separate work has a positional value in relation to a sequence'.[19] For instance, *La Trahison des images* (1928-9) marks the culmination of a pictorial line of reasoning spanning several years, in the course of which verbal elements became oppositions to and contradictions of the pictorial depiction. Yet, in a painting executed as early as 1923, *La Pipe*, not only was Magritte exploring this same concept, but he was doing so in practically identical terms. Just like *La Trahison des images*, the earlier *La Pipe* contains the depiction of a pipe, albeit in a rudimentary form, which is placed in opposition to its verbal equivalent. The phrase 'la pipe', appearing in heavy impasto next to the silhouette of a pipe, emerges as tautological and, thus, superfluous. As in the later work, the presence of the written word renders the image redundant. Clearly, as early as 1923, Magritte had already formulated the notion of negating images by means of words.

Before examining the disassembly of the visual construct to which Magritte devoted his early oeuvre, however, this study turns to a survey of the period in his career immediately following his training at the Academy of Arts, during which he became involved with avant-garde thinkers and artists from whom he derived insights into Abstraction, Cubism and Dada. These anti-art movements acted as catalysts that prompted Magritte's radical probing of the canons of art and led to an iconoclastic subversion that deconstructed the pictorial paradigm into a fully articulated *code*.

---

[1] André Blavier suggests that Michel Foucault had 'misinterpreted' Magritte, in René Magritte, *Écrits complets* (Paris, 1979), p. 521, unnumbered footnote. Also, Magritte had criticized Achille Chavée for having taken 'the liberty to interpret my paintings', in Magritte, *Écrits complets*, pp. 596-7.

[2] Magritte, *Écrits complets*, p. 597.

[3] Suzi Gablik, 'A Conversation with René Magritte', *Studio International*, 173/887 (Mar. 1967): 28.

[4] Magritte, in Georges d'Amphoux, 'Magritte, prince des surréalistes belges', *Phare Dimanche* (Brussels, 23 Feb. 1958): 9. All citations from French texts are translated by the author.

[5] Magritte on Paul Nougé, in Magritte, *Écrits complets*, p. 110.

[6] Magritte, *Écrits complets*, p. 376.

[7] André Breton, in *Magritte*, exhibition catalogue Obelisk Gallery (London, 1961), p. 26. Magritte, *Écrits complets*, p. 552.

[8] Magritte, *Écrits complets*, p. 552. Édouard Mesens, 'The World of René Magritte', *The Saturday Book*, 19 (London, 1959): 274. André Blavier, in Magritte, *Écrits complets*, p. 369.

[9] Patrick Waldberg, *René Magritte* (Brussels, 1965), pp. 82 & 88.

[10] David Sylvester, *René Magritte: Catalogue Raisonné Volume 1: Oil Paintings 1916-1930* (London, 1992), p. 13.

[11] José Vovelle, *Le Surréalisme en Belgique* (Brussels, 1972), pp. 77-81. Louis Scutenaire, *Avec Magritte* (Brussels, 1977), p. 160.

[12] Scutenaire, *Avec Magritte*, p. 161.

[13] Scutenaire, *Avec Magritte*, p. 161.

[14] Sarah Whitfield, *Magritte* (London, 1992), p. 17.

[15] Scutenaire, *Avec Magritte*, p. 161.

[16] Magritte, *Écrits complets*, p. 19.

[17] John Berger, 'A Way to Magritte', *New Society*, 338 (20 Mar. 1969): 450.

[18] Suzi Gablik, *Magritte*, (London, 1971), p. 15.

[19] Gablik, *Magritte*, p. 15.

REBEL IN THE MAKING
1919-1924

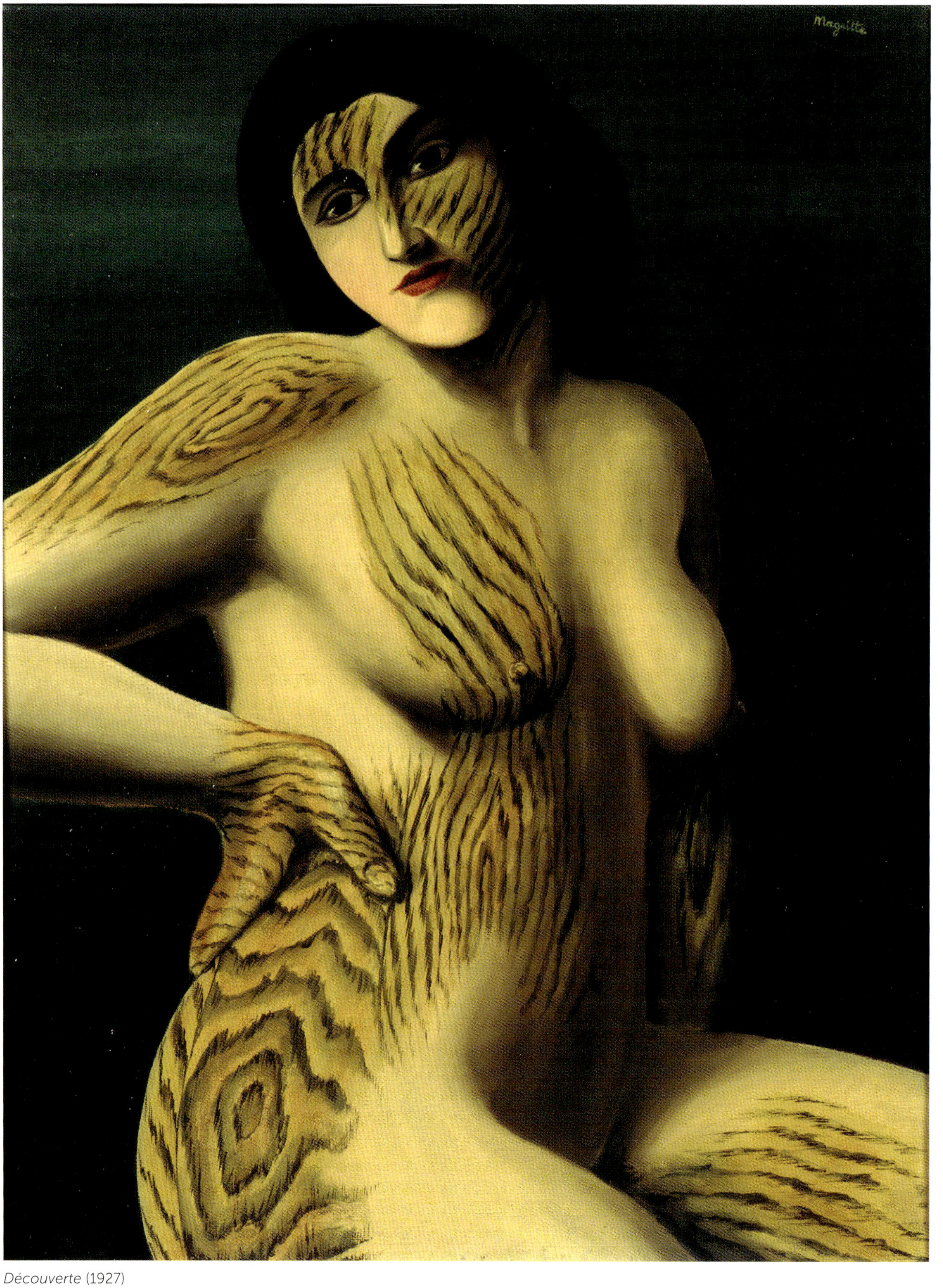

Découverte (1927)

Rebel Artist

Analysing Magritte's works as a critique of the principles meted out by an early twentieth-century formal art education becomes all the more plausible when it is considered in an historical context. This would not only reflect the preoccupations of the artists and writers with whom Magritte was in close contact, but also the general trends of the time. At the start of Magritte's career, the Brussels artistic *milieu* was charged with a desire for change. Traditional methods of teaching art had generally remained unchanged for generations and the Académie Royale des Beaux-Arts et École des Arts Décoratifs, founded in 1768, was offering such courses as 'Flora, Fauna and Landscape', 'Ornamental Composition', 'Decorative Painting', 'Anatomy' and 'Perspective', all of which Magritte attended during his intermittent time as an officially enrolled art student between 1916 and 1920. The overall pedagogical framework was formal and prescriptive, with the notion of timeworn 'rules' at the forefront. As with all art academies, the standards were, in essence, founded on the exacting geometric precepts first propounded by Leon Battista Alberti.

Alberti's systemization of the various construction stages of painting and sculpture is generally acknowledged as fundamental to formal art:

> Alberti's 'della pittura' is the prophetic book of academism. There is practically no part of academic teaching during the next four hundred years which does not lie, compressed but calculated, in its pages.[1]

A flavour of the rigour of Alberti's canons is given by his instructions regarding the 'orthogonals' and the 'transversals' of his complex perspectival formulae. To establish the orthogonals, he states, one begins by drawing a quadrangle whose base-line is divided into 'braccia' measuring one third of the height of the figures in the painting. Then, a 'centric point' needs to be established at the eye level of the observer and in the centre of the panel. In this way, Alberti continues, the observer and the painted figures will appear to occupy the same spatial setting. The orthogonals are then to be drawn from the divisions in the base line to the centric point. With similar rigour, Alberti stipulates that the transversals must progressively diminish by one third. The distance of the first transversal from the base and so the actual distance between the subsequent transversals is to be established by first dividing a horizontal line into *braccia*. Then, another horizontal line is to be drawn above the first line and parallel to it at a vertical distance from the base equal to the distance of the centric point from its base. The distance of the eye of the observer to the panel is then marked on the parallel line from a point above the first *braccio* marking.[2] Subsequently, lines are drawn from the eye distance mark to the baseline markings and the divisions established on the vertical line are taken to be equal to the distances between the transversals. Finally, transversals are drawn on the original panel on this basis.

It was such exactitude and pedantry that was under attack after the Great War, when an emerging notion of a 'modern' conception of art gave rise to the formation of groups of young intellectuals who advocated the dynamic avant-garde of the time. To this end, a magazine called *Au Volant: Art et littérature* was launched in 1919 by the brothers Victor and Pierre Bourgeois, with whom Magritte became acquainted towards the end of his course at the Academy, and in whose gallery, Le Centre d'Art, at 6 rue Coudenberg in Brussels, he was to exhibit for the first time.[3] As the title of the magazine implies, the editors sought to extend the changing attitudes of the 'modern' era to the realm of art and literature. In the manifesto 'Vers la plénitude par la dictature de la Conscience' (Guided to Fulfilment by the Diktats of Consciousness), appearing in the first issue of April 1919, a stand was made against the subjugation of the creative act to external reality, as convention is said to have favoured at that time.[4] The artist is urged away from 'a creative submissiveness', which is said to entail 'the engulfment of the Creator by Things [...] the submersion of the individual by Reality [...] the Supremacy of the Elements over the Maker, of materials over the Builder'. What is regarded as more appropriate for the *artistic* creator is determinism. The article champions personal strength of character and resourcefulness and implies that such traits should be echoed in the creative act: 'the premise of aesthetic creation is [...] the individual's ability to dominate himself and the world'. Somewhat melodramatically, it asks: 'Does not this uplifting term, "Master", charged with sumptuousness, encapsulate the supreme state to which you aspire?' Leaving aside the hyperbolic style, what comes across in the text is the emphasis on the drastic nature of the proposed change in attitudes towards the role of the artist. The modern view of art is presented as an upheaval of accepted ideas. In contrast to what is implied to be current practice, art is directed towards a keener use of the senses and a more imperious, even arrogant, responsibility for fashioning the way in which the world is conceptualized:

> The inner enthusiasm that presides over the execution of works of art, which we habitually term 'inspiration' is, in the final analysis, no more than a passionate propensity of Consciousness to absorb the ephemeral form of things in order to change them, through sparks of lucidity, into concrete sounds or shapes. Essentially, we confuse inspiration with the workings of Consciousness, which endeavours to tap internal or external forces in order to recreate them as beauty.

Au Volant put forward that the new principle from which art is said to emanate, 'Consciousness', engenders what can be termed a 'direct comprehension' that penetrates immediate appearances to reveal the core of things. With such 'mastery', the article argues, the artist is charged with the task of

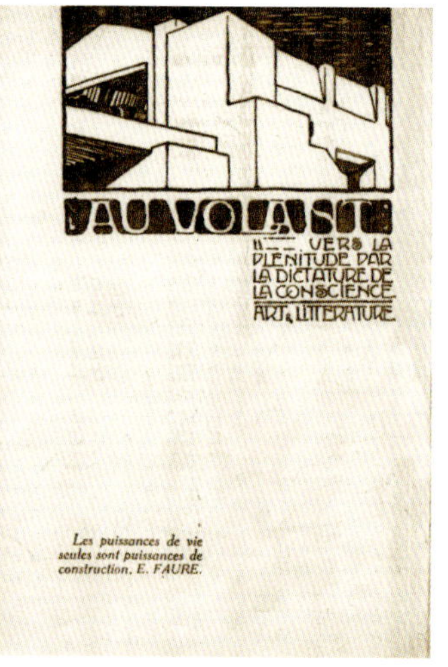

Au Volant. Art et littérature, 1 (Apr. 1919)

overriding the given order and moulding visible phenomena in a 'conscious' manner, a trajectory, as it turned out, that was to be subsumed within Magritte's oeuvre of the twenties in an unwavering and literal manner. As the manifesto spells out, in a manner that uncannily anticipates the basic tenets of surrealism, the task of the artist is to capture the internal and external worlds in order to transform them, thereby attesting to the artist's 'liberty', a term that Magritte was to adopt as a central tenet in his later treatises on the meaning of painting:

> Slaves of Consciousness – that's the only route for free artists, for, as such, they acquire the regal capacity of seizing the full extent and intensity of the world and of their dreams, as well as the god-like ability to mould them according to their own image through expressive form.

The modern artist is said no longer to need to pay lip service to an awe-inspiring 'Creation'. Rather, s/he is to be 'conscious', cogently absorbing Creation and regulating the world. With an image that accounts for the title of the magazine, the article concludes:

> Being conscious does not mean refusing to sit in a racing car; it means only accepting a seat in it as the driver.

The symbol of the motor car, which encapsulated modernity, the new machine age and speed, stands for the rejection of the traditional and the espousal of new values. *Au Volant* (at the steering wheel) urges the artist to take an active part in the modern world. Decorative painting and sculpture, we are told, are to be 'reintegrated into their context', that is to say are to be determined by the artist, as opposed to hackneyed convention. In a challenge against the conservative limitations traditionally imposed on the role of art, the creative artist is urged to place him/herself 'at the steering wheel' of a fast moving world, rather than acquiesce to the prescriptions of the backward-looking formal art institutions.

The fourth issue of *Au Volant* makes just this point. Its editorial, 'Prolegomena', explicitly criticizes 'the training of artists', leaving no doubt that the focus of its disapprobation is academic pedagogy.[5] Yet, we are told that this is nothing new and that the methods of art instruction had for some time been the subject of controversy; some of its critics had even suggested its abolition – 'demolish all the academies'. *Au Volant* itself does not go quite that far. Whilst denouncing the way in which the Brussels Academy was conducted, it also advocates its conservation. It supports proposals instigated by Victor Horta some years earlier that had called for 'the reorganization of courses at the Brussels Fine Arts Academy'. This is not to say that *Au Volant*'s 'art of Consciousness' is not drastically at odds with the expectations of traditional academic art. Indeed, the journal demands reformulations that are both extreme and radical. The inconsistency of this stance, however, is not lost on the editors, who openly admit: 'what a paradox – an avant-garde review upholding an official establishment'. Nevertheless, for Magritte this very point was to prove pivotal. Particularly during the 1920s, his work was to abide by the broad lines of his training at the Brussels Fine Arts Academy, whilst fundamentally reformulating it. In accord with the hopes of *Au Volant*, Magritte was to 'liberate' painting from the precise formulae of academic orthodoxy whilst never straying from the general framework of concepts that constitute formal art. For him, this was no contradiction in terms.

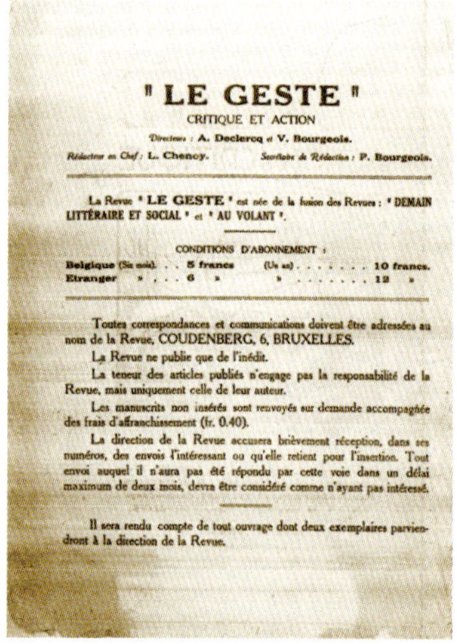

" LE GESTE "
CRITIQUE ET ACTION
Directeurs : A. Declercq et V. Bourgeois.
Rédacteur en Chef : L. Chenoy. Secrétaire de Rédaction : P. Bourgeois.

La Revue " LE GESTE " est née de la fusion des Revues : " DEMAIN LITTÉRAIRE ET SOCIAL " et " AU VOLANT ".

CONDITIONS D'ABONNEMENT :

Belgique (Six mois)	5 francs	(Un an)	10 francs.
Etranger »	6 »	»	12 »

Toutes correspondances et communications doivent être adressées au nom de la Revue, COUDENBERG, 6, BRUXELLES.

La Revue ne publie que de l'inédit.

La teneur des articles publiés n'engage pas la responsabilité de la Revue, mais uniquement celle de leur auteur.

Les manuscrits non insérés sont renvoyés sur demande accompagnée des frais d'affranchissement (fr. 0.40).

La direction de la Revue accusera brièvement réception, dans ses numéros, des envois l'intéressant ou qu'elle retient pour l'insertion. Tout envoi auquel il n'aura pas été répondu par cette voie dans un délai maximum de deux mois, devra être considéré comme n'ayant pas intéressé.

Il sera rendu compte de tout ouvrage dont deux exemplaires parviendront à la direction de la Revue.

Le Geste. Critique et action, 1 (Dec. 1919)

Yet another prophetic notion in *Au Volant*, as far as Magritte's later work is concerned, is its insistence on 'integral teaching [...] a shrewd alliance of all the sciences to achieve a fully-rounded aesthetic' or in other words, the formation of links between the various art forms. It is suggested that 'the poet and the musician draw on all the verbal and sonorous richness that exists in the plastic arts'. It would not be too long, as it turned out, before Magritte was to experiment with the inverse proposition, namely the plastic treatment of music and words; his paintings were to incorporate both words and sheet music. What is not clear, however, is whether he was in any way directly responsible for the formulation of the magazine's position on art, which he clearly endorsed. His name appears under the heading of 'Board of Directors', but his named contributions to the publication are solely pictorial: he illustrated Pierre Bourgeois' poems *Ciel et terril* and *Ouverte et Fermée* and designed an ex libris.[6] All that can be said, therefore, is that Magritte's works of the early twenties concur with the principles of the Brussels avant-garde in a general sense. *Le Geste: Critique et action*, an avant-garde magazine formed in 1919 by the merger of *Au Volant* and *Demain littéraire et social*, champions his work and describes his exhibition, jointly-held with Pierre-Louis Flouquet at the Centre d'Art on 10 January 1920, as a 'successful innovation'.[7] Magritte is clearly counted among the 'innovators' whom the magazine promotes.[8] The classification 'new' in this context signifies the idea of surpassing the artistic traditions of the past, and it is this aspect of Magritte's work that is brought out in the review of the exhibition; 'such noble experiments – to break away from the objective literality that previous generations had prescribed'.[9] Magritte's work is held up as the essence of the 'modern' conception of art, being said to convey 'the real perception of what lies at the heart of life', an achievement that dovetails with *Au Volant*'s aspiration to the 'diktats of Consciousness'.[10]

Not only can Magritte rightly be said to have 'emerged in the midst of this stream of theorising', but his work maps directly onto it.[11] It is not surprising, therefore, that he was chosen as one of the Belgian representatives at the *Exposition internationale d'art moderne* in Geneva from 26 December 1920 to 25 January 1921, an event at which the emphasis was on 'radical renewal'.[12] From the preface of the 1921 exhibition catalogue, it becomes clear that the insistence of the Brussels avant-garde magazines on the replacement of the established conventions of art represented a widely held view:

> We are on the verge of an unknown order, but the way forward is cluttered by the deeply decadent ways of the previous order. But the disintegration of decadence spawns the long-awaited system.[13]

According to *Au Volant*, the Paris Academy had led the way with changes that it saw as forming 'a perfect model'.[14] Perhaps the main reason for the general belief in the possibility of institutionalized 'modern' art instruction was the foundation in 1919 by Walter Gropius of the progressive Bauhaus School of architecture and design at Weimar.[15] This was seen as inaugurating empirical methods that exemplified the modern, 'conscious', approach to creativity:

> Painting studios have been replaced by laboratories, where students are put through an intensive training through all the senses, all the mental faculties involved in creation.[16]

Nevertheless, the hopes of the young Bruxellois were to remain unsatisfied throughout the decade. In 1924, the magazine *L'Esprit nouveau* was still expressing the same hopes of change in attitudes:

> Before achieving a new work of art, a complete work of art capable of satisfying complete men, we must fashion new men.[17]

Even as late as 1930, the position had remained unchanged and pedagogic practice was still seen as incompatible with the ideals of the modern movements; 'the modern vision' was still 'a challenge [...] to the norm'.[18] Indeed, *Le Centaure*, published by the gallery of the same name and in which Magritte had held his first solo exhibition in 1927, makes the point that the academic curriculum was as archaic then as it had been in 1920:

> Nothing is more absurd than continuing to insist on a formal language belonging to another age, as is done in certain academies. If we want to instigate a veritably effectual training, we need ruthlessly to do away with all the outdated formulae, to do away with anatomy and perspective classes [...] which are still taught in our art schools.[19]

This statement simply reiterates the stand made by *Au Volant* a decade earlier. Progress was clearly an uphill struggle for the Brussels avant-garde who, despite persistent calls for modernization, increasingly realized that academic tradition was well and truly entrenched, particularly at the Brussels Academy, where Magritte had received his training between 1916 and 1918. It is not surprising therefore that the disgruntled former student, who actively decried academic pedagogy, should have engaged in what has been termed a 'revolt that puts

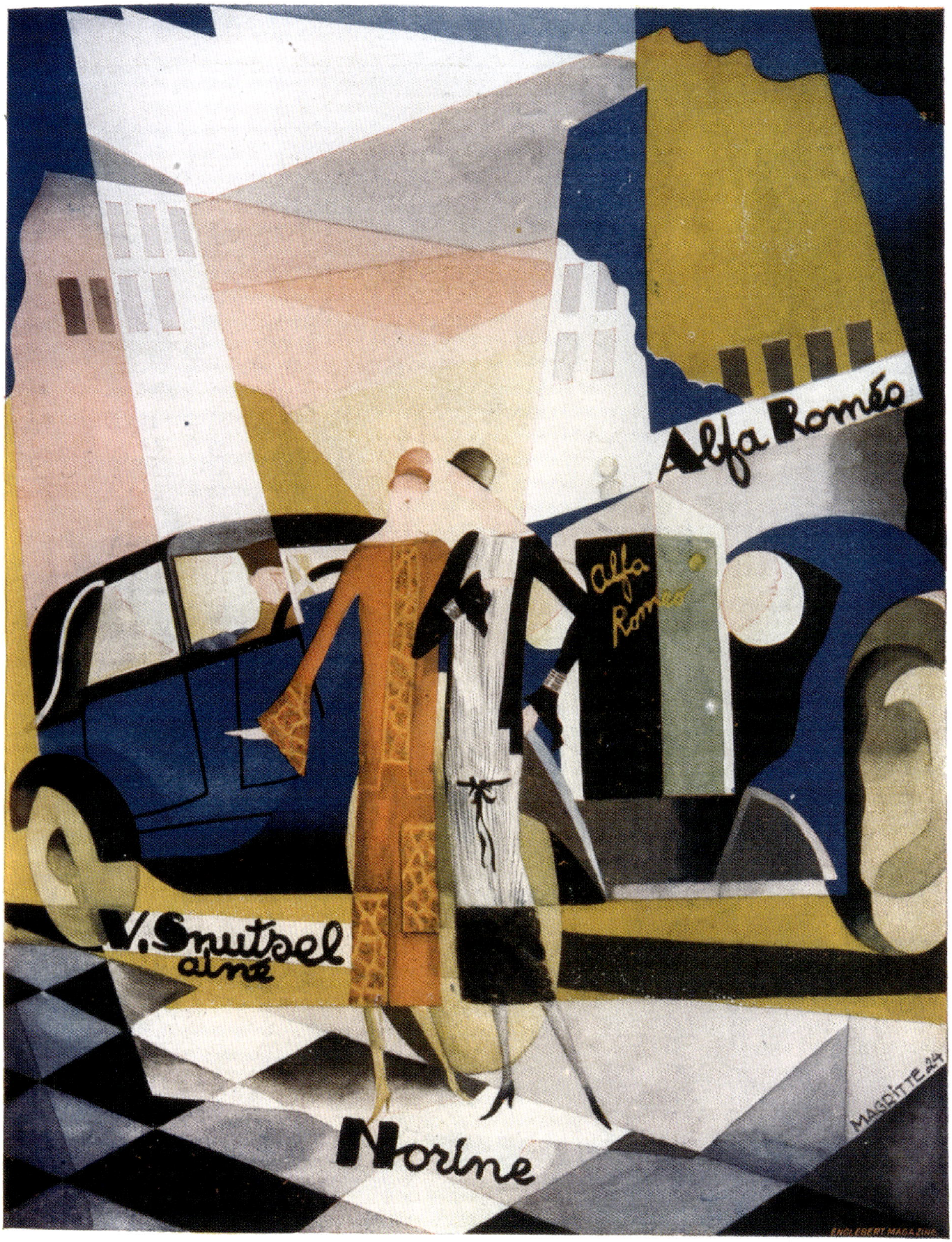

Harmonie moderne (1924)

him at odds with the academism of still-life and traditional composition'.[20] Of course, this is precisely what Gropius had advocated and, rather tellingly, an advertisement appeared in Magritte and Mesens' 1925 journal *Œsophage* for the gallery Cabinet Maldoror, that announced exhibitions by, amongst others, Klee, Schlemmer, Kandinsky, Feininger, Moholy-Nagy and Georg Grosz, all of whom were teachers at the Bauhaus.

Magritte himself is included in the list of 'the most daring painters' and, indeed, particularly during the 1920s, his work openly paralleled the experiments of the German school.[21] What the Bauhaus set out to provide was an alternative to the conventional academic formation of art students. It eliminated, for instance, the distinction between fine art and crafts; Gropius stated that 'the Bauhaus is consciously formulating a new coordination of the means of construction and expression'.[22] Rather than observe the world with preconceived ideas, he wanted students to investigate and re-examine the visible world. He questioned the relationships, the properties and the potential of objects. His vision combined the analytical visual skill of the artist with the practical dexterity of the craftsman. A typical class exercise would have involved the contradiction of the inherent properties of certain substances: wood would be carved so as to appear as pliable as a spiral of apple peel, paper would be folded in such a way that it would become rigid and three-dimensional. It was precisely such contradictions of the properties of materials that featured heavily in Magritte's work of the time – *L'Esprit comique* (1927) gives a paper cut-out of the voluminosity of a lurching human figure and *Découverte* (1927) endows wood with the softness and pliability of female flesh. Magritte's paradoxes blatantly echo the Bauhaus curriculum and even relate directly to one of its core courses; just as in 'The Analysis of Materials' classes, which aimed at isolating the 'elements that constitute the "grammar" of creation', Magritte strove to reduce representation to its elements.[23] But it wasn't just Magritte's restructuring of 'anatomy' that found its equivalent in the Bauhaus curriculum; his defiance of conventional 'perspective' was also paralleled by the new thinking. One of Gropius's chief concerns in 'The Theory of Space' was the redefinition of composition itself. 'What is space, how can it be understood and given a form?' were some of the questions he posed.[24] Kandinsky, for his part, developed the concept of 'tensions in a composition'.[25] Space, for him, was conceived as the convergence of forces on various foci, an approach, again, that Magritte's work of the twenties would closely reflect. *Cinéma bleu* (1925), for instance, depicts linear trajectories along which objects appear to travel and, similarly, *Harmonie moderne*, an advertisement of 1924, 'extends' objects in the composition in a way that brings to mind Feininger's *Gothen* (1919).[26] Here, the trajectory of lines that should logically terminate within the circumscription of objects is continued beyond individual forms.

That such parallels abound is not that surprising however; Magritte's dual role as commercial artist and painter was bound to blur the distinction between fine art and crafts, a key precept for Gropius. As wallpaper designer and advertisement illustrator, Magritte would have acquired the 'applied' techniques that Gropius was attempting to blend with fine art. Gropius set great store by 'practical training in the industrial world', providing workshops for display design, stage design and typography and layout, all of which resonated with Magritte's hands-on experience as poster artist and theatre scenery designer, as well as his exploitation of shop window display techniques.[27] Whilst Magritte cannot be said to have drawn directly from Gropius, his early experimentation was arguably analogous to the rebellious reformulation of artistic expression that the Bauhaus had been propounding.

---

1 Kenneth Clark, 'Leon Battista Alberti on Painting', *Annual Italian Lecture of the British Academy*, 30 (1944): 10.

2 Alberti neither explains how to determine the distance of the eye to the panel nor how to locate the vertical line on which values for the transversals are established.

3 The magazine was to have four issues, not three, as indicated in José Vovelle, *Le Surréalisme en Belgique* (Brussels, 1972), p. 75, note 26. These are dated April 1919, May 1919, August 1919 and 1919, the fourth issue not bearing a month of publication. Vovelle states that Magritte had left the Academy by 1919, p. 66.

4 *Au Volant. Art et littérature*, 1 (Apr. 1919): 1-3. The translation 'Towards plenitude through the dictates of conscience' is proposed in David Sylvester, *René Magritte: Catalogue Raisonné Volume 1: Oil Paintings 1916-1930* (London, 1992), p. 15, but this does not convey the importance accorded by the avant-garde of the early twentieth century to the notion of the supremacy of the senses, which would have been intended here. The term 'consciousness' is used in the sense of 'alertness of the senses'. Among the members of the editorial board is listed a certain 'René Maguerit'.

5 *Au Volant. Art et littérature*, 4 (1919): 49-52.

6 The title is not 'Ciel et Terre', as stated in Patrick Waldberg, *René Magritte* (Brussels, 1965), p. 286.

7 Pol Stievenart, untitled review, *Le Geste. Critique et action*, 2 (Jan. 1920): 15.

8 *Le Geste. Critique et action*, 1 (Dec. 1919): 1.

9 Stievenart, untitled review.

10 *Le Geste. Critique et action*, 2 (Jan. 1920): 31.

11 E.L.T. Mesens, 'The World of René Magritte', *The Saturday Book*, 19, (1959): 274.

12 Élie Faure, 'Preface', exhibition catalogue *Exposition internationale d'art moderne*, Bâtiment Electoral (Geneva, 1920), p. 5.

13 Faure, 'Preface', *Exposition internationale d'art moderne*, p. 6.

14 *Au Volant. Art et littérature*, 4 (1919): 61.

15 In 1925, the school moved to Dessau and then to Berlin. In 1933, it was closed down by the Nazis. The New Bauhaus was started in Chicago in 1937 by Laszlo Moholy-Nagy.

[16] Georges Marlier, 'Du Métier et de l'enseignement artistique', *Le Centaure*, 9-10 (June-July 1930): 182.

[17] Amédée Ozenfant & Édouard Jeanneret, 'Destinée de la peinture', *L'Esprit Nouveau*, 22 (1924): n. pag.

[18] Waldemar George, 'Morphologie du Baroque', *Variétés*, 5 (15 Sept. 1929): 342.

[19] Marlier, 'Du Métier et de l'enseignement artistique': 181-2.

[20] Paul Caso, 'René Magritte : fils de Fantômas ou peintre du merveilleux', *Le Soir*, (20 Jan. 1966): 10.

[21] *Œsophage*, 1 (Mar. 1925): n. pag.

[22] Walter Gropius, in Herbert Bayer, Walter Gropius & Ise Gropius (eds), *Bauhaus 1919-1928* (London, 1979), p. 26.

[23] Gropius, *Bauhaus 1919-1928*, p. 27.

[24] Gropius, *Bauhaus 1919-1928*, p. 20.

[25] Bayer *et al. Bauhaus 1919-1928*, p. 168.

[26] Magritte's work appeared in the January-February 1925 and March-April 1925 issues of *Englebert Magazine*.

[27] Gropius, *Bauhaus 1919-1928*, p. 29.

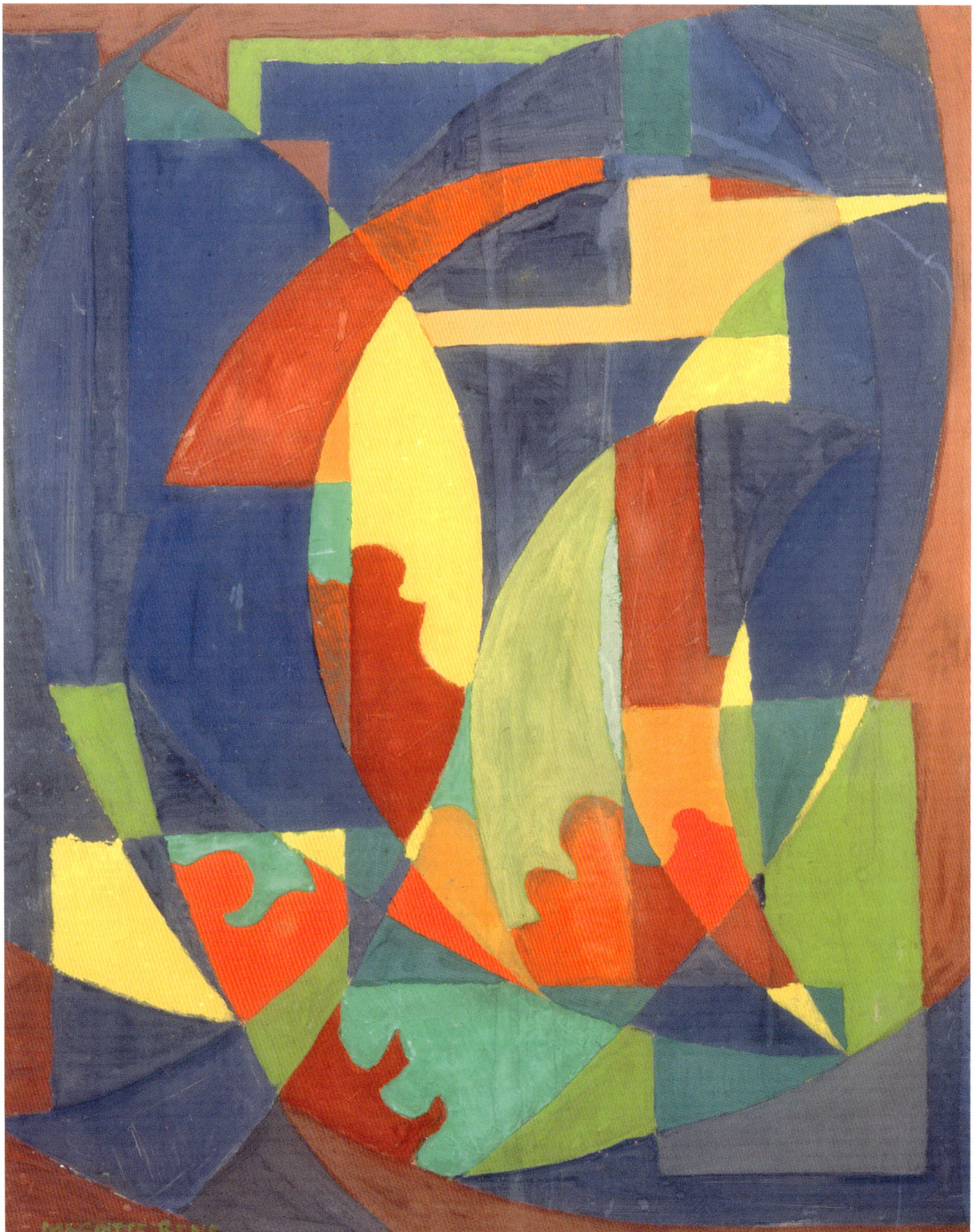

Fleurs devant une fenêtre (1920)

Pure Art and Abstraction

Magritte's first published text, 'L'Art pur : Défence de l'esthétique' (Pure Art: Defence of Aesthetics), written with Victor Servranckx, a former fellow student at the Academy and destined to become one of the leading Belgian abstract artists, has much in common with declarations that appeared in *Au Volant. Art et littérature.*[1] Although 'L'Art pur' is dated 1922, Magritte's year of military service in 1921 effectively situates the piece immediately after his association with Le Centre d'Art.

With a stance that is anti-decorative and advocates basic pictorial forms inspired by modern machinery, the text begins by making a distinction between architecture and art, the former being said to have the purpose of designing constructions according to purely practical considerations. Like the engineer, the text continues, the architect should ideally determine forms in accordance with the purpose they are intended to serve: an edifice should be conceived in mechanical terms without recourse to aesthetic dictates. The ideal building, it is argued, results from scientific and technical calculation, just like tools and machines, and particularly aeroplanes: 'in harmony with the approach to building a machine, the approach to building a house should, in every detail, only be concerned with order, precision, efficacy'. The point is made that 'architecture is not an art' and that it should solely aim at producing an efficient, habitable space: 'the architect must be purely scientific'.

Whilst the architect is seen as bound by practical principles, the artist is regarded as less constrained. For Magritte and Servranckx, the ways in which, as they put it, 'savages' transform their bodies by tattooing represent the initial manifestations of 'the creative instinct'. Art, unlike architecture, is not felt to arise from the necessities of physical laws but, rather, is to be conceived in 'the imagination'. It is only then that it is applied to reality. External stimuli serve only to trigger 'an internal form that develops on the inside, like a foetus'. Essentially, the creative act is described as an egression of 'what the artist carries within, in a latent state', a point on which 'L'Art pur' corresponds quite closely to the principles of *Au Volant*. Indeed, with terminology not dissimilar to that of *Au Volant*, Magritte and Servranckx observe that the artist should be 'conscious', 'free' and 'master of his craft and not its slave'.

A point on which 'L'Art pur' does diverge from the precepts of *Au Volant* is in its condemnation of decorative art. Whereas *Au Volant* had exclaimed 'long live decorative painting and sculpture', 'L'Art pur' maintained that any type of decoration or ornamentation has a secondary role and consequently debases art.[2] 'Painting and sculpture', it argued, 'are not there to demonstrate the beauty of materials or to decorate cups.' Because decoration is inevitably

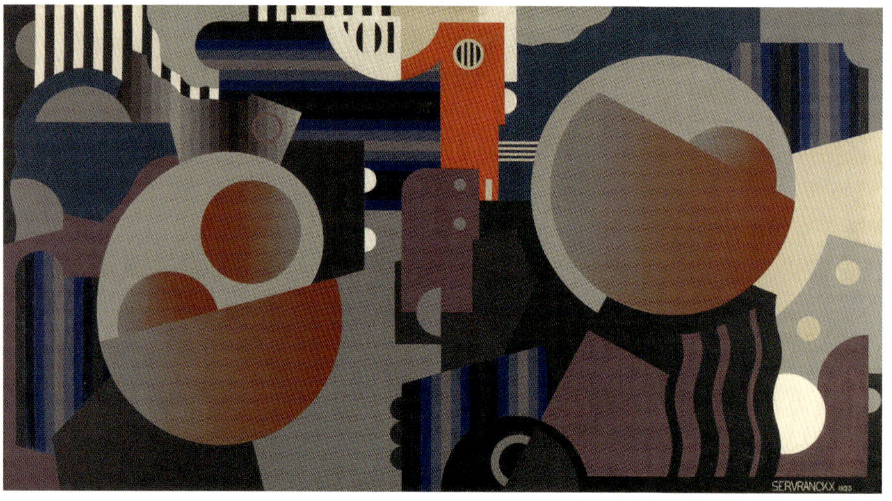

Victor Servranckx, *Opus 47. Exaltation du machinisme*, 1923. Musées Royaux des Beaux-Arts de Belgique, Brussels. Oil on canvas, © 2015. Photo. J. Geleyns / Ro scan. DACS, London 2015

subject to the limitations of given dimensions and shapes, applied art is seen to be incompatible with 'pure art'. Magritte and Servranckx clearly aligned themselves with the postwar avant-garde Purist movement and advocated the theories expounded in 1918 by the painter Amédée Ozenfant and the architect Édouard Jeanneret (Le Corbusier), whose central principle, set out in *Après le Cubisme*, was the rejection of ornamentation and superfluous detail in favour of objectivity and the finite forms of machines, stripped of detail.[3] In concert, 'L'Art pur' specified 'exactitude, logic, economy, veracity' as necessities of painting. Both art and architecture, the piece concludes, should aspire to 'the perfection [...] already possessed by machinery'.

Historically, Purism had little impact and is even said to have 'produced no art at all'.[4] This is not strictly accurate, however, and Servranckx, for one, was certainly an ardent advocate of the style. His *Opus 47. Exaltation du machinisme* (1923), executed in the year following 'L'Art pur', is clearly based on the Purist concept of machine forms devoid of all detail. Shapes are minimal, being delineated by just straight lines and simple curves in a sort of reductionist geometric style, whilst colour is limited to juxtaposed bands of single tones. In places, colour actually disappears altogether and is replaced by monochrome. The theme of the machine, however, remains evident despite this oversimplification of structures. There may be no explicit cogs, levers or gears and yet the superimposition of planes gives the impression of distinct surfaces capable of relative movement. A series of buttons or lubrication holes and two large, circular forms more than hint at mechanization in the form of a kinetic complex of hubs and flywheels interconnected with oscillating pistons. Of course, at the wallpaper factory where he was employed at the time, Servranckx would have been observing

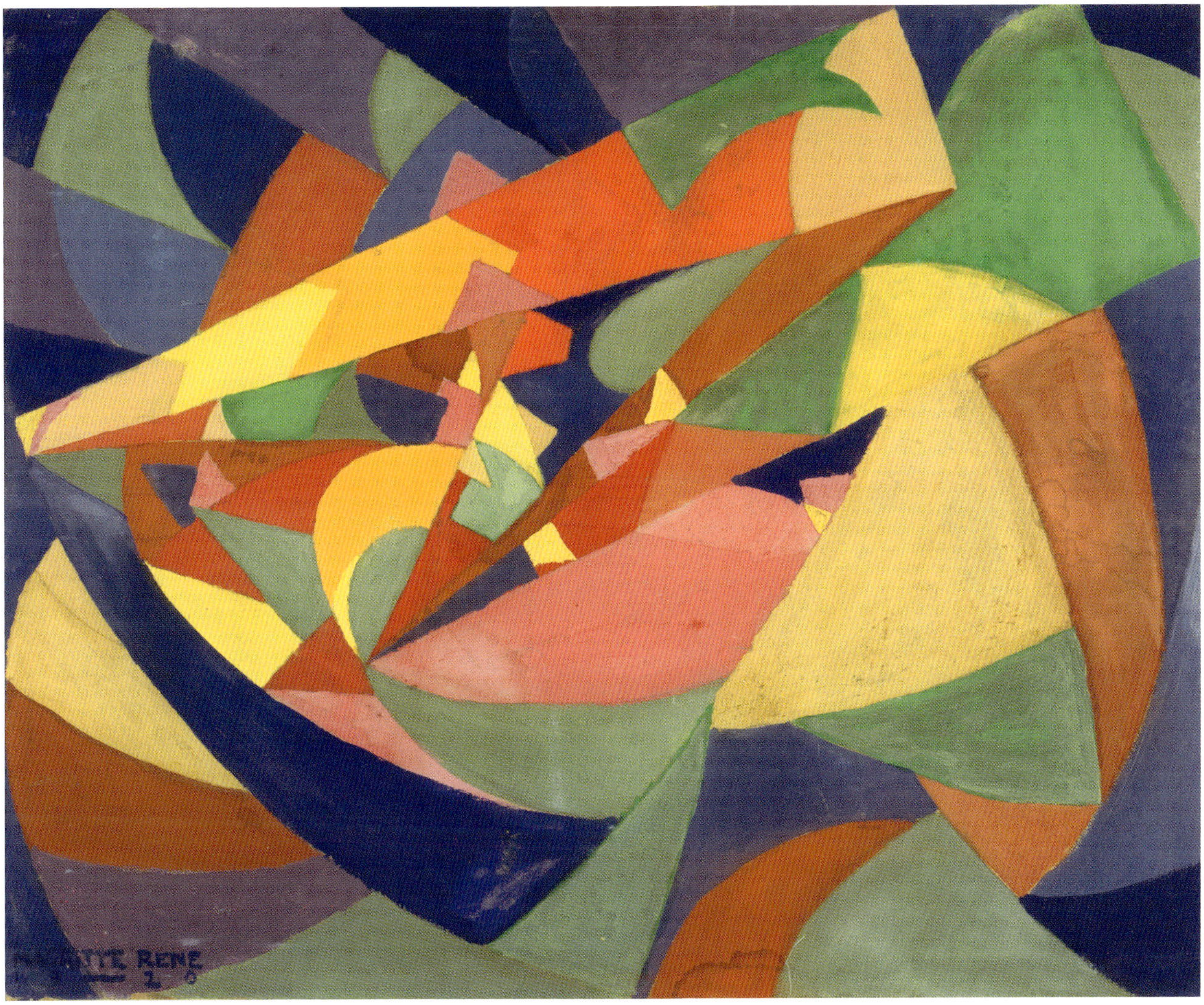

La Retraite militaire (1920)

paper-printing machinery at close quarters and *Opus 47* could well be seen as an abstracted wallpaper machine, with revolving rollers that are spewing out reams of printed paper. Servranckx, nevertheless, does more than to depict a mechanized production line; his evocation of the elegance of the modish machine comes across as stylistically economical, logical and simple, that is to say Purist.

The extent to which Magritte himself had adopted 'pure art' is not clear, however. No evidence has been found of a 'mechanical' style in his paintings of the early twenties and not even the titles of works for which no reproductions have been found indicate any Purist leanings. Yet, there is doubt about his belief in a concept fundamental to 'L'Art pur', the condemnation of applied art. Although in a later autobiography he was to express contempt for his time as a commercial artist, a letter written to Flouquet in 1921 shows that, at the time, he had a keen curiosity about the techniques of industrial design.[5] Not only does Magritte give detailed descriptions of the niceties of wallpaper design, showing his engrossment in the subject, but the fact that he discussed the question at all with a fellow artist suggests that he did not dismiss the notion of a 'decorative' fine art out of hand. Indeed, it was not too long before he began to draw heavily on the techniques of the specific commercial art of window display. All too easily overlooked is the fact that, in commercial art, Magritte would have found the realization of the principal aspiration of the avant-garde, that is a coherent alternative to formal art. This, after all, is precisely what Purism itself had intended. By its nature, wallpaper design disregards formal, painterly academic rules; on the contrary, it is governed by alternative forms of pictorial expression and has its own, autonomous rationale. As Magritte had pointed out to Flouquet, wallpaper patterns had their own 'rules [...] which are strictly determined laws of harmony'.[6] As he was well aware, these 'rules' lent weight to, rather than opposed, a main theme of 'L'Art pur', the rejection of academic formulae. Wallpaper design clearly defies 'anatomy, perspective, the photographic image (faithful drawing)', which 'L'Art pur' had, after all, contested and which Magritte himself was to contest through his painterly modus operandi during the 1920s. Whilst his paintings did not have the overt trappings of Purism, they did adhere to its underlying approach of reducing representation to essential, primary constituents. Like the Purists, Magritte was to challenge academic rules by dismantling the pictorial construct as though it were a machine. Indeed, he had written that 'the painting is a constructed object'. What 'L'Art pur' does is to set out, inadvertently perhaps, the principles of Magritte's paintings for the following decade: as he insisted, 'what is needed is the anatomy of painting and not the medical anatomy of the model'. In Magritte's early work it is the process of painting itself, just as much as the objects he painted, that is subdivided and dismantled.

Yet, this disassembly of the pictorial construct was not to be embarked upon for another two or three years, during which Magritte's sole preoccupation was with what he described as 'paintings that are currently termed "abstract" or "non-figurative"'.[7] By that measure, his essays turned out to be unremarkable, amounting to mere pastiches of somewhat passé Cubist and Futurist vocabularies.

Within his oeuvre as a whole, however, his paintings *circa* 1920 emerge as the seeds of a more significant and enduring rationale that Michel Foucault was to regard as underpinning Magritte's subsequent methodology. As Foucault saw it, the radical principles of Abstraction, with which Magritte's early abstract works inevitably align themselves, are what lie behind paintings that were to negate pictorial assertion.[8] Just like Kandinsky, Foucault argued, Magritte extricated 'resemblance' from 'pictorial affirmation'. Kandinsky achieved this in a twofold manner: firstly, and most obviously, he departed from representation and secondly he imbued lines and colours with significance in their own right, giving them autonomous pictorial status. The result was that the constituents of pictorial representation were no longer bound to a primarily referential function. In a similar vein, according to Foucault, Magritte's subjects were accompanied by their own contradiction and thus ceased to function as affirming signifiers. For Magritte, just as for Kandinsky, referential resemblance ceased to exist. All that Magritte's painted objects can be said to be capable of is referring to themselves in just the same way as Kandinsky's lines and colours call to mind nothing but their own physical reality.[9] Magritte, in Foucault's view, severed the direct link between the image and the model.[10] In other words, he arrested the ties with tangible reality and his work, like that of Kandinsky, exists in terms of 'similitudes', rather than being grounded in 'resemblance', that is the subordination of the pictorial to the actual. Both Magritte and Kandinsky are said to have developed a self-sufficient visual language independent of external reality.

Conversely, André Blavier feels that Foucault, who had based his conclusions on Magritte's philosophical texts, had 'misinterpreted what Magritte was writing'.[11] Magritte had, after all, commented that 'representation derived from the senses' is 'essential to art', which situates his work far from Expressionism, as does his acknowledgment of his reliance on 'Cubism, Futurism'.[12] Magritte even went as far as to place on record that in about 1915 he had become enthused not so much with Kandinsky as with 'Mondrian', whose conception of abstract painting stemmed from the analysis of concrete form.[13] Arguably, Magritte's abstract works are in sharp contrast to Kandinsky's free-flowing, lyrical abstract expressionism. *La Retraite militaire* (1920), for example, firmly belongs to the tradition of geometric abstraction and, whilst not presenting the formal analytical rigour of Picasso and Braque, it does resemble the less mathematical Orphic experiments of Robert Delaunay and Kupka, particularly the latter's *Amorpha, Fugue in Two Colours* (1912).[14] In his 1920 painting, Magritte uses the abstract vehicles of pure colour and non-representational line to convey the concrete notion of dynamism. As in Balla's *Abstract Speed the Car has Passed* (1913), the depiction of the object is replaced by a suggestion of the lines of force that result from its energy. What is captured is movement itself, rather than an object in motion. In parallel with his Orphic predecessors, Magritte paints rhythm and luminosity, but does so within the bounds of a geometric style grounded in a contact with material experience. Less obviously than Picasso's Cubism, his patterns and contrasting colours do emerge from the world of natural appearances. As with Delaunay's pictorial experiments with light, which Apollinaire had described as inseparable from 'réalité', Magritte painted commentaries on sense data.[15]

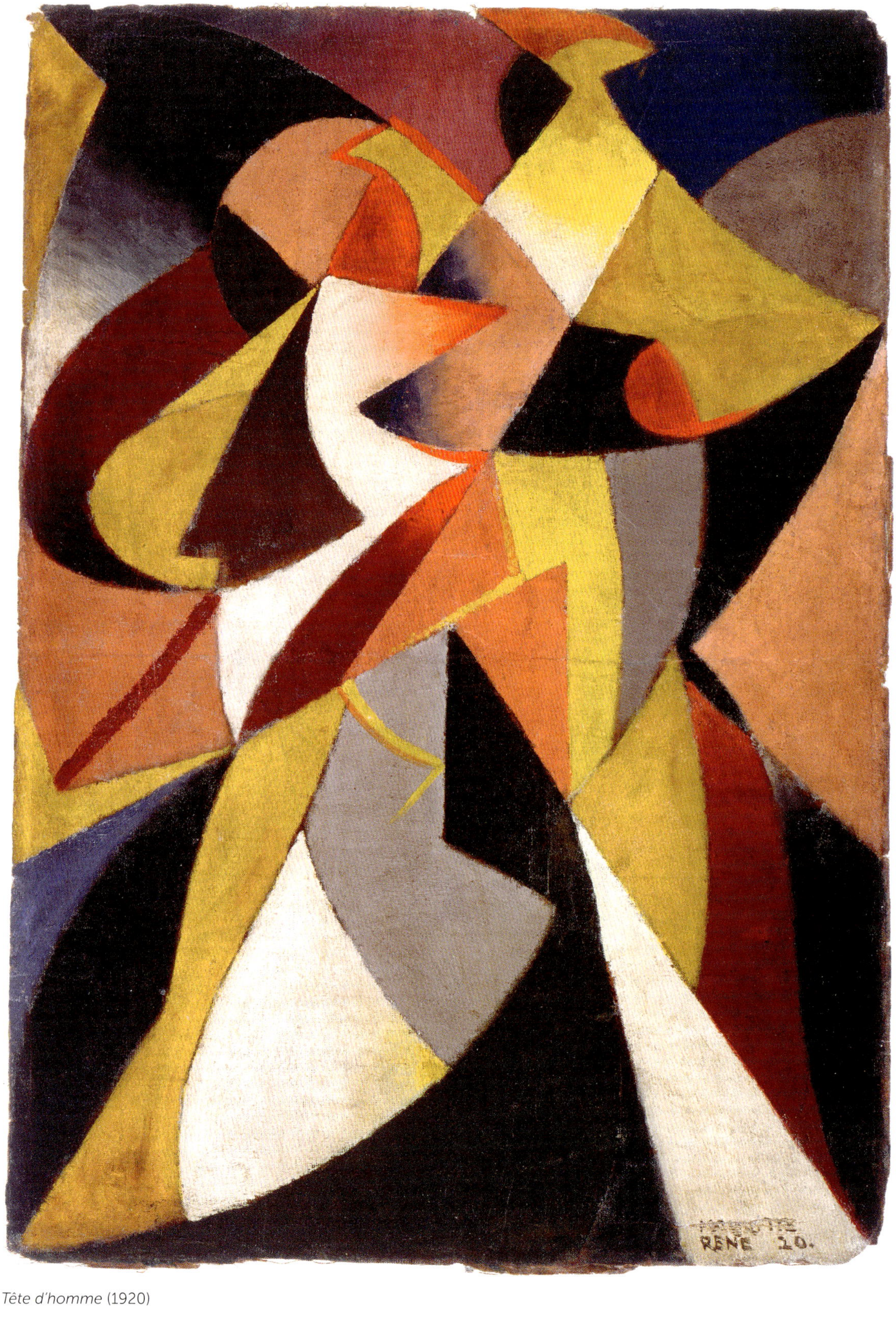

Tête d'homme (1920)

Whilst what could be termed Magritte's 'Neo-Orphism', his abstraction based on physical phenomena, appears somewhat unformulated in *La Retraite militaire*, it emerges in a more consolidated form in *Tête d'homme*, also of 1920. The work unambiguously makes the connection with 'reality', that Apollinaire had deemed so important. Being patently based on a human head, the abstracting 'transformation' illustrates Delaunay's principle that appearances are continually subject to distortion and fragmentation. Not only are the facial features and outline broken up into distinct planes, which are elongated and simplified to create a mosaic of coloured patches, the form is also generally stylized and fractioned into prismic-like subdivisions of light. As in Delaunay's transition from *The City, First Study* to the later *The City No.2*, figurative representation is sacrificed for the sake of 'pure' aspects – light, colour, movement, immediacy, geometric pattern.

Notwithstanding, working seven or eight years after the birth of Orphism, Magritte, it must be said, produced nothing particularly novel with his abstract paintings. Indeed, *La Retraite militaire* could easily have resulted from his having seen *La Couturière* by the Belgian Prosper de Troyer at the 1920 *Exposition internationale d'art moderne*.[16] At most, what can be said is that, through his abstract essays, Magritte identified with the rational and analytical methodology that underlay both Cubism and Mondrian's 'reductionist' rationale. Moreover, like Mondrian, Magritte was to go on to focus on a protracted breaking up of visual vocabulary. More so than the Cubists, who readily reassembled the fragments of their analyses into coherent structures, Magritte was to proceed by reduction alone in what would turn out to be a single-minded 'dissolution' of conventional pictorial language. Mondrian may have proceeded by means of abstraction and Magritte by means of figuration, but both persisted in a systematic and relentless form of artistic reductionism. In parallel, they exploited Cubism as a point of departure for a searching analysis of visual reality. Mondrian, for his part, is said to have used 'the methods of composition' of Cubism but not 'the spirit'; he attempted to capture the internal make-up of objects, while Cubism focused on their surface structures.[17] Mondrian's analysis was bent on reducing objects to their fundamental framework, to their 'interior structure', as is shown by his 'Trees Cycle' (1909-11), in which he progressively transformed the external appearance of a tree to mere linear relationships. From surface randomness he derived internal consistent relationships – vertical and horizontal, presence and absence. To him, the 'very structure' of a tree, its 'pure reality' resulted from the 'necess[ity] to reduce natural forms to the constant elements of form'.[18] This is precisely the trajectory that Magritte was to pursue a decade later. Quickly departing from the Cubist focus on surface structure, his attention turned to the penetration of form, to the revelation of elemental constituents. In unison with Mondrian, Magritte was to eat away at the pictorial object, particularly in the form of the human body, in order to arrive, in his own way, at the 'pure pictorial elements'.[19]

In themselves, Magritte's abstract works only minimally anticipated such developments. All that can be said is that they engaged with a frame of reference within which these developments were to be possible. Magritte himself was never to acknowledge the formative stimulus of his abstract work, going as far as to say that the 'so-called non-figurative art has no more meaning than a school that does no teaching, cooking that produces no food'.[20] In a letter to Paul Bourgoignie he even wrote: 'I hope you will write against "abstract art"'. Later, he would state that 'the point of the act of painting is to reveal poetry and not to reduce the world into its various material constituents'.[21] Notwithstanding, it is precisely such a 'reduction' of visual appearances into its material 'constituents', that takes form in Magritte's abstract period at the beginning of the 1920s and sets his trajectory for at least the remainder of the decade.[22]

---

[1] René Magritte, *Écrits complets* (Paris, 1979), pp. 15-20. Unless otherwise indicated, citations in this chapter are from this text.

[2] 'Vers la Plénitude par la dictature de la conscience', *Au Volant. Art et littérature*, 1 (Apr. 1919): 3.

[3] Amédée Ozenfant & Édouard Jeanneret, *Après le Cubisme* (Paris, 1918).

[4] Peter & Linda Murray, *A Dictionary of Art and Artists* (Harmondsworth, 1975), p. 344.

[5] 'René Magritte found the factory as hard to endure as the barracks', in Magritte, *Écrits complets*, p. 366.

[6] René Magritte, letter to Pierre-Louis Flouquet, 1921.

[7] Magritte, *Écrits complets*, p. 367.

[8] Michel Foucault, *Ceci n'est pas une pipe* (Montpellier, 1973), p. 45.

[9] Patricia Allmer states that 'Copies are copies of previous copies, the affirmative in similitude is denied. Representations of objects stay locked up in representation and relate to other representations, never reaching outside of themselves'. Patricia Allmer, *René Magritte: Beyond Painting* (Manchester, 2009), p. 139.

[10] Foucault, *Ceci n'est pas une pipe*, p. 61.

[11] In Magritte, *Écrits complets*, p. 521.

[12] Magritte, *Écrits complets*, pp. 561 & 591.

[13] Magritte, *Écrits complets*, p. 585.

[14] In the year of this painting Magritte took part in the *Exposition internationale d'art moderne* in Geneva and there came in contact with both geometric abstractionists, such as van Doesburg, and expressionists, such as Jawlensky. His adherence to the former faction must have been a conscious choice. *Abstraction* (1923) reinforces this view.

[15] Guillaume Apollinaire, 'Commencement du cubisme. Réalité, peinture pure' (previously unpublished text of 1912), in Robert Delaunay, *Du Cubisme à l'art abstrait, documents inédits publiés par Pierre Francastel, École Pratique des Hautes Études – VIe section* (Paris, 1957), p. 157. In *Les Peintres cubistes : méditations esthétiques* (Geneva, 1950) Apollinaire is more specific about 'pure painting' (p. 14), pointing out the apparent paradox of a style which is based on an observation of reality and which nevertheless employs 'elements not borrowed from visual reality, but entirely created by the artist'. (p. 27) 'Works of Orphic artists', he writes, 'must simultaneously present a pure aesthetic charm, a construction that can be immediately perceived and a sublime meaning, that is to say the subject. This is pure art.' (p. 27).

[16] In an undated letter (Archives de l'art contemporain de Belgique, 36359) probably of 1920, Magritte writes 'My masterpiece *La Couturière* is a marvellous work'. There is no suggestion of a link with de Troyer, but the possibility does exist.

[17] Marcelin Pleynet, 'Mondrian vingt-cinq ans après', in *L'Enseignement de la peinture* (Paris, 1971), p. 109.

[18] Italo Tomassoni, *Mondrian* (London, 1970), p. 10. Mondrian, in Adrian Heath, *Abstract Painting: Its Origin and its Meaning* (London, 1953), p. 11.

[19] Peter Vergo, 'Introduction', exhibition catalogue *Abstraction: Towards a New Art*, Tate Gallery (London, 1980), p. 18.

[20] Magritte, *Écrits complets*, p. 576.

[21] Undated letter in 'Lettres à Paul Bourgoinie', *Le Fait Accompli*, 49 (Mar. 1971): n. pag. Magritte, *Écrits complets*, p. 585.

[22] Irène Hamoir, in conversation with the author (Brussels, 1981), warns against too literal an interpretation of Magritte's views on his work: 'He did not have the means to develop philosophical arguments, but he loved doing so'.

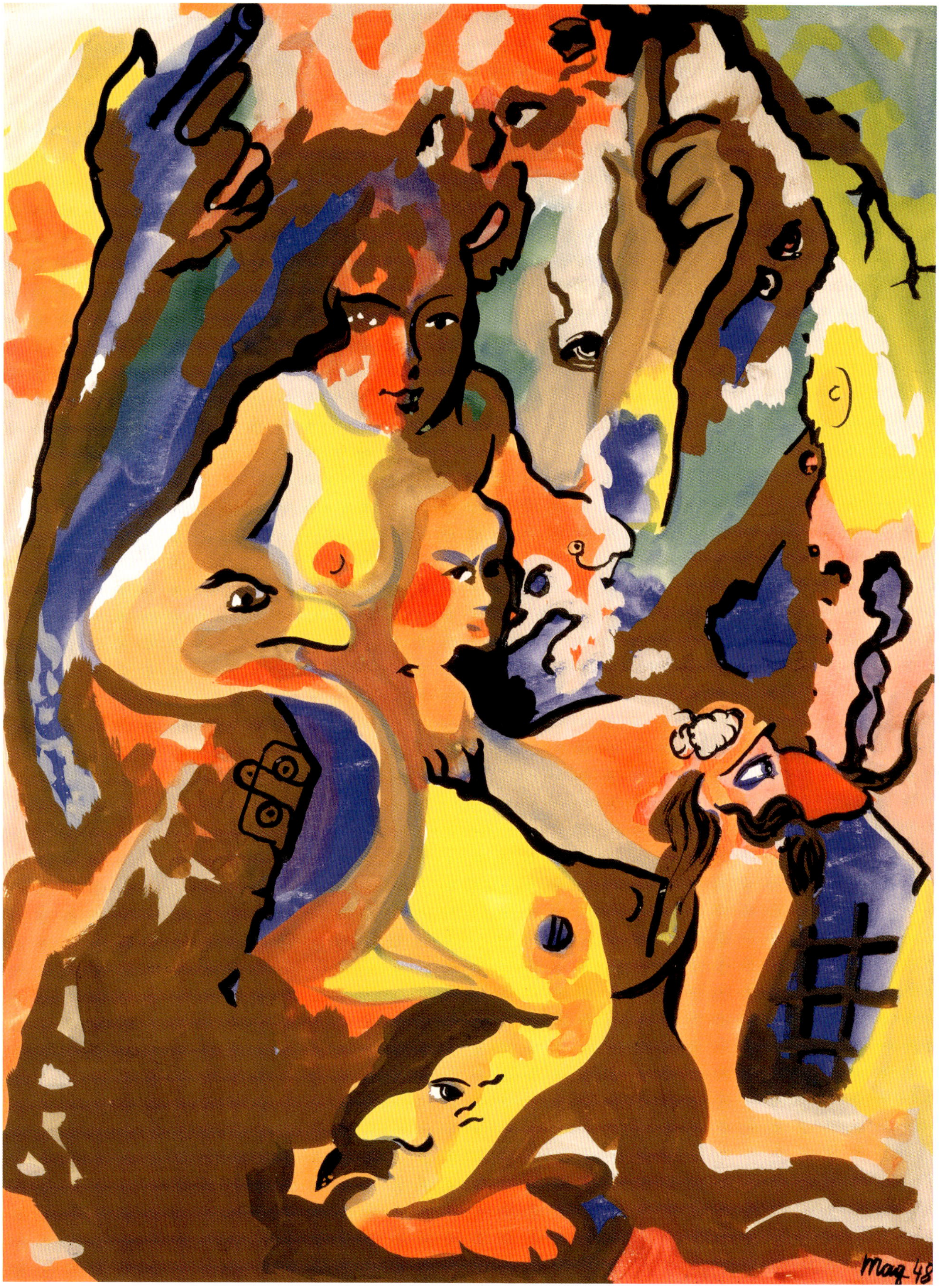

Titania (1948)

Vile paintings

What is significant about Magritte's Purist and Abstract essays is that they reveal the iconoclastic tendencies underlying his oeuvre as a whole. This is equally true of a small number of works executed in 1948, which have come to be known as the 'Vache', or 'vile', paintings.

Wholly out of keeping with the rest of his output, this phase in Magritte's work has been described as 'an unusual pictorial adventure'.[1] The paintings in question, fifteen oils and ten gouaches, were shown at a single exhibition in 1948 and, at the time, gave rise to considerable public disapproval.[2] 'Ridiculous' was one of the comments in the visitors' book according to Mariën, who further recalled that the set of paintings was condemned as 'something absolutely mad' and 'wholly inadmissible'.[3] From the outset, the works were branded as 'Vache', that is to say vulgar and offensive to good taste. They instantly provoked 'a scandalous effect on public and critics alike', according to Gablik.[4]

Significantly, the term 'Vache' had been coined by Magritte himself as a description of his own paintings and it is clear that the incitement of public outrage was not unintentional. Indeed, it was a deliberate 'way of irritating the French', according to George Melly.[5] Mariën, for his part, was convinced that Magritte had long resented the absence of recognition within France:

> It came as an act of defiance, because he was known without being known. He had never had a solo exhibition in Paris. Out of the blue, when he was fifty, a Parisian dealer offered him an exhibition [...] So, solely for this exhibition, he dreamt up the entire Vache period.[6]

Similarly, Scutenaire points out that 'he didn't have good memories of France or the French and he wanted to upset them'.[7]

The tactics that Magritte employed in this 'punitive foray' were surprising in themselves; he purposely undertook what can only be described as self-abasement.[8] By completely deviating from the expectations of his Parisian public, by (in their eyes) 'blundering', he insulted them. He made it clear that their approval and opinions were of little consequence. The execution of these works was 'in such fantastic bad taste' and demonstrated 'such absurd negligence' that they amounted to 'a total destruction of everything he stood for'.[9] Magritte's posture was made abundantly clear in the exhibition catalogue, where even the title of Scutenaire's text, 'Les Pieds dans le plat', which conveys the idea of an excessive, vulgar or inappropriate candour that embarrasses or infuriates, made the point that the exhibition was intended to be tasteless, gauche and discomforting.[10] In his text, Scutenaire is at pains to point out that the paintings on display are alien to the true nature of Magritte's work by design and amount to a 'coup'. The 'attack' was, of course, against the aesthetic sensibility of the Parisian art connoisseurs. Scutenaire not only defiantly taunted the public with the declaration that 'you've been beaten', but he also reminded his readers that the conquest had taken place 'on your own home ground'. With more than a tinge of disrespectful sarcasm, Scutenaire assured the public that 'we don't want to hurt you, disconcert you, frighten you' and went on to make clear that the whole exhibition was just a spoof. Very much in Marx Brothers' style, with an intermingling of discourtesy and conventional etiquette intended to mock and confuse, the dignity of the unsuspecting guests of a formal vernissage at a Parisian gallery was outrageously attacked: 'we have every intention', they were informed, 'of politely saying shit'.[11]

Scutenaire went on to introduce the Vache works themselves as an intentional, tongue-in-cheek spurning of conventional taste: 'you will vomit when you see them'.[12] What was probably seen as most shocking, however, was that they were an extreme departure from Magritte's habitual work and, as such, they acted as a measure of the principles underlying Magritte's more typical work. Scutenaire was in no doubt that the Vache works were discordant with the rest of Magritte's output 'as much', as he writes, 'by their outward appearance as by their inward motivation'.[13] Without exception, they were based on a gaudy use of colour, straight from the tube, that gave an overall sense of crudity. The technique in, say, *Titania* (1948), with its visibly rough paint texture, has a hurried, incomplete and botched look which wholly disregards craftsmanship. What is more, Magritte coupled this unseemly execution with vulgar and objectionable content – the naked 'female' figure suggestively oozes deformed faces from various parts of her anatomy, as if afflicted with some sort of grisly ailment. These caricatural 'facial expressions' are excreted from her breast, arm, knee and calf and appear to be bringing about a degeneration of the entire body into formlessness. As though to compound the viewer's repugnance, Magritte surrounded his putrid Titania with a viscous area the colour of faeces.

Another Vache painting, *L'Arc-en-ciel* (1948), is more explicitly provocative. In one compartment, the inscription 'L'Avarié', a euphemism for 'syphilitic', is accompanied by a facial form with vertical lips that indelicately call to mind a vulva; in another division the caption 'the Apostle' is illustrated by an embracing or copulating couple; and in a third partition 'the pleasure-seeker' is depicted as a nut and bolt being driven into a mechanism or even a cranium, with faint sadistic allusions. Finally, 'the Godly person' emerges as a scatological form within which a demonic face can be made out. The overall impression is that of mess and confusion and to the visitors of the exhibition, who were expecting to see a more controlled style, the work would have appeared frustratingly devoid of skill and painterly concerns. What they were

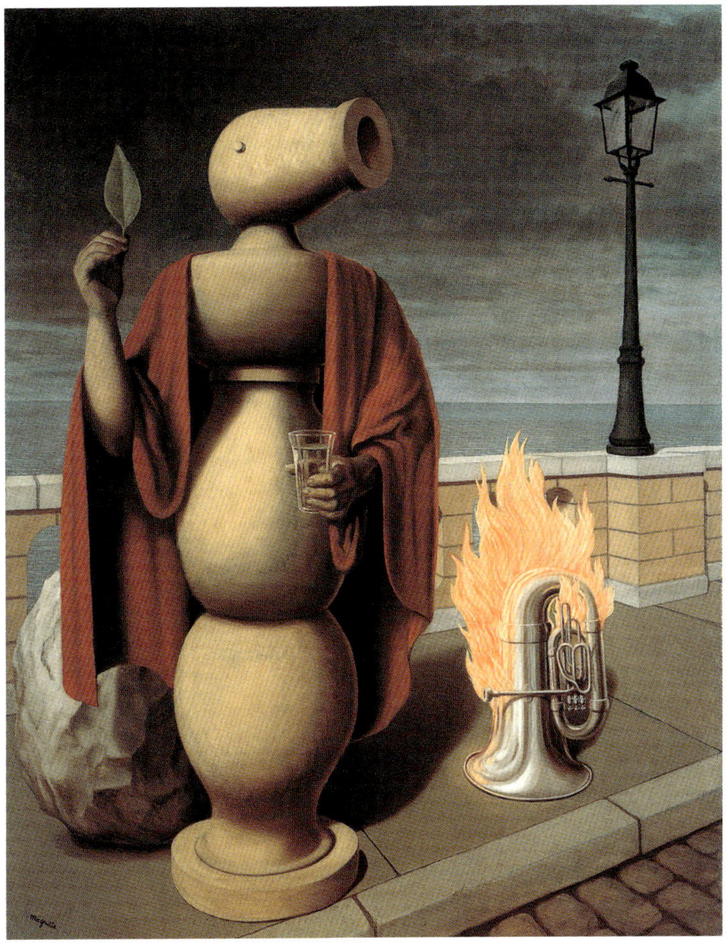

Les Droits de l'homme (1948)

expecting were the academic execution, control and overt mastery of materials that Magritte had been employing up to then and had continued to employ, even at that time, in works such as *Les Droits de l'homme* (1948). This almost contemporaneous work displays precisely the qualities that were lacking in the Vache series: accomplished technique and exacting execution. In this carefully calculated composition, Magritte paints an anthropomorph in accordance with the laws of perspective and chiaroscuro. Not only does the heavy shadow firmly position the figure on a foreground pavement, but also, the entire space of the picture is consistent and comprehensible. Nothing is left plastically unresolved and every object is painstakingly executed with geometric accuracy. The central figure itself is depicted with particular precision and coherent modelling in the round. Like a giant chess-piece, it is made up of mathematically perfect forms, cylinders and spheres. The surfaces are flawless and regular and even the drape that partially covers it is neatly hung. The contrast with the untidy, asymmetrical and plastically imprecise *Titania* could not be greater.

The distinction between the two styles is, to recall Scutenaire's words, equally apparent on the level of 'intention'. *L'Arc-en-ciel*, *Titania* and the rest of the Galerie du Faubourg works, with their undisciplined and facile use of colour and line, have a predominantly makeshift and spontaneous conception that was, as Scutenaire pointed out, deliberately calculated to be 'repulsive'.[14] *Les Droits de l'homme* represented Magritte's controlled and 'aesthetic' approach. Beyond these overt differences, moreover, the two modes of painting may not be quite so incompatible. In different ways, they both engage with formal art, albeit to bring about its derangement. In one case there is outright mockery, whilst in the other a more subtle subversion takes place in which the rules of painting are only selectively adhered to and so set in disharmony with themselves. Unwittingly perhaps, the Vache exhibition had unmasked Magritte by showing his iconoclasm in its unbridled state. It is openly defiant and disrespectful. It is unquestionable, moreover, that, in more understated ways, his entire oeuvre can be said to be a defiance: it consistently scrutinizes and disputes the rules and principles of formal art. In other words, the Parisian exhibits, in their unconcealed violence, had simply put technical execution on a par with latent intention. As Scutenaire had explained, 'his oeuvre is wholly violent: even in Magritte's calmest canvas there is violence'.[15] The Vache exhibition, therefore, entailed an irony; the public may have rejected the works, but it had been only too happy to celebrate Magritte's rule-breaking in the guise of a tongue-in-cheek academism. George Melly appositely described the Vache exhibition as 'a good joke' and Paul Éluard had written in the visitors' book that 'he who laughs last, laughs the loudest'.[16] What was not lost on them was that, whether Magritte painted in the 'vile' manner or in his more 'acceptable' style, he would be showing equal 'aggression towards good painting'.[17]

---

1 Marcel Mariën, *L'Activité surréaliste en Belgique* (Brussels, 1979), p. 440.

2 Galerie du Faubourg, Paris, 11 May-5 June 1948.

3 Marcel Mariën, conversation with the author, Brussels, 9 March 1981.

4 Suzi Gablik, *Magritte* (London, 1971), p. 152.

5 George Melly, conversation with the author, London, April 1981.

6 Marcel Mariën, conversation with the author, Brussels, 9 March 1981.

7 Louis Scutenaire, conversation with the author, Brussels, March 1981.

8 Scutenaire, conversation with the author, Brussels, March 1981.

9 Melly, conversation with the author, London, April 1981.

10 This French expression means to bring up a delicate subject without any delicacy at all, or to discuss a topic that everyone else is avoiding, thus embarrassing them in the process. The text is reprinted in Mariën, pp. 438-9.

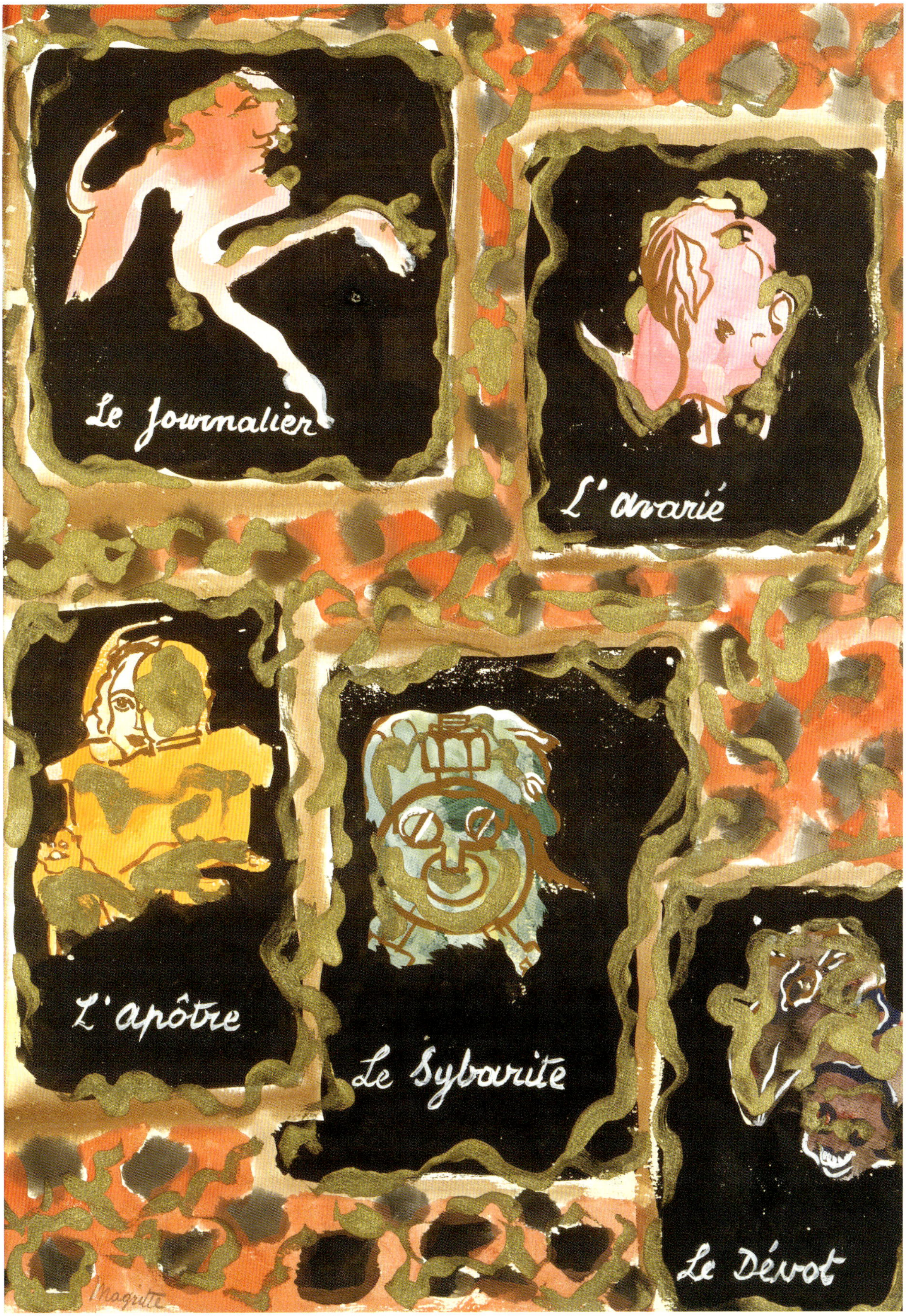

L'Arc-en-ciel (1948)

[11] Louis Scutenaire, 'Les Pieds dans le plat', in Louis Scutenaire, *Avec Magritte* (Brussels, 1977), p. 111. In a letter to Scutenaire, dated 13 June 1948, Magritte had written that 'Picabia shat on a blank canvas and stuck his visiting card in the paste (Magritte, *Écrits complets*, p. 192).

[12] Scutenaire, 'Les Pieds dans le plat', p. 111.

[13] Scutenaire, 'Les Pieds dans le plat', p. 111.

[14] Louis Scutenaire, 'Gloser à Propos de l'Exposition parisienne à Paris des œuvres de René Magritte est prématuré. Allons-y donc', *Au Miroir d'Elisabeth*, tract, (Brussels, 1948), reproduced in Scutenaire, *Avec Magritte*, p. 115. Gablik, *Magritte*, p. 149.

[15] Scutenaire, conversation with the author, Brussels, March 1981.

[16] Mariën, conversation with the author, Brussels, 9 March 1981.

[17] José Vovelle, 'Magritte à Paris', exhibition catalogue *Magritte*, C.A.P.C., (Bordeaux, 1977), n. pag.

Dada

Contemporaneous with Magritte's association with the avant-garde was his friendship with E.L.T. Mesens, who was the first to introduce the young painter to Dada, whose objectives rang true with an already iconoclastic outlook. The two had met in 1919 at Le Centre d'Art, when Mesens was 17 and, by 1921, they had established contact with the Parisian dadaist circle. This occurred when the avant-garde singer Evelyne Brélia, who, in 1922, was the first to buy a work by Magritte, introduced Mesens to Erik Satie.[1] 'On Satie's insistence', according to George Melly, Mesens had gone to Paris, where he met Tzara, Man Ray, Duchamp, Picabia and Soupault.[2] Before long Mesens began to collaborate with the Parisians, setting to music in 1921 *Garage*, a poem by Soupault, which was published with a cover by Man Ray.[3] Mesens' role became that of 'an ambassador between Brussels and Paris', bringing back dadaist publications and modern music to Brussels.[4] Georgette Magritte recalled that 'he often went to Paris [...] to see Erik Satie and would return with his musical compositions'.[5] Mesens quickly became a committed dadaist and, predictably enough, impressed his enthusiasm on Magritte, who readily espoused the movement's unruly spirit of discontent and troublemaking.[6] The mainly stylistic contestation of formal art proposed by the avant-garde must have seemed rather tame in comparison with the unmitigatingly anti-art spirit of Dada. In Dada, Magritte found an uncompromising transgressiveness which gave him the means to thwart pictorial representation itself. Dada made no exceptions in its attack on convention: 'Dada [...] opposed not only all academicisms, but also all the avant-garde schools which claimed to be releasing art from the limits which confined it'.[7] Nothing could have chimed in better with Magritte's opposition to conventional art.

Initially however, Magritte's involvement in the dadaist venture was tentative. Well after the official dissolution of Paris Dada in 1922, he collaborated, together with Mesens, in the last issue of Picabia's *391*.[8] Both Belgians contributed a series of brief nonsensical aphorisms – 'I like beer and hollyhocks / A man in his birthday suit', wrote Magritte, echoing Tzara's poems made of snippets randomly cut from newspapers, while Mesens disrespectfully informed us that 'holy images have a vague cheesy smell'.[9] Such were the dadaist beginnings that marked an increasing polemic that eventually gave rise to an ideological division in the Brussels intellectual group of the mid-1920s, comprising Mesens, Marcel Lecomte, Camille Goemans, Magritte and Paul Nougé. When in October 1924 Mesens published a prospectus for a new magazine, *Période*, Nougé disapproved and produced a counter tract, resulting in the group's 'split[ting] in two', as Magritte later recalled, with each faction taking a divergent stand.[10] On the one hand, Nougé with Lecomte and Goemans, the latter of whom Nougé had dissuaded from continuing with the *Période* enterprise, turned towards surrealism, which had just been established in Paris, with the publication of *Correspondance* in November 1924.[11] On the other hand, Magritte and Mesens maintained their 'public advocacy of the Dada spirit'.[12] Due to Nougé's interference, the appearance of *Période* was delayed for some months and when it finally was published, in March 1925, it was renamed *Œsophage*. Despite these executive hindrances, however, the magazine did not attenuate Magritte and Mesens' commitment to Dada.

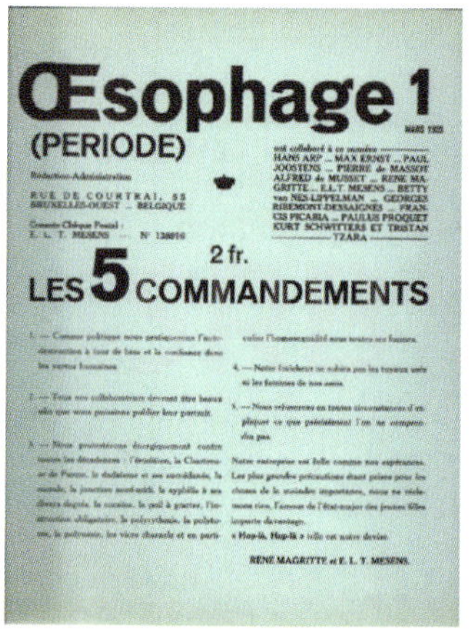
Œsophage 1
(PERIODE)
2 fr.
LES 5 COMMANDEMENTS

Œsophage, 1 (Mar. 1925)

In no uncertain way, *Œsophage* set out to be a mainstay for Dada. Its tone was nihilistic, provocative and contentious throughout and, more significantly, its list of contributors included the foremost exponents of Dada – Hans Arp, Ernst, Picabia, Schwitters and Tzara. This alone puts paid to Christian Bussy's suggestion that, as far as Belgian surrealism was concerned, 'Dada had had no preparatory role at all'.[13] Indeed, quite the contrary could be said of *Œsophage*, which, in an openly defiant manner, clearly stood for the dadaist view, pulling no punches when it came to decrying the emergent and rival surrealist movement. Pride of place was given to a vitriolic statement by Tzara that declared that 'realism is shit; surrealism is the smell of shit'.[14] Equally derisory of surrealism is a drawing by Picabia entitled *Superréaliste* in which a figure, probably intended to portray the surrealist poet, only manages to register a moderate temperature on a 'thermomètre Rimbaud' even though, as the drawing indicates, the figure is under the influence of a muse of 'hyperpoésie'. The attitude towards Breton is one of derision and ridicule.

As well as being discernible in the content and literary style of *Œsophage*, the dadaist bent is patently reflected in its typography. Emulating *391* and other Dada publications, its fifth page, for instance, is laid out in the form of an erratic maze of print, with type size that alters illogically such that the page begins with small letters and ends with the largest type. The effect is one of total disorientation and incoherence; words are indiscriminately scattered across the page, some areas are left blank, others are crammed full of type and text is set perpendicularly to the rest of the page. The disorder and senselessness aptly convey Dada's characteristic 'abolition of logic [...] intertwining contradictions [...] non sequiturs'.[15] In a particularly striking approbation of Dada, the magazine is illustrated with the interior of a public urinal, which is presented as an important statement of the magazine's ideology, being labelled 'Do not discard: an œsobiliphagist document'. The allusions to Duchamp's *Fountain* of 1917 and to the fact that the 1920 Cologne Bräuhaus exhibition incorporated a public lavatory are blatant. It would also not have escaped the editors' attention that Tzara had demanded the right to 'shit in different colours', and had described art as 'a pretension warmed in the timidity of a piss-pot'.[16]

For their own part, Magritte and Mesens did not omit to register their own credo, which they set out in the form of a manifesto, 'Les 5 Commandements' (The 5 Commandments), sardonically presented in the form of a royal decree, complete with a crown motif.[17] In concert with Tzara's paradoxical assertion that 'real dadas are anti-DADA', the Belgian duo announced that 'as a policy we shall practise self-destruction with all our might' and they then proceeded to reiterate Dada's anti-intellectualism in their third 'commandment', which states that they 'protest vehemently against all forms of decadence: learning, the Charterhouse of Parma, Dadaism and its substitutes'.[18] Tzara had, after all, wanted to 'destroy the drawers of the brain and of social organisation', as well as advocate 'the institution of the idiotic everywhere'.[19] In its perverse mission, *Œsophage* not only cultivated the imbecilic, but it also set out deliberately to baffle the reader – 'We refuse to explain under any circumstances precisely those things which won't be understood'. Such obfuscation and deliberate contrariness precisely reflects the tactics used by Tzara to eliminate all intellectual points of reference: 'I am [...] in favour of continual contradiction, and in favour of affirmation; I am neither for nor against; and I won't explain anything as I hate common sense'.[20] For Magritte, and Mesens too, any notion of certainty and comprehensibility had to be purged and replaced by alignment to the fact that 'DADA doubts everything'.[21] Just about every commandment is a negation and the declaration concludes with a refusal to take anything seriously, including themselves:

> Our undertaking is mad, like our ambitions. The greatest precautions are taken over affairs of the slightest importance, we ask for nothing... Giddy up! Giddy up! That's our motto.

To all effects, 'Les 5 Commandements' represent an alignment with the nihilistic manifestos of Tzara, who had proclaimed: 'I am writing a manifesto and I don't want anything, I however say certain things and I am in principle against manifestos, just as I am against principles'.[22]

Yet, the view that Magritte's co-authorship of 'Les 5 Commandements' demonstrates a commitment to Dada principles is contested by Mariën. He puts forward that *Œsophage* as a whole reveals a rather different undercurrent that has more in common with surrealism: 'Despite the dadaist tone, which at this time (March 1925) is already dated, there are remarks by Magritte which show obvious perspicacity'.[23] This, we are told, is particularly evident in an article entitled 'Jusqu'où l'Évolution peut mener' (How far can evolution lead), which, although obscure in places, does, in fact, appear to advocate an alternative vision, based more on an exploration of 'the marvellous' than on

Tzara's derision and negativity.[24] Indeed, Magritte wrote 'When the will is no longer the slave of things, all seems lost and it becomes possible to form images of a marvellous universe – creation', which is in stark contrast to the generalized disaffection of 'Les 5 Commandements'. The stance appears more in keeping with the surrealist trajectory of Nougé's *Correspondance*, which had, by this time, set itself in opposition to *Œsophage*. As Lecomte wrote, *Correspondance* concerned itself 'with moral philosophy, as one might put it, which characterized French surrealism, but which we had formulated in our own distinct manner'.[25]

Such dovetailing with the Parisians was a deliberate intention on Nougé's part and in one issue of *Correspondance* he not only described his Brussels grouping as Breton's 'friends' but he also proclaimed 'that Messrs Breton, Aragon, Éluard and others around them [...] are proceeding in an extremely efficacious manner'.[26] This wish to be identified with the nascent surrealist movement is further suggested by the fact that Nougé and Goemans, as well as *Correspondance* in its own right, were signatories of 'La Révolution d'abord et toujours' which appeared in *La Révolution surréaliste*.[27] That *Correspondance*, in conformity with these professed allegiances, should have extolled 'the marvellous' rather than, as was the case for *Œsophage*, attacked established values, is borne out by the tone of Camille Goemans' article 'À la Recherche du temps perdu'.[28] In considering the nature of Proust's novel, Goemans proposed that the events it recounts cannot be interpreted with any sensitivity solely by recourse to what he described as 'explanations with which we can be satisfied'. For him, Proust's narrative was not simply a 'reliving' or mimesis of past events, but, rather, aspired to a reformulation of the real on another level of consciousness that reached beyond the certain, the known and the logical:

> Rather, we dream of some new way of thinking and writing, of a world that we hold to be arbitrary, the more it bases itself solely on itself, the less it grasps this other world that it is said to imitate and which, however, more veritably imitates it.

Goemans' 'other world' is almost certainly a thinly veiled reference to Breton's axiom 'existence is elsewhere', announced only months earlier.[29]

It is this penchant that, according to Mariën, characterizes some of Magritte's contributions to *Œsophage*. Certainly, his 'Jusqu'où l'Évolution peut mener' would, at face value, place Magritte more than mildly at loggerheads with Dada. The text itself begins with a note of warning: 'liberty', Magritte says, can lead to an entrenchment in the 'pictorial problem'. In other words, he is wary of purely formalistic considerations and goes on to give the examples of 'impressionism, renaissance, copyism, ornamentalism', which he sees as lacking in originality or, at best, as refinements of extant art forms. As an alternative, the same concept of 'liberty' could, Magritte continues, equally lead to 'a rapid individual evolution', by which, as 'L'Art pur' clarifies, he means a progression towards pictorial reductionism. At the same time, Magritte comments that this 'beauty', as he puts it, has its limitations and is equally 'unbearable'. For him, reductionism is self-defeating: 'mere destroyers cannot develop any further as they have nothing left to defeat'. What Magritte appears to be condemning, therefore, is an intellectual outlook bent on wrecking and undermining, which, of course, was precisely how Dada saw itself. His concluding criticism of reductionism is that it stems from 'anarchy', which, tellingly, was one of Dada's mainstays. Moreover, whilst conceding that the only worthwhile kind of pictorial 'evolution' does involve reductionism, Magritte also insists that the process needs to be brought under control before it goes too far: 'careful people check themselves, thinking it necessary to represent something'. He certainly advocates the negation of existing conventions, but also maintains that this course can only be justified when it results in some sort of 'creation'. Crucially to Mariën's point, Magritte insists that the essential value of 'liberty' is that it opens the door to 'images of a marvellous universe', thus rejecting the notion of iconoclasm ad absurdum in favour of formative actualization. In this sense, he could well be seen to be advocating Breton's surreality, just as much as Nougé does in *Correspondance*.

It would be too simplistic, however, to conclude that 'Jusqu'où l'Évolution peut mener' sets its author against Dada in every respect. It is far from beside the point that, as a painter, Magritte would have found himself in a problematical position in relation to the movement's tenets. According to Tzara, 'any pictorial work of art is worthless', and yet, during this period, Magritte had been at his most productive.[30] What does emerge on closer scrutiny of 'Les 5 Commandements' rather is a subtext that addresses this precise dilemma of subscribing to two apparently inimical directions. Unsurprisingly, Magritte's text advocates 'creation', which ostensibly stands in diametric opposition to Dada. Notwithstanding, it then goes on to maintain that there is a distinction between 'destroyers', whom it considers to be retrograde, and 'negation', which is seen as the basis of an 'evolution'. Magritte's contention was that a negating form of iconoclasm could be regarded as a process and that, therefore, it could be realized by means of an evolving productiveness, rather than being seen as straightforward stagnation. In other words, he argued that it was more appropriate and fertile for painting to evolve towards negation than to be reined in and ultimately effaced, as Tzara would have had it. By making this distinction, Magritte endeavoured to justify the act of painting within the context of his commitment to dadaist iconoclasm. At the same time, he was only too conscious that he was sailing close to the wind and that he was grappling with discordance and contradictions; in an interview some forty years later, he reiterated the dilemma of rejecting constructiveness, whilst acknowledging that destruction was inherently futile:

> We can't go on destroying the idea of art because it's been destroyed now [...] How to go on? It's a delicate matter. To be in a situation which does not involve us in destruction or construction either.[31]

As it turned out, Magritte was vindicated by the course taken by his paintings. The concept of a 'negative painting' was precisely what was borne out by his work in the years that were to follow and, from the mid- to the late 1920s, he undertook what can be termed as a progressive deconstruction of painting, that is to say he effected an evolution towards negation. To all effects, he was to paint in the Dada spirit – his was an act of painting executed in defiance of the very canons of painting.

Magritte was, of course, not alone in his somewhat passé nod towards Dada. Mesens, his close collaborator, was himself a fervent champion of anti-tradition and in *Œsophage* he too had blatantly and provocatively attacked accepted values: 'Just as long as one doesn't bore an imbecile', he had written, 'one can try to be an accountant or a scholar'. His dadaist defiance of the conventional, however, is most apparent in his visual works, which generally took the form of collages. During the mid-1920s especially, he produced deliberately jarring and 'unaesthetic' compositions, which showed awkward, unworkable pieces of machinery, fragmented and distorted anthropomorphic shapes and displaced objects, usually assembled in senseless ways and in disorientating settings. His *Projet de monument aux suicidés de tous les temps* of 1925, the year of *Œsophage*, for instance, senselessly depicts a disembodied man's jacket which, nevertheless, 'sits' on a stool and is flanked by a gas cylinder. The influence on this and other collages of the period is patently that of Ernst, who, at the time Mesens discovered him, was resolutely dadaist. In joining forces with this 'thoroughly Dada mentality', Magritte was clearly affirming his own theoretical leanings.[32]

Whilst it is reasonable to argue that Dada had had a preparatory role for the two Belgians, after this formative phase and with the advent of *Marie*, the publication that followed *Œsophage*, Mesens and Magritte's Dada spirit began to lose its vigour. This is not so surprising however, given that four years had elapsed since the collapse of Parisian Dada and surrealism had, by then, been active for two.[33] Yet, Magritte and Mesens' resistance to surrealism was by no means fully extinguished and even in *Marie* they managed, in the first issues at least, to resist totally joining forces with the *Correspondance* group. As far as they were able at that time and without risking being labelled outmoded and recalcitrant, they attempted to continue in the vein of *Œsophage*.

Transparently aspiring to be considered abreast of current trends, *Marie* bore the subtitle 'bi-monthly magazine for beautiful youth'. The need to be seen as up-to-date intellectuals, however, forced Magritte and Mesens to acknowledge the significance of the, by then, established surrealist impetus and, accordingly, *Marie* published contributions from the *Correspondance* group; Lecomte collaborated in the first issue, and in the fourth and final one considerable space was occupied by the writings of Nougé and Goemans. Nevertheless, in the initial issues at least, the tone was decidedly dadaist, especially in the typographical layout of the first issue.[34] The second issue, a double number, 2-3, dated 8 July 1926, reproduced *Optophone*, a drawing by Picabia, and a particularly insistent expression of Dada sentiments in the form of 'Les Hommes' by Georges Ribemont-Dessaignes, which is a statement of disgust and disillusionment with the values of Western society in general:

> It is a waste of time to expect anything. We live in an era of bankruptcy: bankruptcy of science; bankruptcy of intelligence; bankruptcy of instinct; bankruptcy of morality; bankruptcy of fine arts; the bankruptcy of the notion of bankruptcy itself.

Yet, there is also an admission in the article that such a view of life can only be maintained up to a certain point. Negation in itself, as Magritte had pointed out in 'Jusqu'où l'Évolution peut mener', is seen eventually to undermine the very object of its attack to such an extent that contestation becomes pointless. Even Ribemont-Dessaignes reached the conclusion, just as Magritte had done, that, although negation cannot be abandoned, it should acquire a formulation that does not result in total destruction:

> It is not a matter of affirming, of building, nor of suddenly singing the praises of life. But my appetite for negation stops where it should. One more instant, it's too late: there is nothing left to negate.

Marie certainly is a statement of Dada, but within that statement there is also the admission that Dada can no longer continue in its original form.

With the last issue of *Marie*, came the end of Mesens and Magritte's overt involvement in Dada and their opposition to *Correspondance*. In 1926 or 1927 the polemic which had existed within the Brussels group waned and Magritte, Mesens, Lecomte, Goemans and Nougé formed 'a new group in Belgium which [was] engaging in activity in parallel with the work of the French surrealists'.[35] The fact remains, nevertheless, that by this time Mesens had been active as a dadaist for some four years and the like-minded Magritte had produced well over one hundred works. Whatever 'modern' trend they may have both followed in print, their oeuvre was to continue to tell a different story. Magritte for one painted with overtly dadaist negational spirit right to the end of the twenties.

1 René Magritte, *Écrits complets* (Paris, 1979), p. 367.

2 George Melly, in *Transformaction*, 10 (Oct. 1979): 11. E.L.T. Mesens, 'I Was in Marvellous Company', *Transformaction*, 10 (Oct. 1979): 11-6.

3 Mesens, 'I Was in Marvellous Company': 12.

4 George Melly, conversation with the author, London, April 1981.

5 Melly, conversation with the author.

6 Several letters are held by the Archives de l'Art contemporain de Belgique, which show that Magritte socialized with Mesens at the time.

7 Sarane Alexandrian, *Surrealist Art* (London, 1969), p. 29.

8 *391*, Paris, 19 (Oct. 1924). The first issue had appeared in January 1917.

9 Tristan Tzara, 'Pour Faire un Poème dadaiste', in 'Dada Manifeste sur l'amour faible et l'amour amer', in *Œuvres complètes, Tome 1, 1912-1924* (Paris, 1975), p. 382. Tzara was in contact with Magritte and contributed to the latter's *Œsophage*.

10 Magritte, *Écrits complets*, p. 367.

11 As is pointed out by José Vovelle, *Le Surréalisme en Belgique* (Brussels, 1972), p. 8. Breton's first 'Manifeste du surréalisme' is dated 1924 and the first issue of *La Révolution surréaliste* appeared in December 1924.

12 Vovelle, *Le Surréalisme en Belgique*, p. 14.

13 Christian Bussy, *Anthologie du surréalisme en Belgique* (Paris, 1972), p. 15.

14 *Œsophage*, 1 (Mar. 1925), n. pag. First published in 391 (May 1924).

15 Tristan Tzara, 'Manifeste Dada 1918', *Œuvres complètes, Tome 1, 1912-1924* (Paris, 1975), p. 367.

16 The affix 'bili' implies that the tone of the magazine is 'bilieux'. The illustration in *Œsophage* is printed on its side, possibly alluding to the fact that Duchamp's *Fountain* is a urinal placed on its side. Tristan Tzara, 'Manifeste de Monsieur Antipyrine' (1916), in *Œuvres complètes, Tome 1, 1912-1924*, p. 357. Tzara, 'Manifeste Dada 1918', p. 369.

17 Belgium, of course, is a monarchy.

18 'Dada Manifeste sur l'amour faible et l'amour amer', p. 381.

19 Tzara, 'Manifeste Dada 1918', p. 363. Tzara, 'Dada Manifeste sur l'amour faible et l'amour amer', p. 384.

20 Tzara, 'Manifeste Dada 1918', p. 360.

21 Tzara, 'Dada Manifeste sur l'amour faible et l'amour amer', p. 381.

22 Tzara, 'Manifeste Dada 1918', pp. 359-60.

23 Marcel Mariën, 'Les Pieds dans les pas', in exhibition catalogue *Magritte*, Centre d'arts plastiques contemporains, Bordeaux (1977), n. pag.

24 *Œsophage*, 1 (Mar. 1925): fourth page. See André Blavier in Magritte, *Écrits complets*, p. 32, note 4.

25 Marcel Lecomte, in Marcel Mariën, *L'Activité surréaliste en Belgique (1924-1950)* (Brussels, 1979), p. 60.

26 *Correspondance*, Vert, 10 (20 Feb. 1925): n. pag.

27 5 (15 Oct. 1925).

28 'Thus Dada was born from a need for independence, for distrust of the community.'

Tzara, 'Manifeste Dada 1918', p. 361. Camille Goemans, 'A la Recherche du temps perdu', *Correspondance*, Nankin, 5 (30 Dec. 1924): n. pag.

[29] André Breton, 'Manifeste du surréalisme' (1924), in *Manifestes du surréalisme* (Paris, 1975), p. 64.

[30] Tzara, 'Manifeste Dada 1918', p. 362.

[31] Suzi Gablik, 'Conversation with René Magritte', *Studio*, London (Mar. 1967): 129.

[32] Vovelle, *Le Surréalisme en Belgique*, p. 240.

[33] Dada had lasted in Paris from 1920 to 1922. The first issue of *Marie* is dated 1 June 1926 and the last is undated. Bussy remarks 'we only know that at the end of January 1927 the issue had not yet appeared and we think that it finally did in February or March', *Anthologie du surréalisme en Belgique*, p. 31, note 2. Vovelle writes 'We can only suggest the date September 1926', *Le Surréalisme en Belgique*, p. 18, note 49. Patrick Waldberg gives 'end of 1926' as the date, *René Magritte* (Brussels, 1965), p. 288.

[34] *Marie*, 1 (1 June 1926): n. pag.

[35] René Magritte, 'Esquisse auto-biographique', in exhibition catalogue *Magritte* (Brussels, 1954), p. 10.

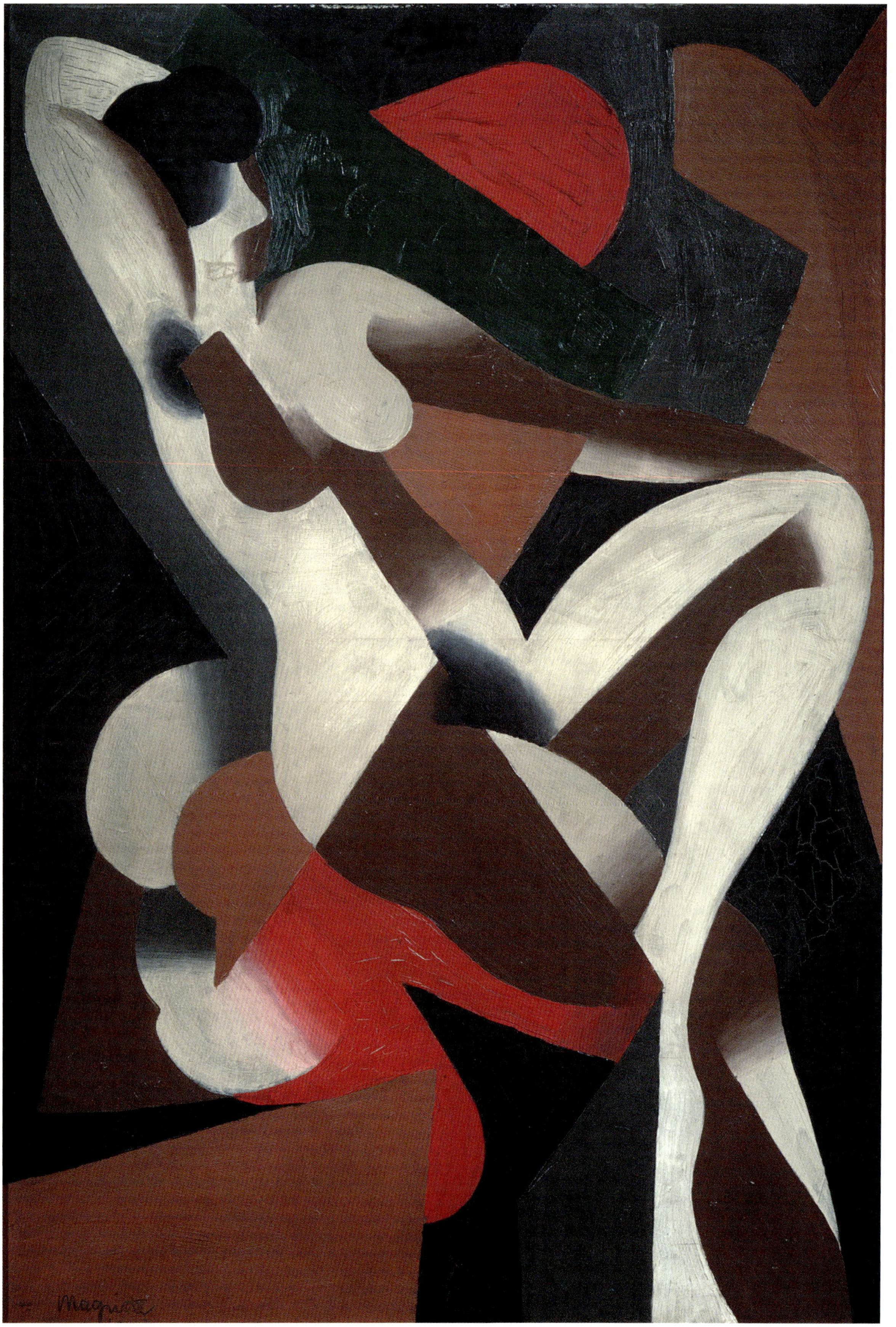

Femme (1923)

Cubism

If Magritte can be viewed as essentially dadaist, he cannot also be said to have had Cubist pretensions. Tzara made it clear that Dada and Cubism were incompatible: 'we have had', he wrote, 'enough of Cubist academies'.[1] Not surprisingly, Magritte's brief contact with Cubism shows neither innovation nor conviction. What is important, however, is that within the spectrum of Cubist experimentation he was able to discern concepts and techniques of composition that, nevertheless, were of relevance to the formulation and execution of his eventual 'dissolution' of painting. His baffling statement that he had been 'strongly influenced by Cubism' can only be seen from this perspective.[2] What can, nevertheless, be said is that Magritte saw parallels between Cubism and Dada and that he drew on the former to further his fundamental allegiance to the latter. Indeed, disregarding Tzara's dismissal of Cubism, Magritte even remarked that Cubism and Dada had had compatible roles in the development of art:

> Cubism is important [...] because it marks the end of the history of art. Up until Picasso, painting had been a matter of construction [...] The Dadaists, on the other hand, were involved in destruction.[3]

What Magritte distilled out of Cubism was its insistence on pictorial disruption; Picasso, after all, had said that 'a picture is a sum of destructions'.[4] It is, therefore, not inconsistent that a whole 'Cubist' phase should have emerged in Magritte's oeuvre from 1920 to 1923 or 1924, during his early experimentations. In themselves, however, these works showed little originality, appearing as little more than attempts to follow in the footsteps of Albert Gleizes and Jean Metzinger. Like them, Magritte based his Cubist works on straightforward depictions of, say, a figure, onto which lines that cut across contours would be superimposed, so as to divide the subject into geometric segments. Magritte invariably began with recognizable forms and would then proceed to divide them up into angled planes, fracturing the continuity of surfaces. The formula is clearly exemplified in *Femme* (1923), in which the schematic silhouette of a nude with crossed legs is broken up by straight lines. The right breast, the torso and the right thigh are all bisected along their axes, as are the right buttock and the left thigh. The resulting segments are then alternatively coloured in brown and cream, with the result that the figure's outer surfaces become disjointed and reduced to geometric planes. The procedure is echoed in Metzinger's *Woman with Mandolin* (*c.* 1913), in which a clearly distinguishable and coherent outline of a female torso contrasts with inner contours that are shattered by fragmentalizing lines. The same is true of Gleizes's *Women Sewing* (1913), which, again, depicts a fractioning of form within the confines of a faithful outline; the three figures are cleaved by straight lines that split them into disjointed planar fragments.

Magritte did not shy from acknowledging his debt to Gleizes, noting in 'L'Art pur' that his forerunner had 'in his "Study on Cubism" clearly defined the role of the work of art'.[5] The significance of Gleizes's text, *Du Cubisme et les moyens de le comprendre*, is that it presents Cubism as a systematic rebuttal of established painting, a sentiment that struck a chord with Magritte in 1922 and the immediately ensuing years.[6] It advocates 'a break with greco-roman classicism' and decries formal art instruction as worthless: 'The Fine Art Academy [...] Art school teaching does not exist, or, if it does, it amounts to no more than the wailings of an old man regressing to childhood'.[7] Of course, Picasso and Braque would have expressed the same opinion about the traditions of the past, since they too aimed at 'a breach with the conventions of Renaissance art' and employed methods in which 'the object was broken down, examined and distilled to elements of structure'.[8] What did distinguish Gleizes and Metzinger though, was that their 'decomposition of form' did not stop at examining the object in terms of its various external facets, but sought to delve beyond surface appearances.[9] Instead of being a consideration of the surface aspects of objects, for them, Cubism was more a matter of analyzing objects on the basis of their 'internal structure'.[10] Crucially, the rationale behind their methods of painting centred on a reduction of the object. In their case, the disruption of surface structure, the stripping away of superficial details was the prerequisite for a more imperative 'internal' analysis: 'Painting is not therefore an imitation of objects. The reality of the external world acts as a point of departure, but painting takes the skin off this reality in order to touch the mind'.[11]

Such a view of Cubism, as a penetrative deconstruction, was to prove pivotal for the subsequent course of Magritte's work. He too would proceed by way of an 'erosion' of the integrity of the object. Just as Gleizes and Metzinger had employed Cubist techniques to reveal what lay below the surface, so Magritte was to embark on a peeling away of the successive layers of form. In fact, Gleizes's appreciation of the Cubist mechanism and its bearing on pictorial 'syntax' maps perfectly onto the notion of 'pictorial agrammatism' that Magritte would be adopting from the mid-twenties: 'The Braque, Picasso trend [...] smashed the *syntactical* validity of the representation of objects [...] to particular essential simplifications'.[12]

As well as analyzing the structure of the independent object, Gleizes considered the nature of visual images themselves. For him, the painting directly corresponded to an anatomical assemblage:

> The internal structure of the pictorial work is like that of all natural, mineral, vegetal and organic formations [...] It has a skeleton which is mapped out by the overall structure given by essential lines, organs which are the divisions of the surface and which are interdependent, a flesh which is the colouration, a core which is substance itself.[13]

It was precisely this parallel between the physical body and the painted canvas that was to impact profoundly on Magritte's own conception of plastic representation and his approach to its demise. When Magritte embarked on his 'disassembly' of painting into its constituents, he did so in terms that resembled an organic dismemberment. Magritte was to 'take apart' what Gleizes had termed 'the body of composition'.[14] The most significant lesson that Magritte would have learnt from Gleizes was that the negation of painting, one of Dada's central preoccupations, need not, as Tzara had insisted, be incompatible with painting per se. Whereas Tzara had called for an end to the plastic work of art, Gleizes proposed that there could be negation within the context of painting, a negation that did not involve obliteration. In Cubist writings therefore, Magritte found a way out of the Dada impasse and a corroboration of the aspiration he had voiced in *Œsophage*, namely that it could be possible to defy painting not so much by discarding it as by utilising it as a self-reflexive tool. As Gleizes had pointed out, 'whilst overturning the way things are presented, [Cubism] retained the descriptive notion of painting'.[15] This was to be the underlying rationale that guided Magritte's early dadaist iconoclasm towards the concept of an 'evolving negation'.

---

[1] Tristan Tzara, 'Manifeste Dada 1918', *Œuvres complètes, Tome 1, 1912-1924* (Paris, 1975), p. 361.
[2] René Magritte, *Écrits complets* (Paris, 1979), p. 561.
[3] Suzi Gablik, 'Conversation with René Magritte', *Studio International*, London, 173(887) (Mar. 1967): 129.
[4] In Dore Aston (ed.), *Picasso on Art* (London, 1972), p. 38.
[5] René Magritte & Victor Servranckx, 'L'Art pur', in Magritte, *Écrits complets*, p. 20.
[6] As André Blavier points out in Magritte, *Écrits complets*, p. 24, note 13.
[7] Albert Gleizes, *Du Cubisme et les moyens de le comprendre* (Paris, 1920), pp. 8 & 11.
[8] Pierre Daix, *Picasso* (London, 1965), p. 88. Paul Waldo Schwartz, *The Cubists* (London, 1971), p. 9.
[9] Daix, *Picasso*, p. 91.
[10] Gleizes, *Du Cubisme et les moyens de le comprendre*, p. 13.
[11] Gleizes, *Du Cubisme et les moyens de le comprendre*, p. 23.
[12] Gleizes, *Du Cubisme et les moyens de le comprendre*, p. 12. Italics my own. This study will argue that in the twenties Magritte severed the links between pictorial elements in a way comparable with the agrammatic aphasics' failure to produce coherent verbal concatenation.
[13] Gleizes, *Du Cubisme et les moyens de le comprendre*, pp. 32-3.
[14] Gleizes, *Du Cubisme et les moyens de le comprendre*, p. 33.
[15] Gleizes, *Du Cubisme et les moyens de le comprendre*, p. 12.

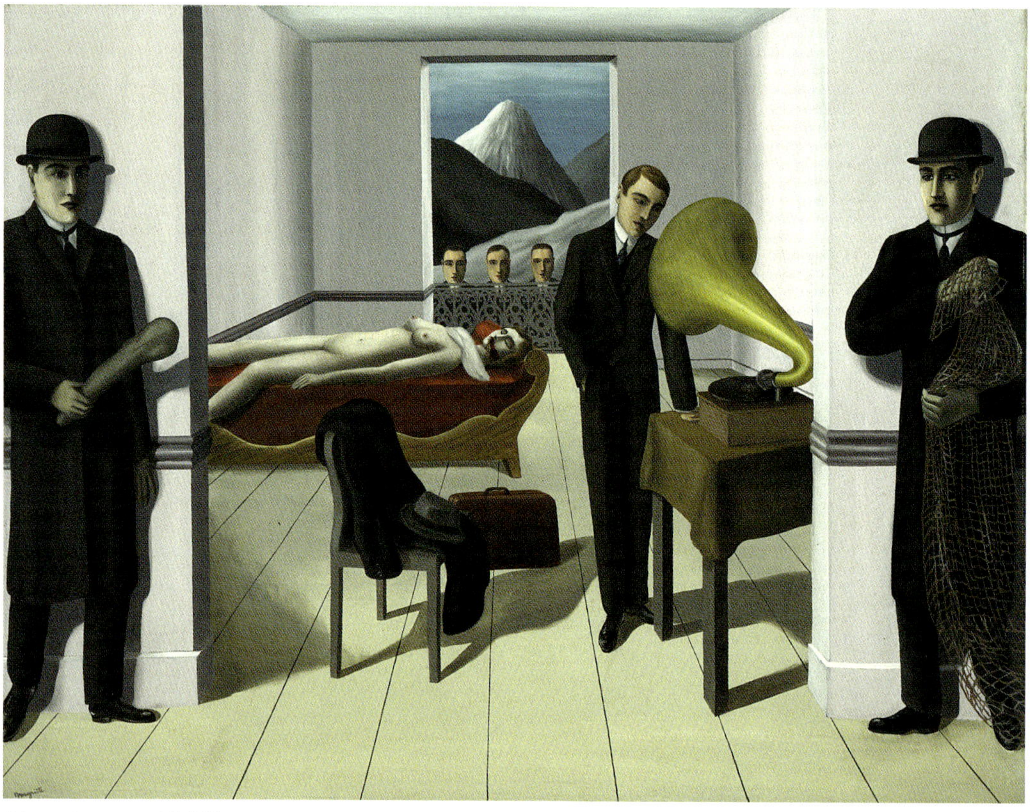

L'Assassin menacé (1927)

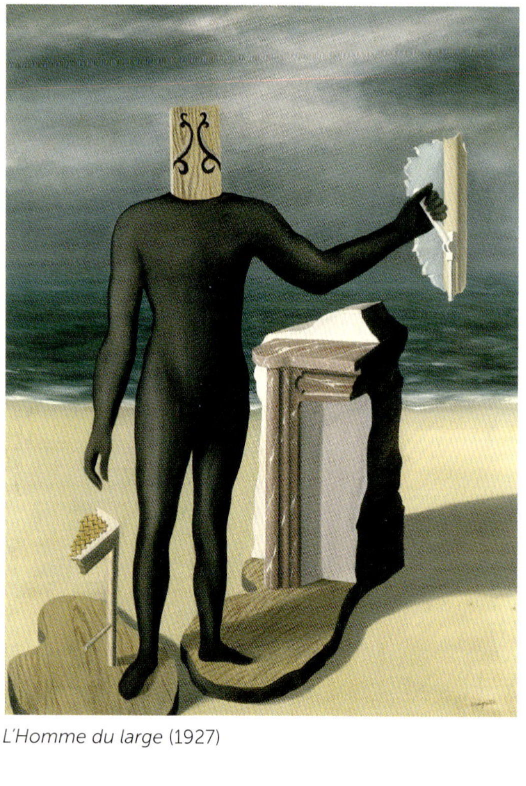

L'Homme du large (1927)

The Spark

Magritte's avowed preceptor was Giorgio de Chirico. 'He was my spark', he acknowledged and Laura Rosenstock went as far as to single out de Chirico as his single most important influence.[1] Magritte himself related that his initial encounter with the work of the Italian painter was no less than an emotionally overwhelming event: 'One of the most moving moments of my life was when I first saw a reproduction of de Chirico's painting *The Song of Love*'.[2]

Exactly when this event occurred and under whose instigation is uncertain. Gablik puts forward the dates 1923-4, whilst James Thrall Soby suggests 'around 1919' and Philippe Roberts-Jones gives a dating of 1922.[3] Blavier, for his part, writes that 'for Mesens, it was after the publication of *Œsophage* that Magritte had the revelation of *The Song of Love*', and Richard Calvocoressi corroborates this with his suggestion of 1925.[4] As for who had been responsible for Magritte's epiphany, most critics credit Lecomte but, according to Blavier, Scutenaire had maintained that 'Édouard – and no one else – showed René Magritte the reproduction of a canvas of Chirico, "Le Chant d'Amour"'.[5] However it had come about, the awareness of de Chirico's work had set a course for Magritte, who saw it as a model for the defiance of the conventions of painting. As he recognized, de Chirico's approach 'replaced the stereotypical effect of traditional painting' and amounted to a 'complete break with mental habits'.[6] Elaborating on this point, Marcel Jean points out that it was specifically the conception of the visible world conceived in the Renaissance that had been defied by de Chirico; his work was a 'perversion of fifteenth century practices', as William Rubin concurs.[7] Indeed, in opposition to the humanist values of the quattrocento, which accorded man primary importance, de Chirico presented a world in which the human element is, at best, fleeting. His townscapes are deserted places where human presences are only hinted at and shadows invariably have more prominence than living figures, which, even when they are portrayed, appear as mere representations of themselves, as statues or mannequins. For Jean, even the apparently assertive figure in *The Child's Brain* (1914) is phantom-like. Time and again the human ingredient is relegated to the inanimate and insubstantial.

Predictably, the early twentieth-century modernist machine-inspired aesthetic of human empowerment was equally undermined by de Chirico. His work turned its back on the fashionable taste for speed and dynamism championed by his Futurist contemporaries and, instead, reduced the emblems of man's mastery over the material, his edifices, his monuments and his tools, to an arid insignificancy. For him, all attempts to rationalize the world were futile and confused. Above all, it was the pictorial endeavours to make sense of space

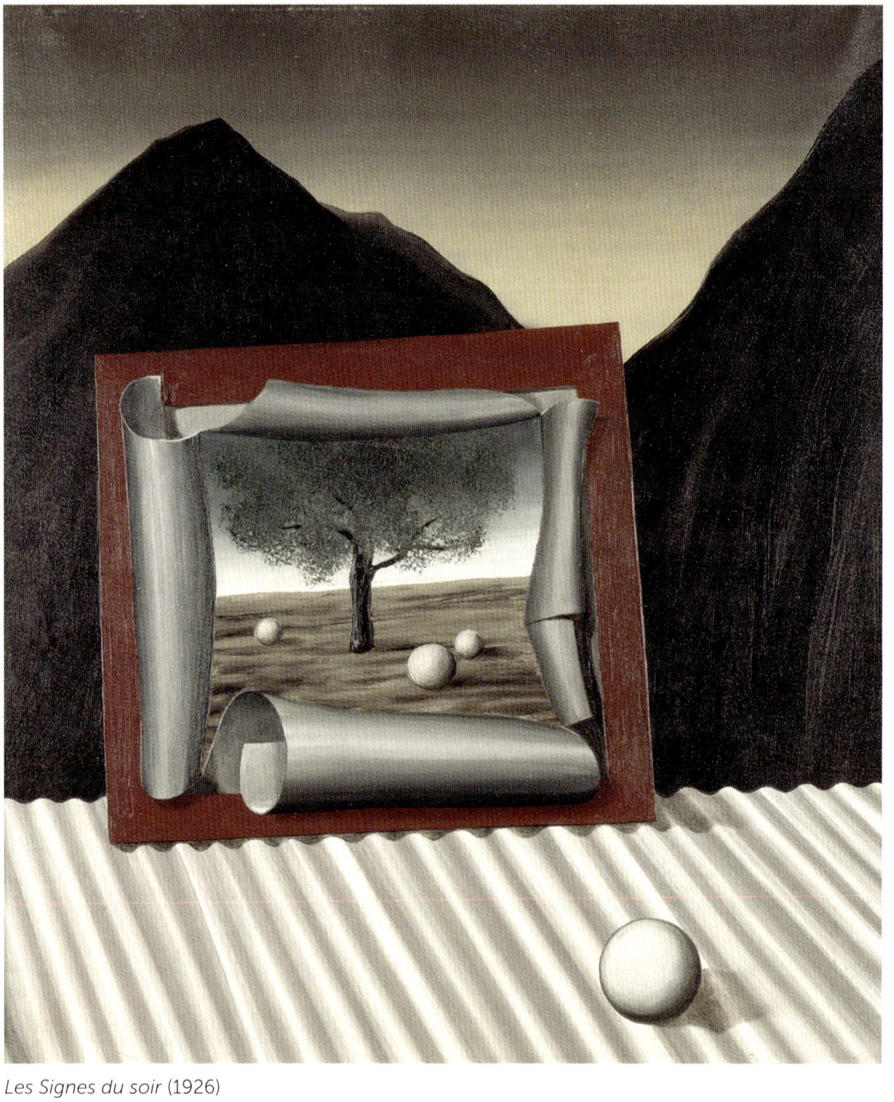

Les Signes du soir (1926)

by means of perspectival formulae that de Chirico attacked. It is because, as Jean further points out, de Chirico distorts rather than ignores perspective that he appears to be pointing out its flaws and limitations. For Jean, de Chirico is intent on undermining not just the conventions of art, but also the fundaments of thinking that brought them about. In a conscious manner, de Chirico took representation beyond the scope of its 'human' rationalization: 'a work of art', he said, 'must go completely beyond the limits of the human: logic and common sense will have to be completely absent'.[8] For de Chirico, art was a rejection of pictorial convention, 'a counter logic' and, even, a 'rebellion from systems of logic'.[9] He wanted to replace the world as it had been seen until then with a new vision, a vision that was to 'rid art of all that has been its familiar content until now'.[10] As he went on to explain, 'a picture must represent something which has no sense in itself, has no subject, which from the point of view of human logic means nothing at all'.[11]

His *Self Portrait* (1913), for instance, is anything but and demonstrates de Chirico's 'ultimatum against the accepted canons of realism'.[12] It depicts an inclined surface on which rest an egg, a scroll and the feet of a marble statue and behind which two distant factory chimneys rise up. Such scenari led Magritte to consider de Chirico as 'the first painter who had thought of making painting speak of something other than painting' and resulted in repeated iconographic borrowings in his own work.[13] Among Magritte's homagistic references are the fluttering pennants in *Le Chevalier du couchant* (1926), the awkward perspective in *Jeune fille* (1924), the theatrical setting of *L'Assassin menacé* (1927) and the recurrent theme of the painting within a painting. In a transparently direct manner, Magritte transposed the lower torso from de Chirico's *The Duo* (1915) to his *L'Homme du large* (1927), the sphere from *The Song of Love* to his *Les Signes du soir* (1926) and the wigs frequently painted by de Chirico to his *Le Mariage de minuit* (1926). Magritte also adopted several of de Chirico's titles – 'Le Duo', 'Le Chant d'amour' and 'Deux Sœurs'.

De Chirico's impact on Magritte, however, goes beyond a straightforward duplication of subject matter. It is not so much de Chirico's choice of pictorial elements that is captured in Magritte's work as their underlying treatment. There is a shift from conventional compositional coherence to a format based on 'dislocations', as Georges Hugnet had remarked in 1936.[14] De Chirico's objects may be seen side by side, but they coexist in an uneasy tension, remaining essentially unrelated within the painting. It was this alternative vision that had made a deep impression on Magritte and would become the model for his own pictorial disruption. In a dual trajectory, he would disarticulate individual pictorial elements, as well as derange the pictorial space that contained them. Crucially for Magritte, de Chirico had subverted the conventional representation of distances and expanses. In direct opposition to the logical space prescribed by Renaissance perspective, his tilted ground planes produced a space that was 'shallow and vertiginous'.[15] As *The Enigma of a Day* (1914) demonstrates, any illusion of a coherent space is immediately shattered by a multiplicity of vanishing points that create mutually contradictory perspective readings. Space is not just indeterminate, according to Rubin, it is positively paradoxical:

> The orthogonals of the arcaded building at the left meet not at, but above, the horizon line, to the left of the lower smoke stack; those of the right-hand building meet at the foot of the other chimney; and the vanishing point of the statue's socle is somewhere far outside the pictorial field.[16]

Moreover, even when architectural spaces are depicted, the impression is no less ambiguous. Perspectival recession is repeatedly challenged, as *Gare*

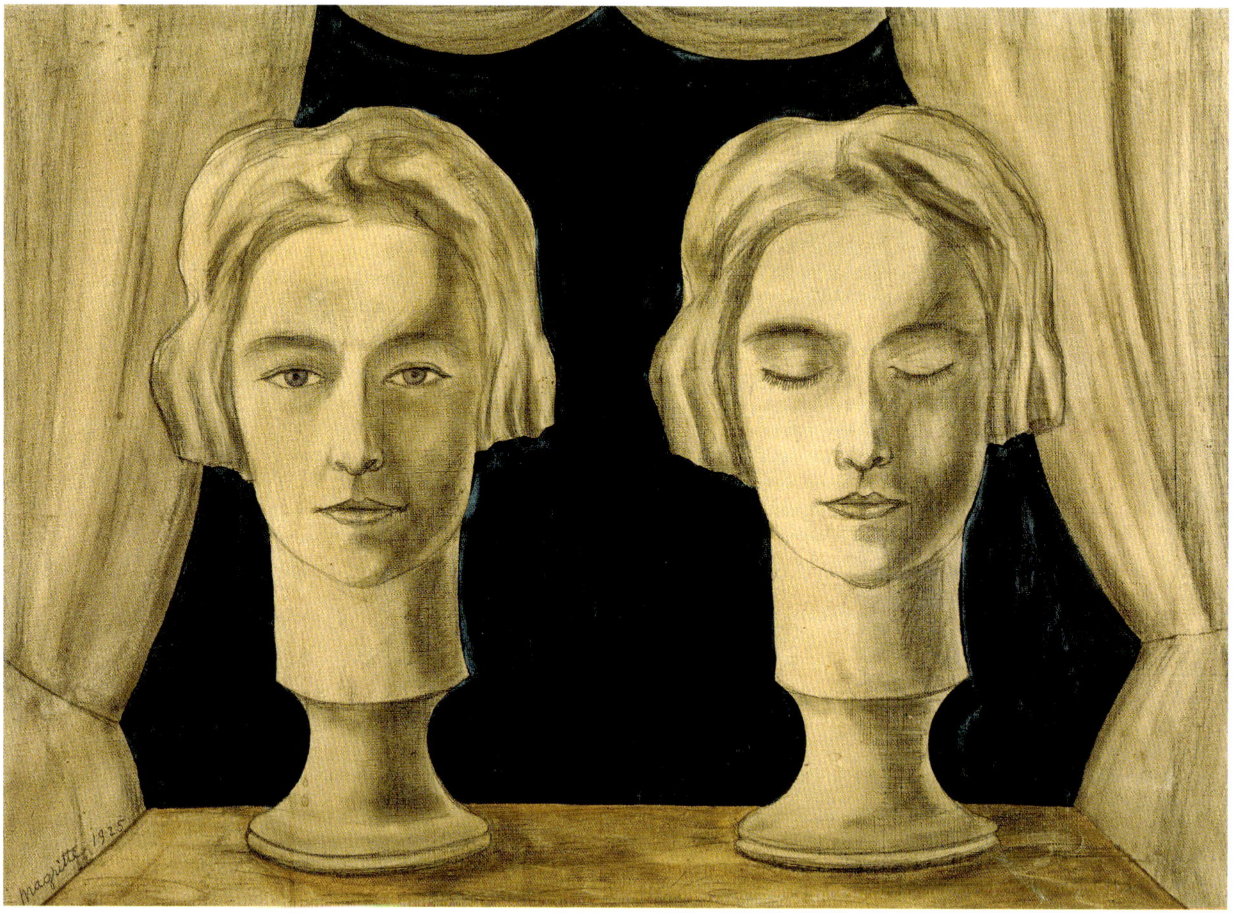

Deux Sœurs (1925)

Montparnasse (The Melancholy of Departure) (1914) shows with its deformation of the ground into a shallow, sharply tilted space that contradicts the dimensions of the upper platform. As Soby concludes, 'the measure of depth is thoroughly ambiguous; geometry has been wilfully altered'.[17]

What de Chirico also erodes is the very substantiality of individual forms. Within his already equivocal spaces he places what are sometimes no more than 'spectral figures and menacing shadows'.[18] Whenever a human element is indicated, it is almost invariably bereft of weight and bulk and, whilst retaining its external contours, it appears disembodied and denuded. De Chirico, we are told by Rubin, 'so diminishes or dissolves the solidity of masses as to finally constitute little more than a decorative convention for articulating the planar surface'.[19] Soby, for his part, observes that the little girl in *Mystery and Melancholy of a Street* (1914) 'is doomed, for she is herself a shadow, perhaps retracing the steps which led to her dissolution'.[20] De Chirico, however,

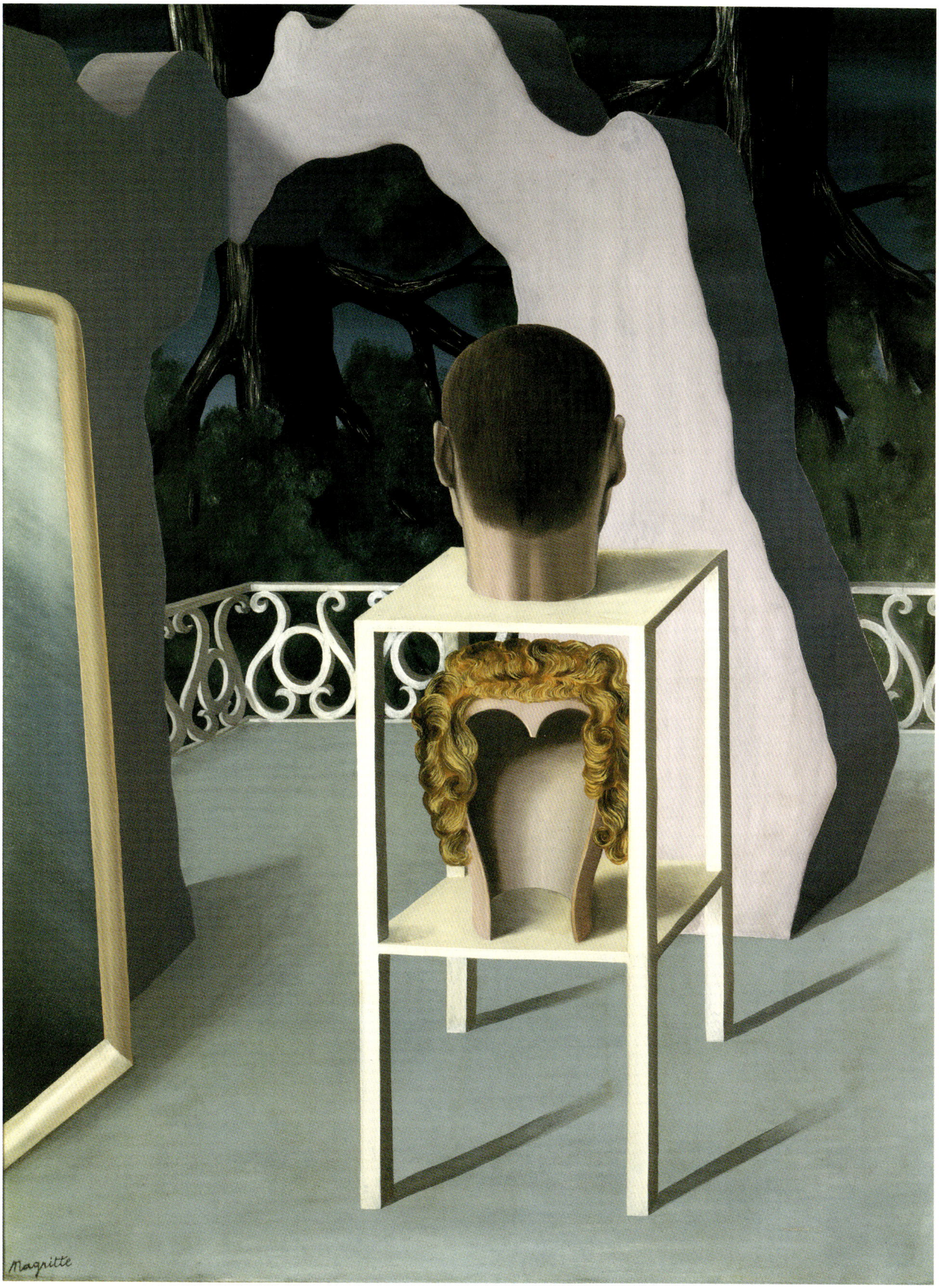

Le Mariage de minuit (1926)

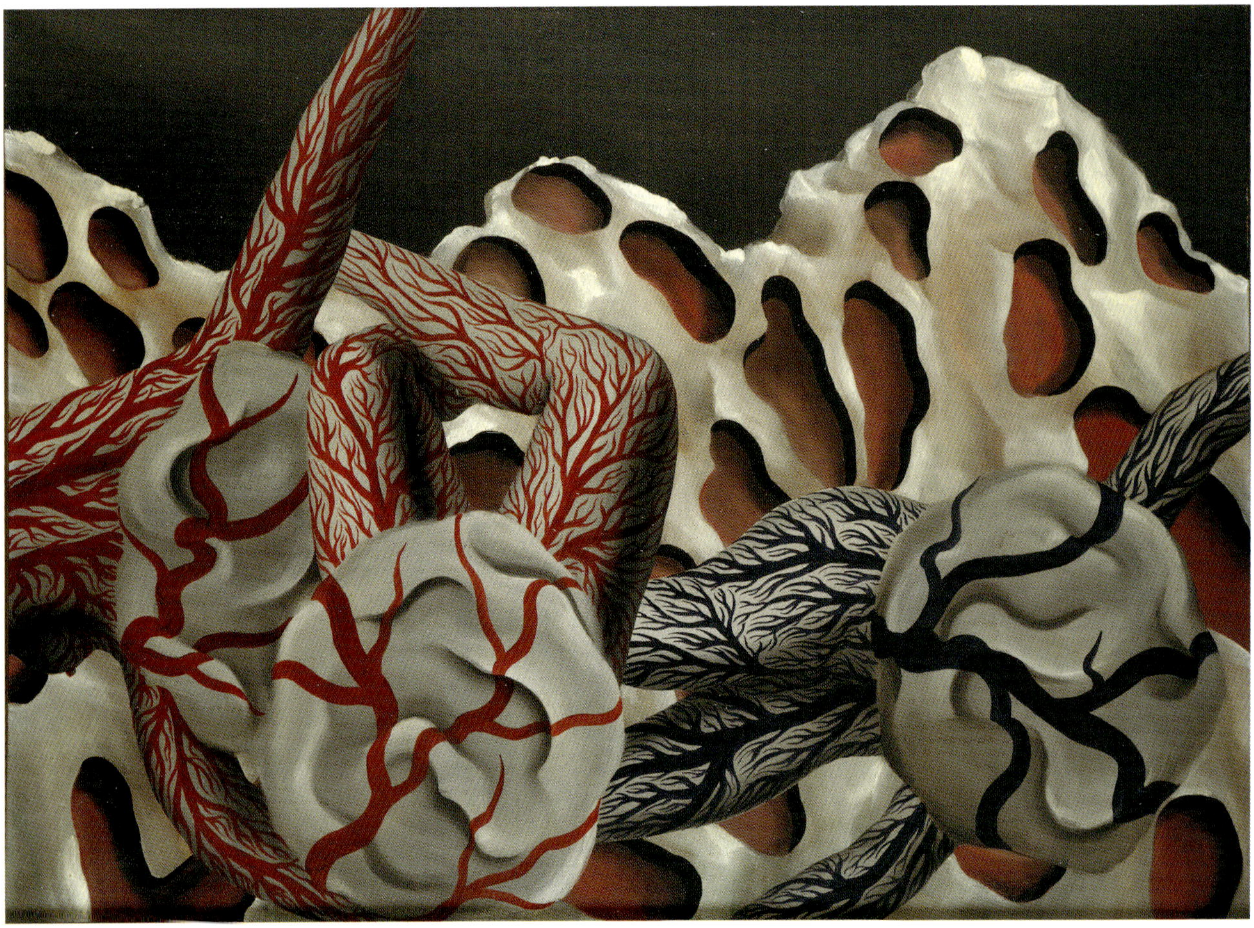

Le Sang du monde (1926-27)

does more than reduce the human form to a spectre: he also challenges it in another, more overtly destructive manner. Alongside his de-substantiation of the body, de Chirico conducts a process akin to dissection. The allusion is explicit in *The Scholar's Playthings* (1917), where diagrams of écorchés expose bones, sinews and veins, all of which suggest that the body's surface layer has been ripped away. *The Span of Black Ladders* (1914) shows this in even more graphic detail, revealing every vessel, bone and muscle of a giant hand. The process does not stop there, however, and extends to de Chirico's pseudo humans, his mannequins, which are cut open, as in *The Inconsistencies of the Thinker* (1915), to reveal inner springs and tubes or as in *The Astronomer* (1915), where the broken mannequin casing exposes a series of loops, resembling a vertebral column. For Magritte, this treatment of the figure was to provide a model, which, in some cases, would be followed literally: *Le Sang du monde* (1926-7) strips away the skin to show the body as écorché, whilst *La Fin des contemplations* (1927) cuts into the body precisely in the manner of *I'll*

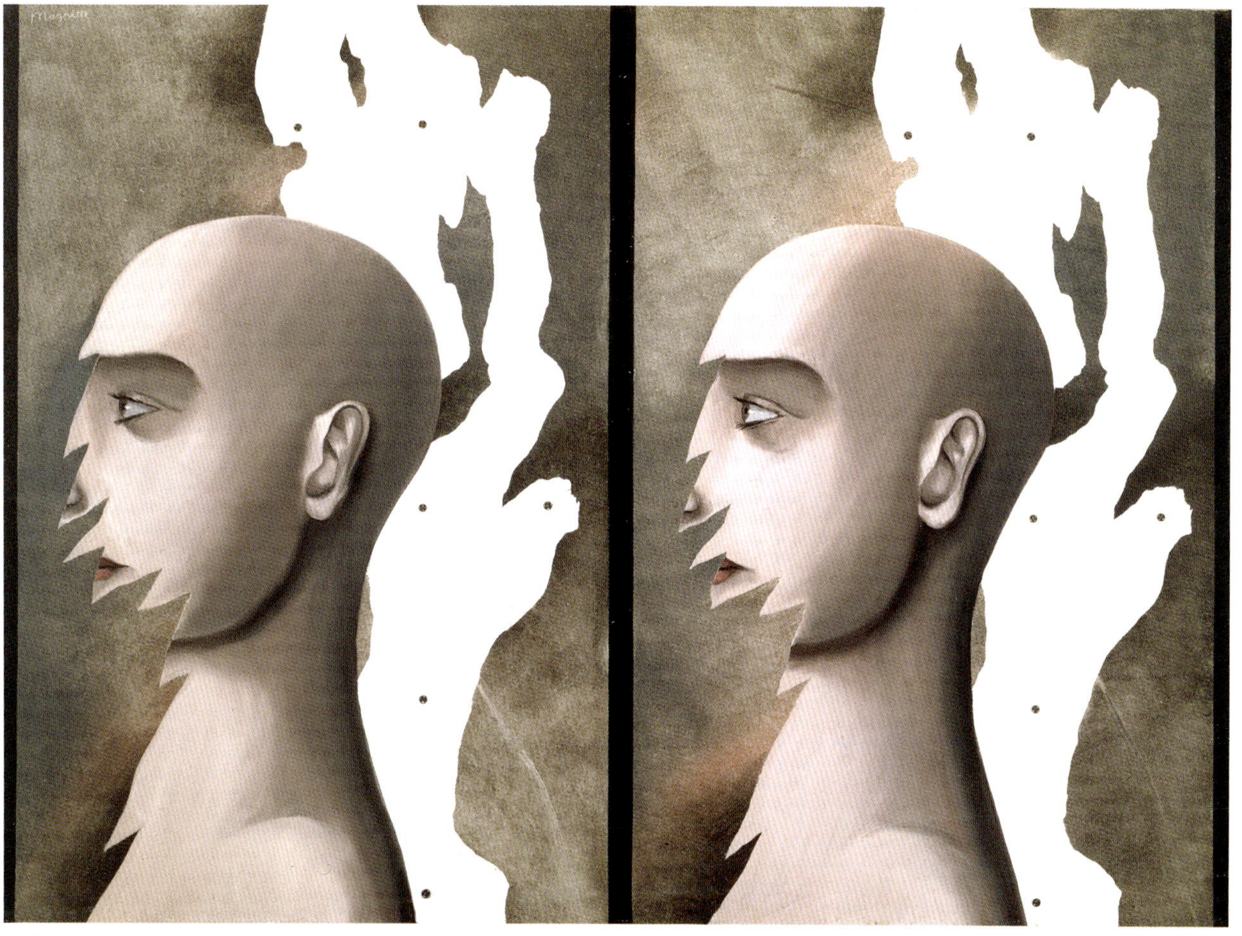

La Fin des contemplations (1927)

be There: The Glass Dog (1914). In the case of both painters the subversion of three-dimensional space is coupled with a systematic 'questioning of the human figure'.[21]

✣ ✣ ✣

The second part of this book will argue that, just like de Chirico, although in a far more rigorous manner, Magritte subjected the two components of traditional pictorial construction, the illusion of space and the modelling of form, to an analytical 'dissolution'. Also like de Chirico, Magritte elaborated this iconoclastic trajectory wholly within the confines of pictorial representation and, inasmuch, he distanced himself from the tenets of Dada. Indeed, Magritte's encounter with de Chirico's paintings has been regarded as the origin of his 'turning towards surrealist painting' and his rejection of Dada's total nihilism.[22] Whilst it can be said that de Chirico's work must have reinforced Magritte's essentially dadaist intention to overthrow traditional art, it also offered an alternative course. Familiarity with de Chirico's oeuvre gave Magritte a way of progressing from the negation on which he had embarked with Mesens to a quest for a 'counter-reality'.[23] By 'questioning the rational world of space and object', de Chirico provided the spark that ignited Magritte's own contestation of the dogmas of formal art.[24]

---

[1] René Magritte, *Écrits complets* (Paris, 1979), p. 642. Laura Rosenstock, 'De Chirico's Influence on the Surrealists', in exhibition catalogue *De Chirico*, Tate Gallery (London, 1982), p. 119.

[2] Magritte, *Écrits complets*, p. 664.

[3] Suzi Gablik, *Magritte* (London, 1971), p. 25. James Thrall Soby, *Giorgio de Chirico* (New York, 1966), p. 76. Philippe Roberts-Jones, *Magritte, poète visible* (Brussels, 1972), p. 14.

[4] André Blavier, in Magritte, *Écrits complets*, p. 370, note 9. Richard Calvocoressi, *Magritte* (Oxford, 1979), p. 8.

[5] Blavier, in Magritte, *Écrits complets*, p. 370, note 9. Louis Scutenaire, 'Mon Ami Mesens', *Transformaction*, 10 (Oct. 1979): 5.

[6] Magritte, *Écrits complets*, p. 116.

[7] Marcel Jean, *Histoire de la peinture surréaliste* (Paris, 1959), pp. 40-55. William Rubin, 'De Chirico and Modernism', in exhibition catalogue *De Chirico* (1982), p. 56.

[8] De Chirico in, Maurizio Fagiolo dell'Arco, 'De Chirico in Paris, 1911-1915', in exhibition catalogue *De Chirico* (1982), p. 31.

[9] Soby, *Giorgio de Chirico*, p. 54. Joan M. Lukach, 'De Chirico and Italian Art Theory, 1915-1920', in exhibition catalogue *De Chirico* (1982), p. 39.

[10] De Chirico, in Soby, *Giorgio de Chirico*, p. 42.

[11] De Chirico, in Soby, *Giorgio de Chirico*, p. 100.

[12] Soby, *Giorgio de Chirico*, p. 42.

[13] Magritte, *Écrits complets*, p. 482.

[14] Georges Hugnet, 'In the Light of Surrealism', in exhibition catalogue *Fantastic Art, Dada and Surrealism*, Museum of Modern Art (New York, 1936), reprinted (New York, 1968), p. 39.

[15] Rubin, 'De Chirico and Modernism', p. 58.

[16] Rubin, 'De Chirico and Modernism', p. 58.

[17] Soby, *Giorgio de Chirico*, p. 71.

[18] Rubin, 'De Chirico and Modernism', p. 56.

[19] Rubin, 'De Chirico and Modernism', p. 59. The concept of 'dissolving' forms is central to the second part of this study.

[20] Soby, *Giorgio de Chirico*, pp. 72 & 74.

[21] José Vovelle, *Le Surréalisme en Belgique* (Brussels, 1972), p. 89.

[22] Vovelle, *Le Surréalisme en Belgique*, p. 86.

[23] Soby, *Giorgio de Chirico*, p. 119.

[24] Lukach, 'De Chirico and Italian Art Theory 1915-1920', p. 112.

THE REBELLION
1924-1930

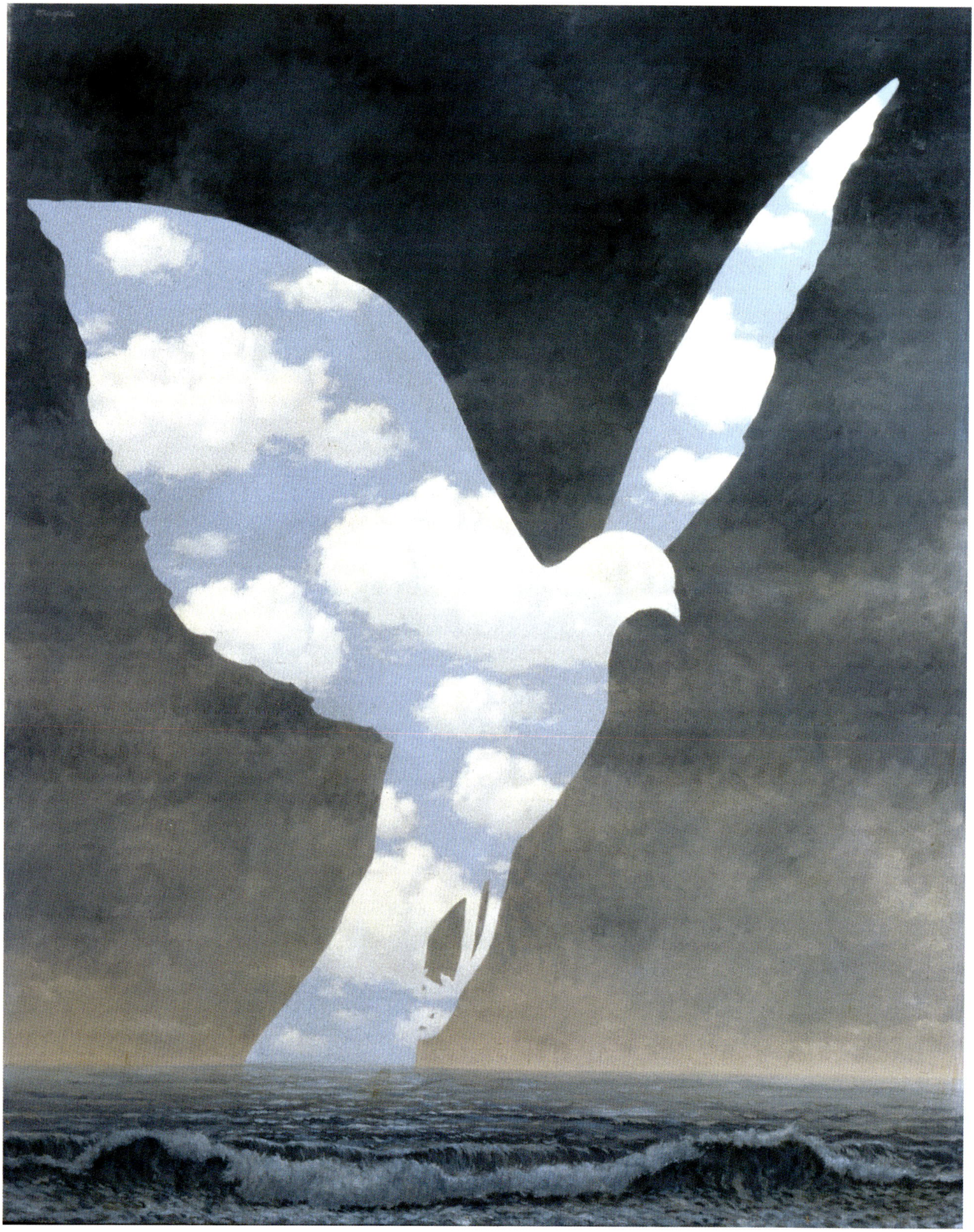

La Grande Famille (1963)

Unlocking the Code

Magritte has been described not only as a 'pictorial poet', but also as one who 'dissolves the untidy picture of the ordinary world'.[1] That he unravels the ways in which pictorial convention organizes visual perception had been apparent from his initial Orphic essays. Even the early work *La Retraite militaire* had been an overt endeavour to break up form and to subdivide light. That this process should have been considered 'poetic' additionally suggests that Magritte's methods rest on essentially verbal principles.

To Magritte himself that would have made perfect sense. Repeatedly, he drew parallels between what is painted and what is written and in 1929 he went as far as to propose that words and images function analogously: 'sometimes', he wrote, 'the name of an object can take the place of an image [...] an image', he continued, 'can take the place of a word'.[2] Central to his thinking was a straightforward interchangeability between the verbal and the visual. The notion was a simple one, but it was far from insignificant. What is important about this 'equivalence' between words and images is that it paves the way for a deep understanding of how Magritte's paintings function. By following his advice of regarding images as words and words as images, we become aware that his plethora of pictorial transpositions, substitutions, amalgamations and segmentations are far from arbitrary. Instead, they emerge as interrelated phases within a coherent rationale. Indeed, not only is Magritte's work underpinned by a 'dissolution' of pictorial convention, as Hammacher had pointed out, but also it is governed by an inner logic that, as will become clearer, mirrors the typology of language.

If, as Magritte himself more than hinted, the inner workings of his paintings find their counterpart in the interplay of words within language, then the key to his 'dissolution' of the picture of the ordinary world may well lie in a dissolution of some sort on the verbal level. This would provide a model, which, on the basis of Magritte's theory of interchangeability, could be mapped onto his paintings to reveal patterns and rationalizations. As it turns out, such a model can, in fact, be deduced from the studies of Roman Jakobson into precisely the ways in which language can break down. In his studies on aphasia, a condition characterized by the loss of the ability to communicate verbally or to use written words, he sets out clear categories of linguistic 'dissolution'. Arguably, these provide templates against which Magritte's stages of pictorial disintegration can be measured. On the basis of an analogy with Jakobson's findings on the aphasic depletion of language, Magritte's system or 'code' can therefore be progressively unlocked.

Aphasia itself is the collective name for various language impairments that a sufferer may possess in various degrees and combinations. The defect is not a loss of words, but a failure in the capacity to use them in communicating meaning. Aphasia has been defined as 'a disturbance in the ability to use a conventional system of symbols to express or comprehend ideas'.[3] Aphasic deviations from the conventions of the verbal system have been classified by Jakobson into two main categories. The first he calls a 'similarity disorder' and corresponds to the difficulty in using words as isolated symbols, or in considering them as substitutes for related symbols.[4] The sufferer in this case is unable to select between alternative symbols in paradigmatic classes. The second defect is termed a 'contiguity disorder' and is marked by difficulty in seeing the interrelations of words in a verbal context.[5] There is an inability to combine different classes of words into syntagmatic sequences.

Clinical observations have confirmed that there are, indeed, two axes of language loss, the main distinction being between grammatical, syntactic errors and lexical, word-finding disorders. In the loss of grammar, termed 'agrammatism', syntactic rules are lost and there is no grammatical coordination or subordination.[6] The opposing loss of names, 'anomia', entails the inability to select or identify concurrent possibilities and alternatives and sometimes leads to neology, the invention of new words or the attribution of new senses to established words. Significantly, aphasia is not a total language loss, but, rather, an impairment of one aspect of language with the relative stability of the other features. Consequently, there is an imbalance that makes aphasic speech stilted rather than incomprehensible. The reason for this becomes clearer when the processes involved in the normal linguistic operations of 'encoding' and 'decoding' a message are considered.[7] The encoder, the initiator of an utterance, first selects words and then combines them into a message. Conversely, the decoder, the receiver of a message, is given an already-combined message, or context, from which s/he selects and classifies words. Thus, for the encoder, selection precedes combination and for the decoder, combination precedes selection. The reason why only partial speech is lost in aphasia is that only the second half of each operation is impaired, the initial stage being retained. Therefore, an encoding-defective aphasic, that is the agrammatic, will be able to select words but fail to place them in a grammatical pattern, whereas the decoding-defective aphasic, the anomic, will be able to produce or identify a grammatical framework, whilst remaining incapable of selecting or recognizing appropriate words to fill it. The encoding-defective aphasia of agrammatism (also known as non-fluent or Broca's aphasia) is exhibited by an inability to combine words into larger linguistic units. A marked absence of prepositions disrupts the interrelation of words and effaces the contextual setting. Jakobson describes the condition as 'the degeneration of the sentence into a mere "word heap"'.[8] As contiguity is in jeopardy, the higher a construction is in the grammatical hierarchy, the more likely it is to disintegrate. The largest unit bound by syntax, the sentence, is, therefore, the most vulnerable construction in agrammatism. The first elements of the sentence that are lost are connectives, articles, pronouns and conjunctions, since these determine grammatical context and hierarchy. However, although syntactic dependence is weakened or dispensed with altogether, selection and vocabulary remain, which results in an imbalance that restricts the utterance to word classes. The effect is pidgin-like and is termed 'style petit nègre' or 'telegraphic speech'. In general terms, it is the 'function' words of grammar that are lost. These words have no meaning but designate condition, subordination, and grammatical relation. Their only purpose is to dictate syntagmatic relations, that is to say positional associations that depend on contiguity. Indeed they are never learnt in isolation but in conjunction with other words. Clearly, conditionals and subordinate clauses become difficult, if not impossible, for the agrammatic aphasic. Equally, the sentence is depleted of dependent words, such as adverbs, adjectives and finite verbs. These types of syntactic dependence, in the form of 'agreements', are nevertheless more resistant in aphasia than the loss of prepositions, which affect government; this is because, whilst agreement marks grammatical similarity, government denotes pure contiguity.

The second level of word loss for the agrammatic is morphological. Despite the persistence of semantic classes in this case, words are not related to grammatical categories. Inflections are lost, again on a selective basis. The more an ending is based on contiguity the more difficult it is. For example, the plural 's' is a semantic modification and so the aphasic is better able to deal with it than the possessive 's', which marks syntactic relation. Similarly, changes of aspect that depend on grammatical context become indistinguishable: cases (he, him, his), derivatives (guarantee, guarantor) and tenses are abolished. The tendency, Jakobson notes, is for words to be reduced to their nominal functions and also to their nominal forms.[9] Characteristically, the nominative case dominates as do verb infinitives and gerunds. In severe cases, however, the phonological level is also impaired and even a sequence of distinctive features becomes difficult. Problematic word construction gives rise to an increase in homonyms and a decrease in vocabulary. Language may finally deteriorate into one-word or one-phoneme utterances, a condition called 'aphasia universalis'. Even when the word does remain, it may be dissociated from its significative function and, whilst grasped as known, it ceases to have meaning attributed to it; the word effectively loses its normal significative function and assumes the purely distinctive function that normally pertains to the phoneme.[10]

A fourth aspect of agrammatic loss of linguistic organization is its impact on perceived interrelations between things. The aphasic's unsystematic linguistic interchange of person, number, gender and personal pronouns indicates an inability to understand that things or people can occupy a place related to a sequence. One patient was reported to have 'failed to distinguish signs that represented positions in the same dimensions – whether time, space or gender'.[11] The problem posed by such concepts, just as by grammar, is that of 'sequences of position' – yesterday, today, tomorrow.[12] Another patient had difficulty in distinguishing parts of the body, since some of their meaning depends on a contrast of sequences of position. The contiguity defect of agrammatism, therefore, affects concatenation and hierarchical organization in a general sense. In the case of words, those that are strong in semantic content are retained, but the links between them, together with the connectives that define them, are lost.

The alternative form of aphasia is a similarity disorder termed 'amnestic', 'Wernicke's', 'fluent' or 'semantic' aphasia. In this condition, the encoding capacity remains intact, whilst decoding is impaired. The grammatical framework of pronouns and conjunctions remains, but there is a marked word-finding difficulty. Nouns become less varied and tend towards group or generalized words, with the suppression of synonyms and antonyms. Consequently, specific nouns are supplanted by words like 'thing' or '*machin*'. The inability to select initially causes the loss of the subject word, since this, above all, is independent of the context; the subject of a sentence arises from conceptual and semantic selection, rather than combination. In other words, the subject is the word with which others combine, not vice versa. Thus, in contrast with the agrammatic, the fluent aphasic has problems with roots, not affixes. Pronouns are more likely to be used than nouns and, although there is sensitivity to differences made by suffixes (editor, edition, editorial), there is a loss of the ability to distinguish roots with the same suffix (editor, auditor, solicitor). The main linguistic aspect that remains is a sense of grammatical relation, and so a 'one track embedding in the context' emerges.[13] The fluent aphasic has difficulty in starting a dialogue, but can react to a context; one aphasic, for instance, could say 'it rains' only if it were actually raining. Equally, there is a tendency to refer to objects by explaining the use to which they are put, a 'knife' being called a 'pencil sharpener' in one case. Any type of definition presents difficulty because it involves the use of a substitution set and, consequently, similarity. The fluent aphasic cannot say what a thing is, but only what it is for or what it goes with; meaning is conveyed through contextualization, rather than identification. It is because substitution is difficult that the amnestic aphasic is unable to grasp the function of naming and this leads to a dissociation of the label from the concept and of one label from a similar one.[14] There is failure to identify constituents of a set of 'concurrent substitutive possibilities'.[15]

This incompetence in the use of a substitution set extends beyond verbal symbols to include pictorial signs. The amnestic aphasic cannot, for instance, attach a label to a visual representation. 'The picture of an object', according to Jakobson, 'will cause the suppression of its name: a verbal sign is supplanted by a pictorial sign.'[16] There is a failure to shift from the icon to the symbol. What the fluent aphasic cannot do, therefore, is to decode, an operation that depends on a similarity jump. Sometimes, this inability extends to simple repetition and progress through word classes becomes impossible. All that remains of language is syntagmatic sequencing. Naming is not achieved through a metalanguage – 'we call this a pencil' – but by relations of contiguity, that is to say by metonymy. For instance, 'fork' is used for 'knife' because 'knife' belongs to 'knife and fork' of which 'fork' is a part. For Jakobson, 'such metonymies may be characterized as projections from the line of habitual context into the line of substitution and selection: a sign (e.g. fork), which usually occurs together with another sign (e.g. knife), may be used instead of this sign'.[17] He sums up this phenomenon as the 'escape from sameness to contiguity'.[18] 'Black', he continues, would be used for 'dead', 'glass' for 'window', 'heaven' for 'God'. This projection from the syntagmatic axis to the paradigmatic can be so pronounced that it may transpose the rules of sentence-building to the construction of words and, thus, result in neology.

An important point for Jakobson is that the two kinds of aphasia reveal not so much different degrees of a language defect, as different facets of language itself. By marking the discrete extremities of the linguistic spectrum, agrammatism and anomia show that language has a fundamental bivalency: 'there is a decided gap', we are told, 'between the very short-phrased Broca's aphasics and the long-phrased fluents'.[19] From this premise, Jakobson goes on to argue that the capacity for verbal combination is independent of the capacity for selection. For him, language functions in terms of the two independent dimensions of the Saussurian model, the paradigmatic and the syntagmatic axes. What studies into aphasia have also shown is that the way in which the two axes intersect need not be equally proportional.

Jakobson goes on to extrapolate that the way in which we speak is an indication of the way in which we think: 'the dichotomy here discussed', he observes, 'appears to be of primal significance and consequence for all verbal behaviour and for human behaviour in general'.[20] Indeed, at the beginning of the twentieth century the neurologist and psychologist Arnold Pick had already concluded that 'certain forms of aphasia can be considered part of a broader disorder of thinking which goes beyond verbalization'.[21] This is Jakobson's point. As he sees it, the interface of the two poles of expression revealed through aphasia can, in varying permutations and degrees of emphasis, act as a paradigm for the articulation of all human thought.

It is logical, therefore, that, in the case of Magritte's visual thought, which centres on dissolution, the structures implicit in aphasic disintegration should offer an apposite model. That is to say, the ways in which aphasia distorts the intermeshing of the axes of combination and selection can be seen as a template for Magritte's disassembly of the pictorial. On this basis, the steps by which Magritte took painting apart would find their linguistic counterparts among the distinct phases by which aphasia proceeds. Both processes, according to Jakobson's rationale, share the same deep structure. It is not simply that aphasia disrupts linguistic relations and that Magritte's work fragments the conventions of pictorial representation; it is more that there is a correlation between the two. Whether they are visual or linguistic, the 'dictionaries' that dictate meaning and the 'grammars' that determine interrelation are, as Jakobson sees it, put together in the same fundamental manner and, thus, he would maintain, they can only come apart in ways that are similar. What can be posited, therefore, is that, analogously with aphasic dichotomic disintegration, Magritte's 'disruptive' paintings function by destabilizing the structures *between* represented objects and also *within* them.

If aphasia, however, is to be a model for the deconstruction of painting, its postulates would have to be transposed from the verbal to the pictorial. There would need to be a visual remapping of Jakobson's schema. For Magritte, this would not have seemed in any way problematical; from their conception in the fifteenth century, the rules of painting that had been drummed into him at the Academy, the Albertian canons, had been formulated in terms of language anyway. As a basic principle, *Della Pittura* had specified that 'youths who first come to painting should do as those who are taught to write'.[22] To Alberti, language was the pre-eminent model for visual representation. It is telling that Magritte should have complained about his art lessons in terms that draw a parallel with verbal language: he had had to 'learn to draw', he said resentfully, 'in the way someone who writes has to learn grammar'.[23] The linguistic schema could be seen as Alberti's very rationale for painting. Indeed, his explications of the pictorial primaries, 'the outlines of planes', for instance, rely on an allusion with the verbal primaries, 'letters'. In other words, the elementary level of picture-making is compared to the elementary level of language, phonetics. The correspondence continues in the next stage of painting, in which these 'elements', as Alberti explains, are joined together to form planes, just as 'letters' are joined to form 'syllables'. Moreover, in language, phonological constraints determine permitted or acceptable sequences of sounds and, correspondingly, Alberti was at pains to point out that pictorial sequencing needs to adhere to the same concept of 'appropriateness': 'in this composition of planes grace and beauty of things should be intensely sought for'.[24] In turn, these combinations result in the depiction of the 'member', that is the smallest part of

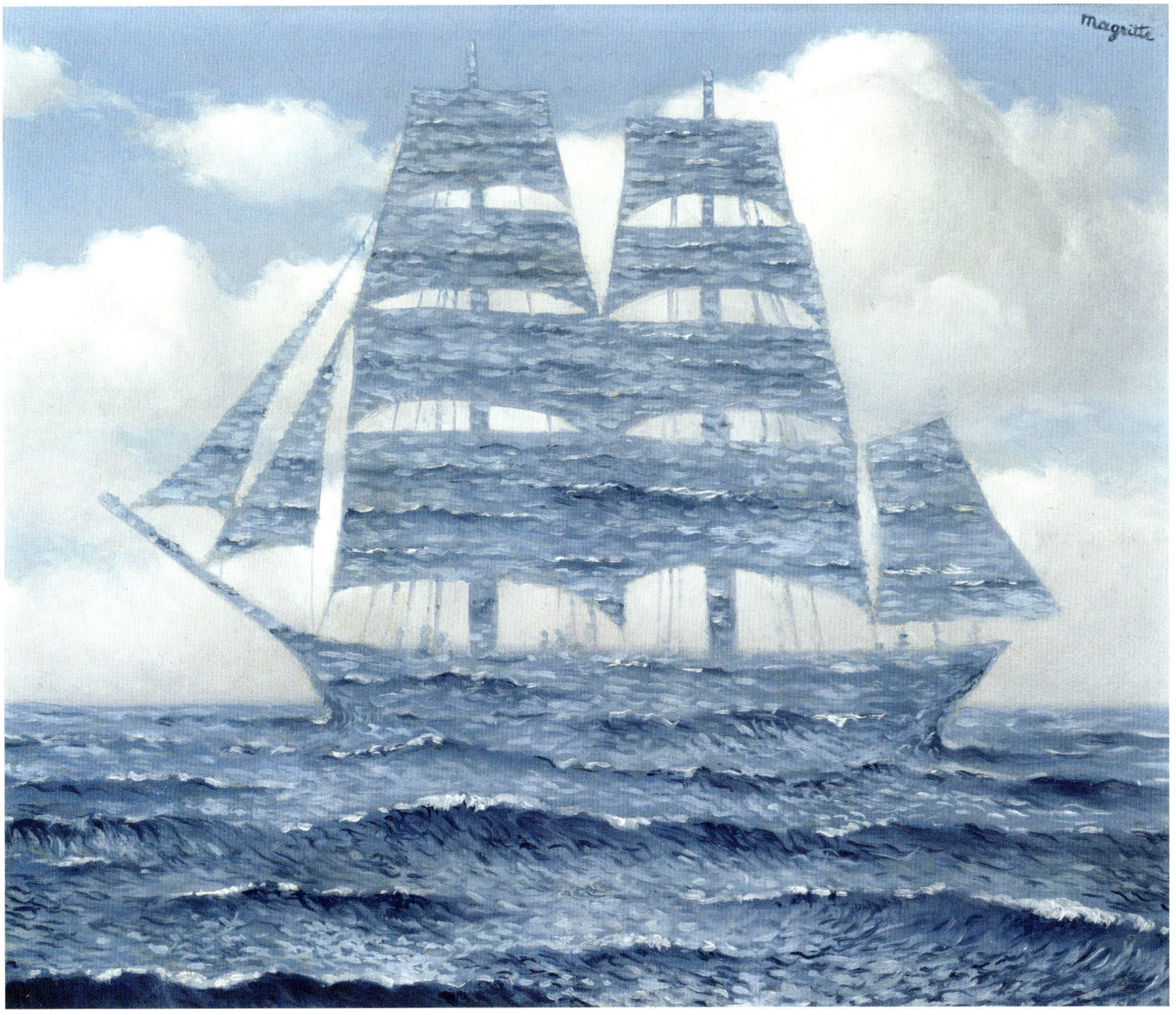

Le Séducteur (1953)

the image that has an autonomous semantic value, which tallies with the notion of the morpheme. What emerges, therefore, is a correlation, far more direct than Jakobson may have envisaged, between the fundamentals of language and the basic principles of an alternative meaningful system, in this case pictorial construction.[25] Indeed, the more advanced stages of painting that Alberti went on to describe emerge as closely comparable to the more complex linguistic strata of lexis and syntax. Clearly, the elementary skill that Alberti required of painters, namely that 'they should learn each distinct form of each member', involves a selection from the various visual possibilities and the capacity to give a unitary shape the identity of an autonomous symbol.[26] Each pictorial shape is part of a class of concurrent alternatives and it is from these alternatives that the appropriate 'kind' of form is expected to be selected. Alberti gave the example of discriminating between 'the rough wool cloak of a soldier' and 'the clothes of a woman'.[27] If this goes wrong and the painter depicts, as Alberti proposed, 'a figure whose face is flesh and full' as having 'muscular arms and fleshless hands', there would be a flawed selection within category sets of body parts, even if the categories themselves are correctly sequenced. In linguistic terms, this inappropriateness of selection echoes aphasic 'similarity disorder', in which nouns are ineptly selected, whilst grammatical relation remains correct.

The distinction between the two facets of painting, selection and combination, is maintained in Alberti's definition of the 'three parts' of picture-making. In these, the notion of interrelation between objects is presented as distinct from the concept of their respective identities.[28] The first of these parts, 'circumscription', is said to involve 'the drawing of the outline' and amounts to a definition in two-dimensional terms of the space occupied on the panel.[29] The outline is therefore seen as a boundary between the internal or 'semantic' description of the object and its external situation or 'syntactic' relations with other objects. This is, of course, true of perception in general, and visual identification begins by 'separating an object from its background'.[30] Magritte himself openly alludes to the principle in works such as *La Grande Famille* (1963) and *Le Séducteur* (1953), in which he mischievously violates the boundary between the interior of a pictorial element and its exterior situational setting. As in the case of neologies, he uses the rules for constructing the grammatical context to formulate the internal structure of the morpheme. In Alberti's second pictorial stage, 'composition', visual concatenation is described as 'that rule in painting by which the parts fit together in the painted work'.[31] This 'grammar' of the picture effectively predetermines a hierarchy of relations: as Alberti continued, 'planes are parts of the members' and 'these members are parts of the bodies'.[32] At a higher level of organization, Alberti placed 'l'istoria', which regulates the various interrelations of each object within the composition, establishing 'the composition of bodies, their relations, their spacing, as determined on the one hand by their actual size and, on the other, by their function'.[33] Composition, therefore, comprises the rules of contiguity, both within objects, thus determining how planes and members are joined, and between them. The final 'part' of painting, for Alberti, was the plastic representation of the object, 'the reception of light', by means of which the object is given 'light and shade', as well as colour and texture.[34] What he describes is semantic definition, by means of which pictorial meaning becomes fixed.

✣ ✣ ✣

From the rationale of picture-making put forward by Alberti, it emerges that there is a broad correlation between the pictorial and linguistic constructions.

It follows, therefore, that the converse could equally be true, namely that a deconstruction of the visual schema could correspond to the ways in which derangement occurs in language when it becomes defective. Since the specific ways in which the verbal construct breaks down are revealed in aphasia, where distinct and discrete categories of verbal organization are progressively deactivated, it is arguable that, once the various parts of language are mapped onto the elements of painting, Magritte's own deconstruction of the visual could appropriately be gauged against an aphasic model. In other words, the topology of language loss would rightly be seen as a pictorial deconstructive template. What this would ultimately determine is whether the relation between normal linguistic usage and the aphasic's unbalanced use of language is analogous to the correlation between Albertian rules of pictorial construction and Magritte's divergence from them. Moreover, given Jakobson's contention that the deep structures of language, as they are revealed by aphasia, are the fundamental model for human expression in all its forms, the corollary of such a decoding of Magritte's oeuvre is that it would be seen as ultimately functioning at the level of 'the permanent structures of the mind'.[35]

---

[1] A. M. Hammacher, *Magritte* (London, 1974), p. 98.

[2] René Magritte, *Écrits complets* (Paris, 1979), p. 60.

[3] Harold Goodglass & Sheila Blumstein (eds), *Psycholinguistics and Aphasia* (London, 1973), p. 3.

[4] Roman Jakobson & Morris Halle, *Fundamentals of Language* (The Hague, 1956), p. 63.

[5] Jakobson & Halle, *Fundamentals of Language*, p. 71.

[6] Described more fully in Harold Goodglass, 'Studies on the Grammar of Aphasics', in Goodglass & Blumstein (eds), *Psycholinguistics and Aphasia*, pp. 183-215.

[7] Roman Jakobson, 'Towards a Linguistic Classification of Aphasic Impairments', in Goodglass & Blumstein (eds), *Psycholinguistics and Aphasia*, p. 45.

[8] Jakobson & Halle, *Fundamentals of Language*, p. 71.

[9] Jakobson, 'Towards a Linguistic Classification of Aphasic Impairments', p. 35.

[10] Jakobson & Halle, *Fundamentals of Language*, p. 75.

[11] Harold Goodglass, 'Studies on the Grammar of Aphasics', in Sheldon Rosenberg & James H. Koplin (eds), *Developments in Applied Psycholinguistic Research* (New York, 1968), p. 204.

[12] Goodglass, 'Studies on the Grammar of Aphasics', p. 204.

[13] Jakobson, 'Towards a Linguistic Classification of Aphasic Impairments', p. 39.

[14] In *La Clef des songes* (1930) Magritte deliberately dissociated the label from the concept.

[15] Jakobson, 'Towards a Linguistic Classification of Aphasic Impairments', p. 41.

[16] Jakobson & Halle, *Fundamentals of Language*, p. 66.

[17] Jakobson & Halle, *Fundamentals of Language*, p. 69.

[18] Jakobson & Halle, *Fundamentals of Language*, p. 70.

[19] Goodglass, 'Studies on the Grammar of Aphasics', p. 197.

[20] Jakobson & Halle, *Fundamentals of Language*, p. 79.

[21] Otfried Spreen, 'Psycholinguistics and Aphasia: The Contribution of Arnold Pick', in Goodglass & Blumstein (eds), *Psycholinguistics and Aphasia*, p. 145.

[22] Leon Battista Alberti, *On Painting* (*Della Pittura*), trans. John R. Spencer (London, 1956), p. 92.

[23] According to Marcel Mariën, conversation with the author, Brussels, 9 March 1981.

[24] Combinations in general are determined by the rules of 'composition', but Alberti specifically mentions that planes are to be joined together in fitting ways. Alberti, *On Painting*, p. 72.

[25] Hans Bellmer endorses this view: 'the different modes of expression: [...] sound, word, graphics [...] all result from the same psychophysiological group of mechanisms [...] they all conform to and derive from a single original principle', in *Petite Anatomie de l'inconscient physique ou l'anatomie de l'image* (Paris, 1957), n. pag.

[26] Alberti, *On Painting*, p. 92.

[27] Alberti, *On Painting*, p. 74.

[28] Alberti, *On Painting*, p. 67.

[29] Alberti, *On Painting*, p. 68.

[30] R. L. Gregory, 'The Confounded Eye', in R. L. Gregory & E. H. Gombrich (eds), *Illusion in Art and Nature* (London, 1973), p. 89.

[31] Alberti, *On Painting*, p. 70.

[32] Alberti, *On Painting*, p. 70.

[33] Jean Clair, in exhibition catalogue *Rétrospective Magritte*, Palais des Beaux-Arts (Brussels, 1978), p. 39.

[34] Alberti, *On Painting*, p. 68.

[35] Fredric Jameson, *The Prison-House of Language: A Critical Account of Structuralism and Russian Formalism* (Princeton, 1972), p. 109.

Crumbling Space

The convention of painting from which Magritte most transparently diverges is that of Alberti's 'composition'. To various degrees, Magritte had always put himself at odds with this fundamental pictorial schema, but it was in 1925, with *Cinéma bleu*, that he set out in earnest on this course.

In this work he disrupts all the pictorial and spatial relations that a spectator could normally expect in a painting. The perspective, which normally has the function of unifying the elements of a composition, is either absent or intermittent. As Pierre Demarne remarked 'it's the relation between these objects that is well and truly puzzling'.[1] What jars is the lack of resolution of depth and space, which renders pictorial context barely defined. For Alberti, the intelligibility of pictorial space was central to the stability of composition, but in *Cinéma bleu* none of the objects can be located spatially with any certainty. This is because Alberti's technique of defining space, 'dividing the pavement', is not only disregarded, but also positively contradicted.[2] The problematic stage-like floor area, for instance, is depicted inconsistently, with the result that any illusion of a flat, horizontal Albertian 'pavement' is undermined.[3] Whilst there is a light source coming from the top right, as the skittle and the columns confirm, no shadows are cast, which leaves the central figure hovering in mid-air. The 'floor' becomes an equivocal space with only contingent possibilities of interpretation. Indeed, at some points the ground can be read as a horizontal plane perpendicular to the picture surface and at others it becomes a vertical plane parallel to it. The visual cues – flanking red curtains, rudimentary classical scenery, poised figure – all point to a theatrical situation and yet the understanding of the lower grey area as a flat, horizontal stage floor is contradicted by other elements, such as the lower folds of the curtain on the right, which are neither vertical nor horizontal but, rather, slope downwards towards the spectator.[4]

The pavement, however, needs to be revised once again when it becomes clear that it is a downward continuation of the bottom riser of the classical façade, which means that, perversely, it must be vertical.[5] The confusion seems endless. Yet, these diverse perspectival readings do not result in a series of competing and clashing interpretations, as occurs in Cubism. Instead, the effect is more that of an informal structure that admits ambivalence. Space in *Cinéma bleu* is inconsistent and, consequently, perspective loses its unifying force. Whereas the exaggeration of perspective in, for example, de Chirico's *Melancholy and Mystery of a Street* brings pictorial elements into a tense, brooding proximity, *Cinéma bleu* appears to reconcile incompatible viewpoints. Wholly disregarding Alberti's insistence on compositional cohesion, Magritte adopts an arbitrary pictorial arrangement that is more akin to the vague, illusory settings found in

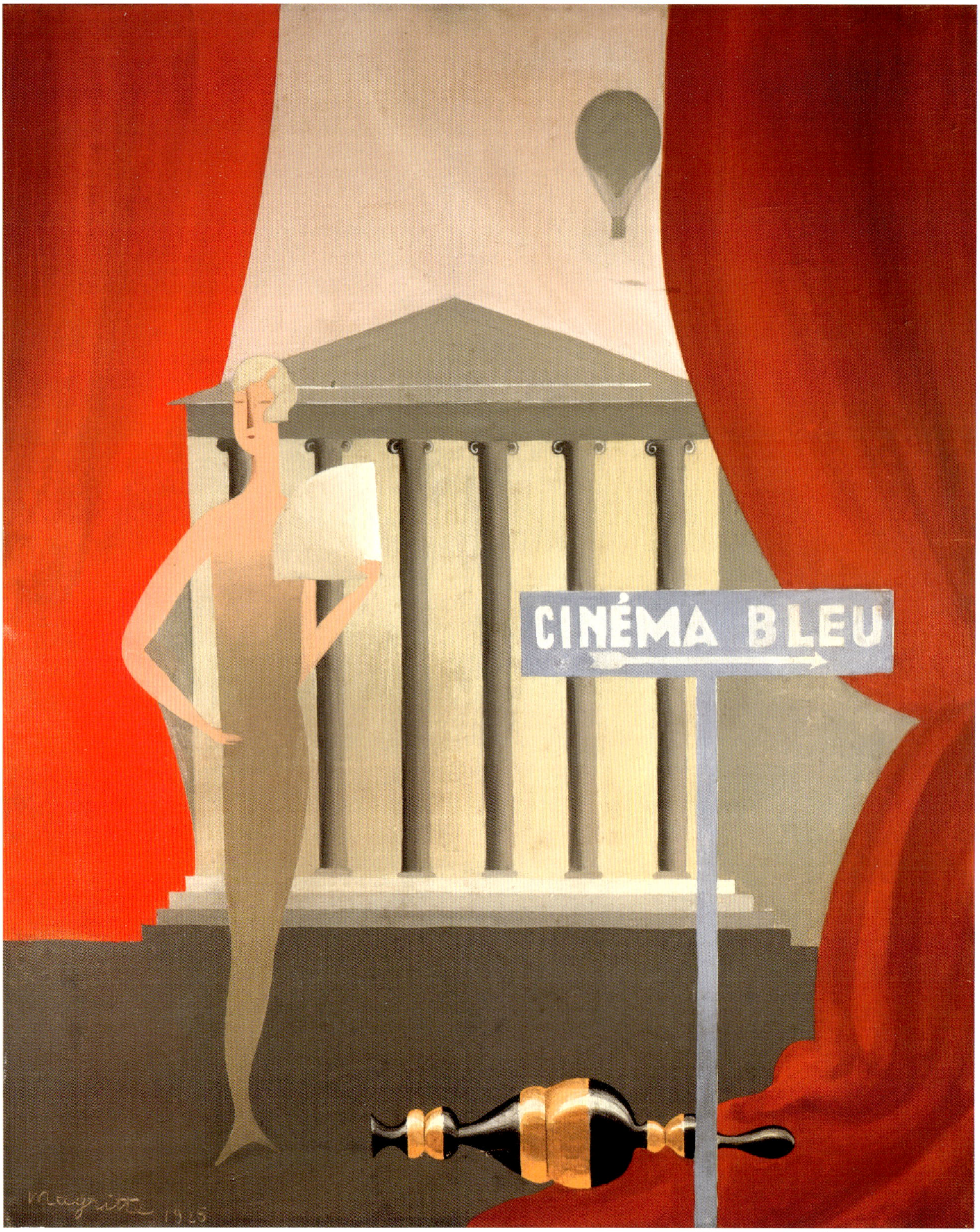

Cinéma bleu (1925)

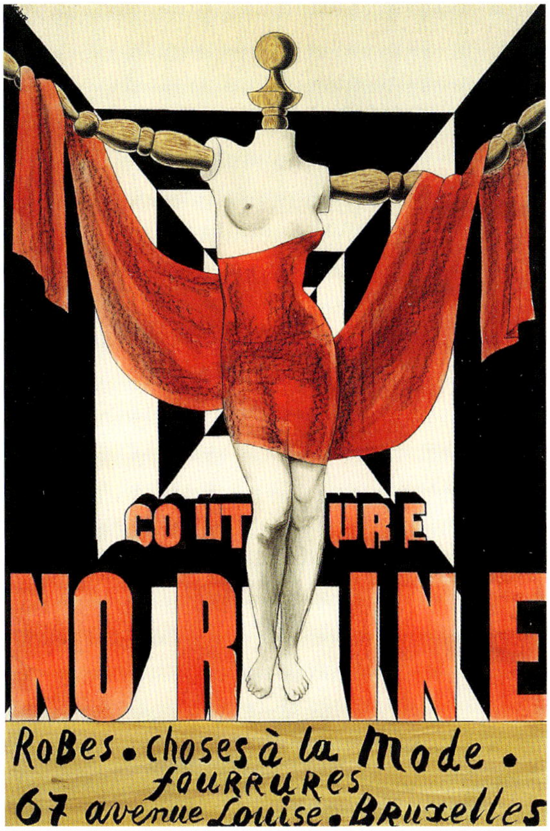

Couture Norine (1926)

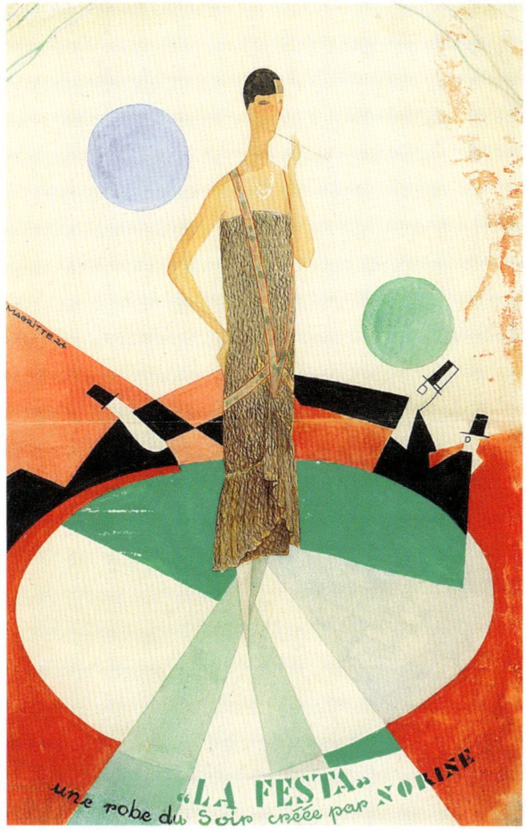

La Festa (1924)

the fashion montages of the time, with which, significantly, Magritte had been closely involved. Particularly known to him was the 'Norine' fashion house, founded during the First World War and known as 'the Chanel of the North', for which he was designing advertisements and catalogue covers during the early twenties.[6] Against this background, *Cinéma bleu* could well be seen as an allusion to a 1920s fashion display, with its schematic objects and overt theatricality. Indeed, the skittle-like object on the floor is drawn directly from one of the commercial designs that Magritte had devised for the Norine fashion house, while the slim, stylish figure at the centre of the work could conceivably be a portrait of the slightly-built, bob-haired Honorine Deschrijuer herself.[7] What these references show about *Cinéma bleu* is its similarity with commercial advertisements and fashion display, reinforcing the view that the painting rests on principles that are independent of formal composition. The analogy points to a divergent blueprint, in which compositional instability and vacillatory relationships are the norm. This is particularly true of the recumbent skittle, which has no shadow and, hence, cannot be spatially fixed; it is not clear whether it sits on the floor or on the curtain or, indeed, whether it is on both or neither. All that can be deduced is that it occupies a position somewhere behind the signpost. In fact, the abandonment of perspective pervades the entire work, and all relative positionings can only be determined in terms of a vague succession of planes, in opposition to the well-defined spatial model that Alberti had elaborated. As Magritte would have known only too well from his Academy classes, Alberti had insisted that, in a correct perspective construction, the transversal closest to the foreground should be carefully calculated, since it is this construction line that determines the subsequent recession markings and, thus, the 'correctness' of the entire picture space. Yet, Magritte appears to sabotage precisely this key point of reference when he plants the foremost element in *Cinéma bleu*, the placard mounted on a post, out of sight, below the lower edge of the painting. This, according to Alberti's formula, would frustrate the primary means of spatial mapping on which the intelligibility of the painting as a whole relies. As such, not only is the composition of *Cinéma bleu* unresolved, it is also irresolvable.[8]

Still more disorientation is brought about by the arrow inscribed on the signpost, which turns an otherwise affirmative label into a pointer towards a context beyond the picture boundary; as it tells us, the words 'Cinéma bleu' have, in fact, nothing to do with what is represented within the painting. The arrow acts as a digressive device and shifts the focus. The other elements do no less; the woman glances to the left, the balloon rises upwards and the skittle tumbles downwards. Together, they disjoin the composition. Instead of being interwoven, the various elements drift apart and appear to be in the process of egressing the depicted space. The same occurs in *La Fatigue de vivre* (1927), where a businessman's suit drifts upwards, beyond the confines of the painting, and in *Le Conquérant* (1925-6), in which only the lower portion of a levitating, eradicated tree remains visible.[9] This is not to say, however, that *Cinéma bleu* conveys a sense of structural integrity that is in the throes of being compromised. It is rather a question of the absence of compositional stability. Objects are no more than loosely grouped and lack any type of finite concatenation. They even remain unresolved internally, within their respective outlines; the architectural façade is three-dimensionally inconsistent and the female figure is flat and unconvincing. In all its aspects, *Cinéma bleu* defies pictorial 'grammar' and replaces compositional clarity with spatial imprecision.

✣ ✣ ✣

Whilst the treatment of the pictorial content in *Cinéma bleu* is tenuous and inconsistent, in *La Fenêtre* (1925) it is unequivocal. The two geometric shapes in this painting, a pyramid and a rectangular cuboid, are unambiguously solid and

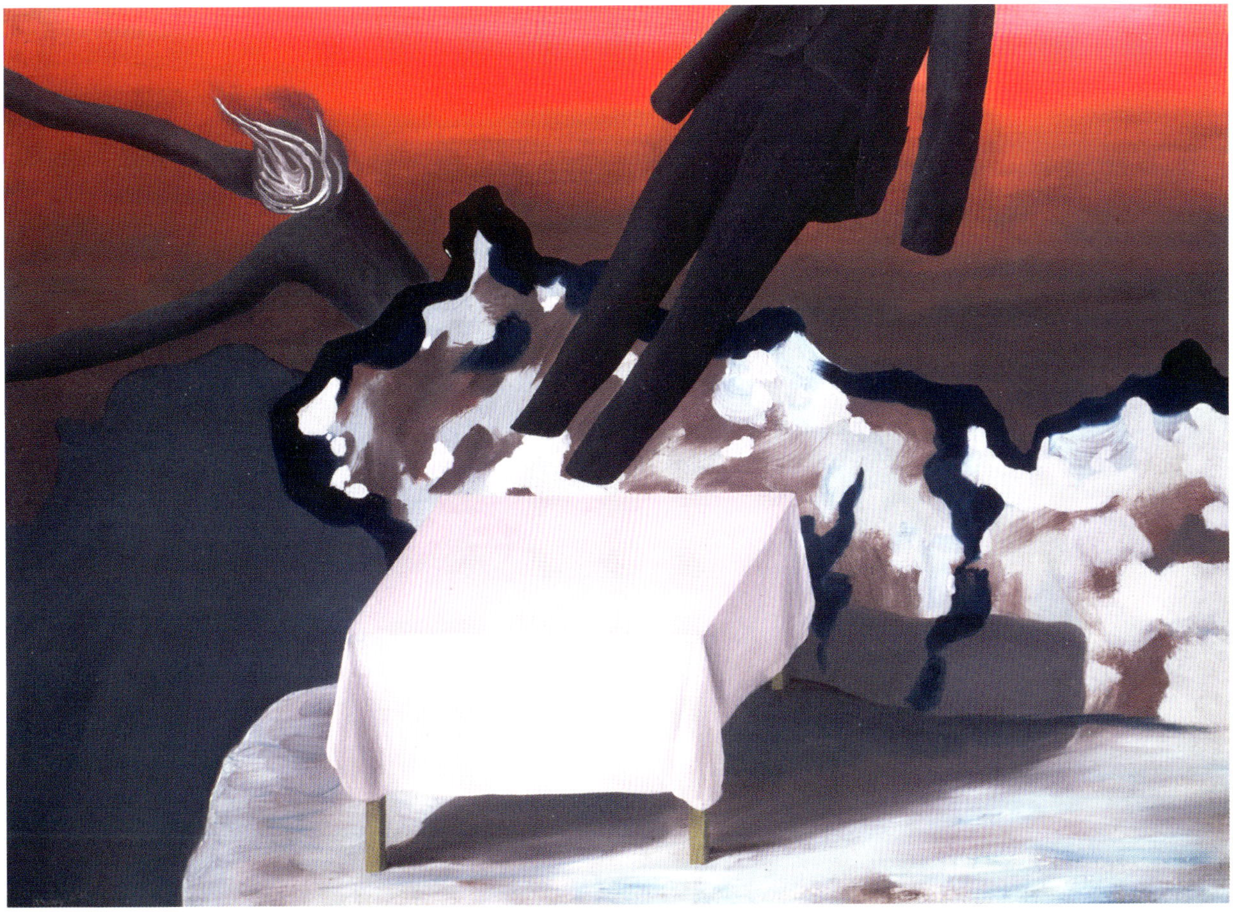

La Fatigue de vivre (1927)

bold, as are the hand, the bird and the curtain. The same, it would seem, is true of the pictorial space, which at first appears as comprehensible as the objects contained within it. For instance, in conformity with the rules of perspective, the pyramid sharply recedes into depth and the uppermost face of the rectangular block correctly slopes towards the vanishing point. Perspectival recession is further reinforced by the succession of fence posts bordering the distant path, which appropriately diminish in size as they become more distant. Indeed, the far-off outdoor scene as a whole is distinguished from the immediate elements inside by being put into a softer focus. Arguably, the landscape in the distance even incorporates textbook aerial perspective in that, as opposed to the clearcut surfaces of the pyramid in the foreground, the hill in the background has a nebulous quality. In much the same way, the crisply modelled hand in front of the window contrasts with the rather more indistinct figure in the distance. Alberti, after all, had stipulated that 'as the distance becomes greater, so the plane seen appears more hazy'.[10] Magritte's adherence to the classical rules, however, is no more than cursory and, whilst the objects he depicts are

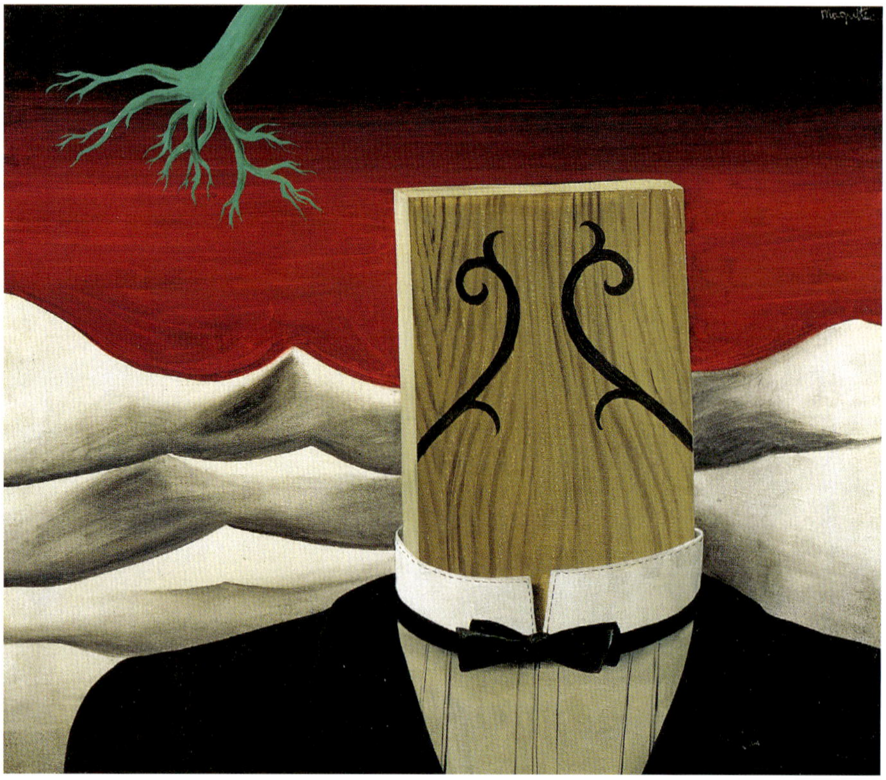

Le Conquérant (1925-6)

themselves accurately portrayed, the space they occupy is, in reality, far from well-defined. The pyramid, for instance, appears as being illuminated from the right, whilst the rectangle close by is illuminated from the left. But it is the awkward relationship between the hand and the bird that causes most disruption to the spatial fabric of the painting. Wholly illogically, the raised hand 'appears to be intent', as Magritte explained, 'on seizing a flying bird', which the rules of perspective should, obviously, have placed it out of reach.[11] With this pictorial solecism Magritte confounds the entire space of the painting; the interior of the room and the distant outside landscape cease to be differentiated and, overall, there is uncertainty about what is close and what is far away.

The same is true of *Une Panique au Moyen Âge* (1927), in which a figure in the foreground appears to be directly connected to a smaller, more distant figure partially outside of a window. As in William Hogarth's *Whoever Makes a Design without the Knowledge of Perspective* (1754), which deliberately confuses planar proximity with distance constructed by perspective, *La Fenêtre* and *Une Panique au Moyen Âge* both create a compositional confusion between two otherwise distinct spatial settings, inside and outside. In a similar manner, in *À la Suite de l'eau, les nuages* (1926) distant clouds from the outside space are shown implausibly to continue through a window into the inside space in

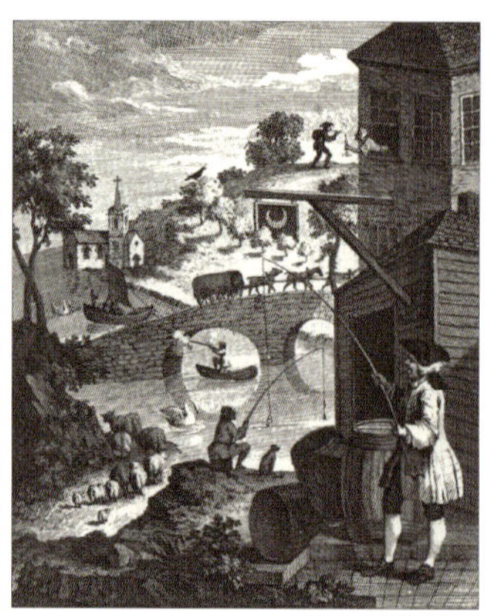

William Hogarth, *Whoever Makes a Design without the Knowledge of Perspective* (1754)

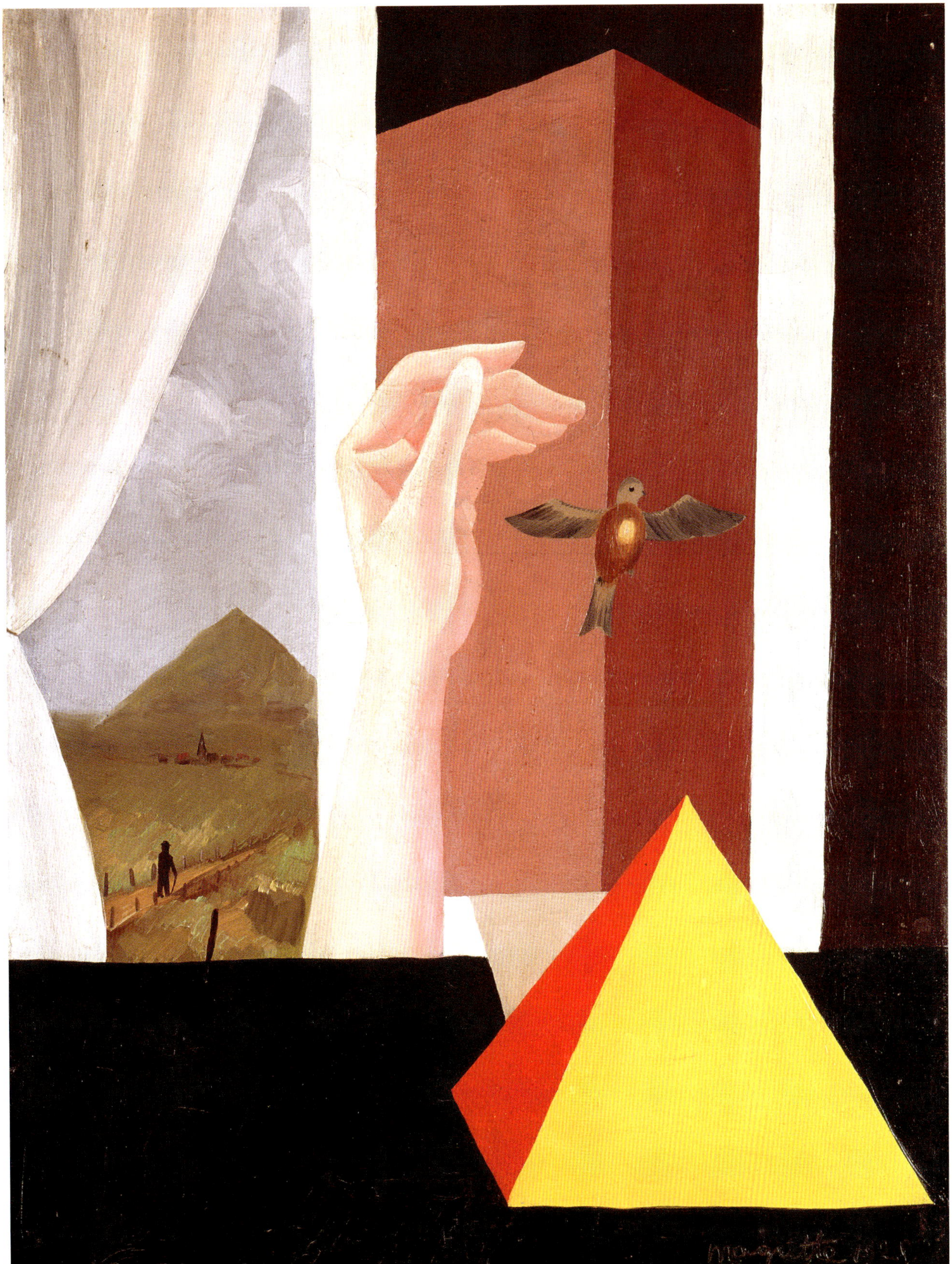

La Fenêtre (1925)

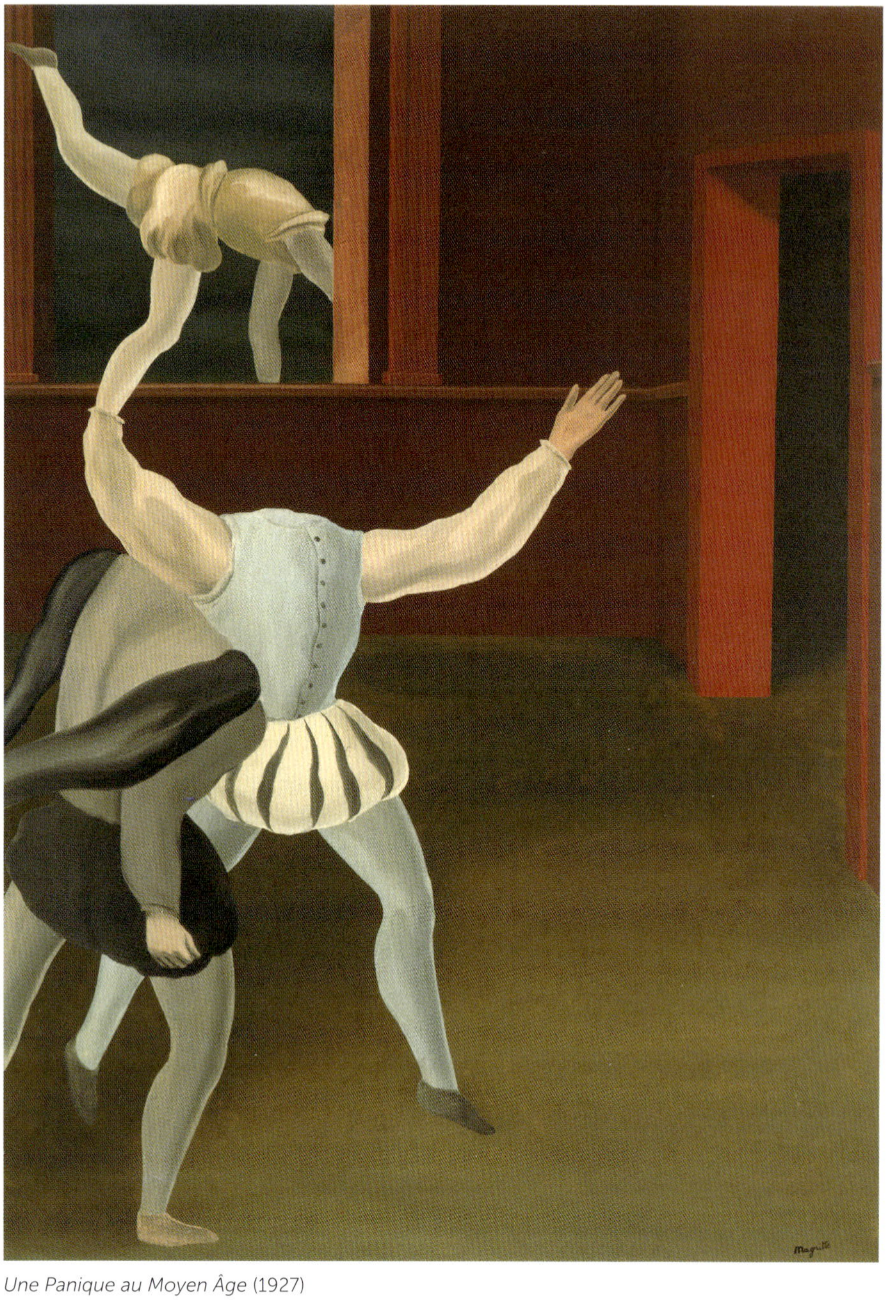

Une Panique au Moyen Âge (1927)

the foreground. This dual interpretation of depth is even present in the limited space visible outside the window of *La Fenêtre*, where the landscape visible from the left pane shows sharp spatial recession, giving the illusion of a penetration of the picture plane, whilst the shape on the right protrudes towards the spectator almost as if the perspective pyramid had been reversed and the orthogonals were intersecting at the foreground, instead of far from it. Any sense of well-defined space is dispensed with and all that is left is three-dimensional incongruity. Even when there are localized areas within which perspective is comprehensible, the concatenations between them are absent. As was the case in *Cinéma bleu*, the spatial setting is not so much disrupted as rendered inconsistent.[12]

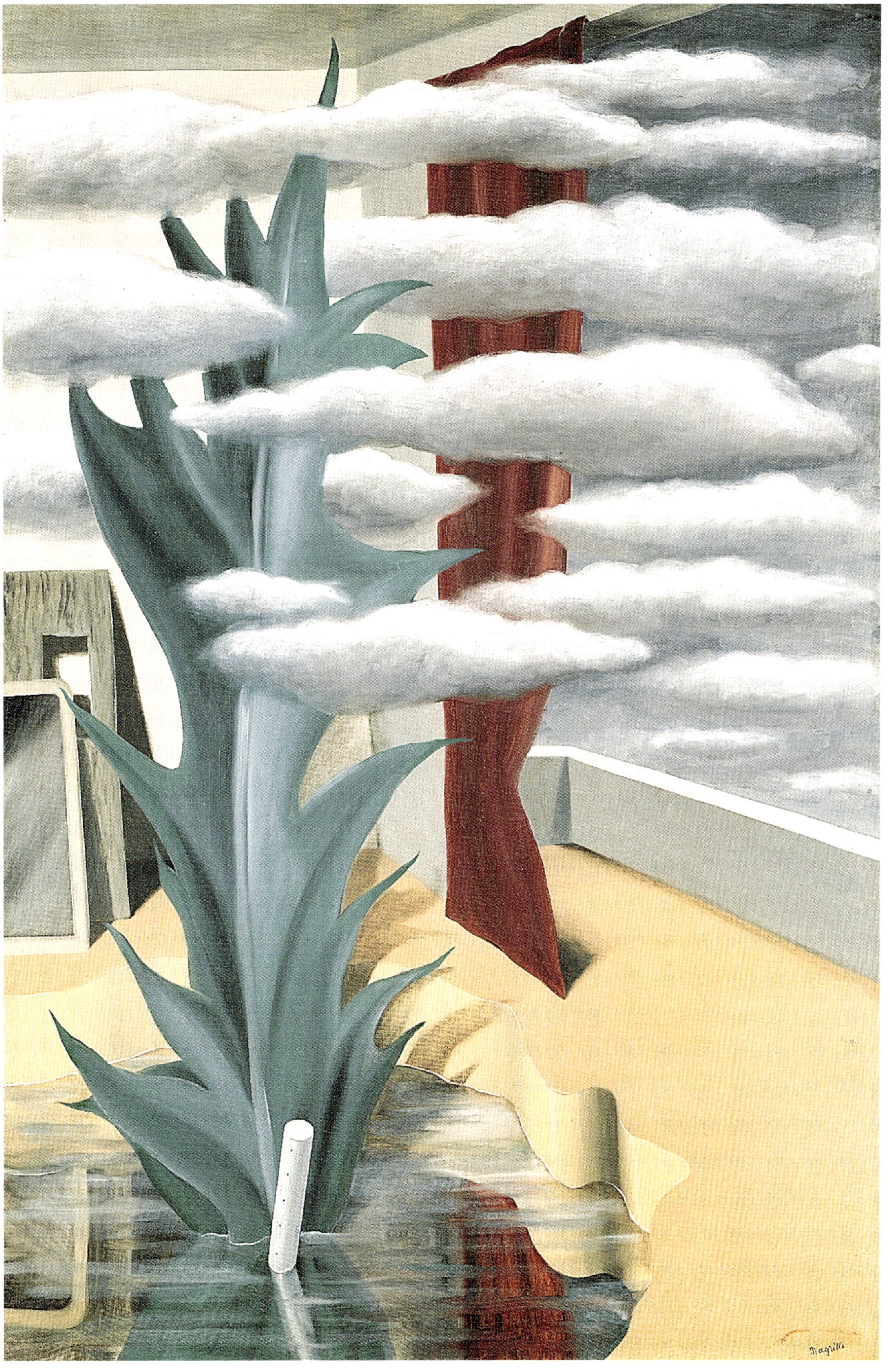

À la Suite de l'eau, les nuages (1926)

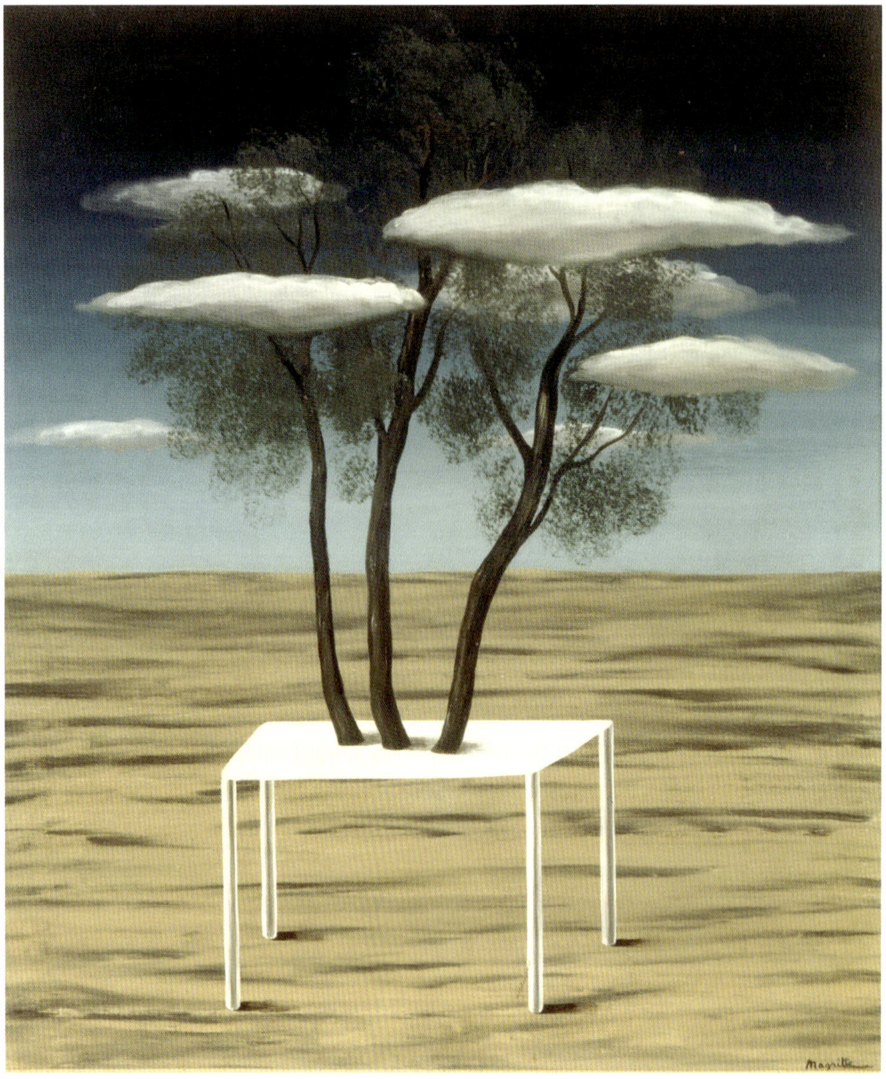

L'Oasis (1926)

The reversal of perspective that had been hinted at in *La Fenêtre* emerges as a recurrent theme in several other paintings of the period. *La Fatigue de vivre*, for example, depicts a table whose misaligned contours tentatively indicate an obverse vanishing point. It is in *L'Oasis* (1926), however, that 'Chinese perspective' is articulated in a particularly flagrant manner. In direct opposition to Alberti's precept that the painting should be a 'cross-section of a visual pyramid', that is a space within which scale decreases as the distance from the viewer increases, the tabletop in *L'Oasis* sharply diminishes towards the foreground.[13] Alberti's system is at once turned on its head and, instead of controlling the representational context, it confuses the sequencing of objects in depth and their relative scale; whereas clouds are normally the largest and most distant elements in a landscape, here they are diminished to mere inches

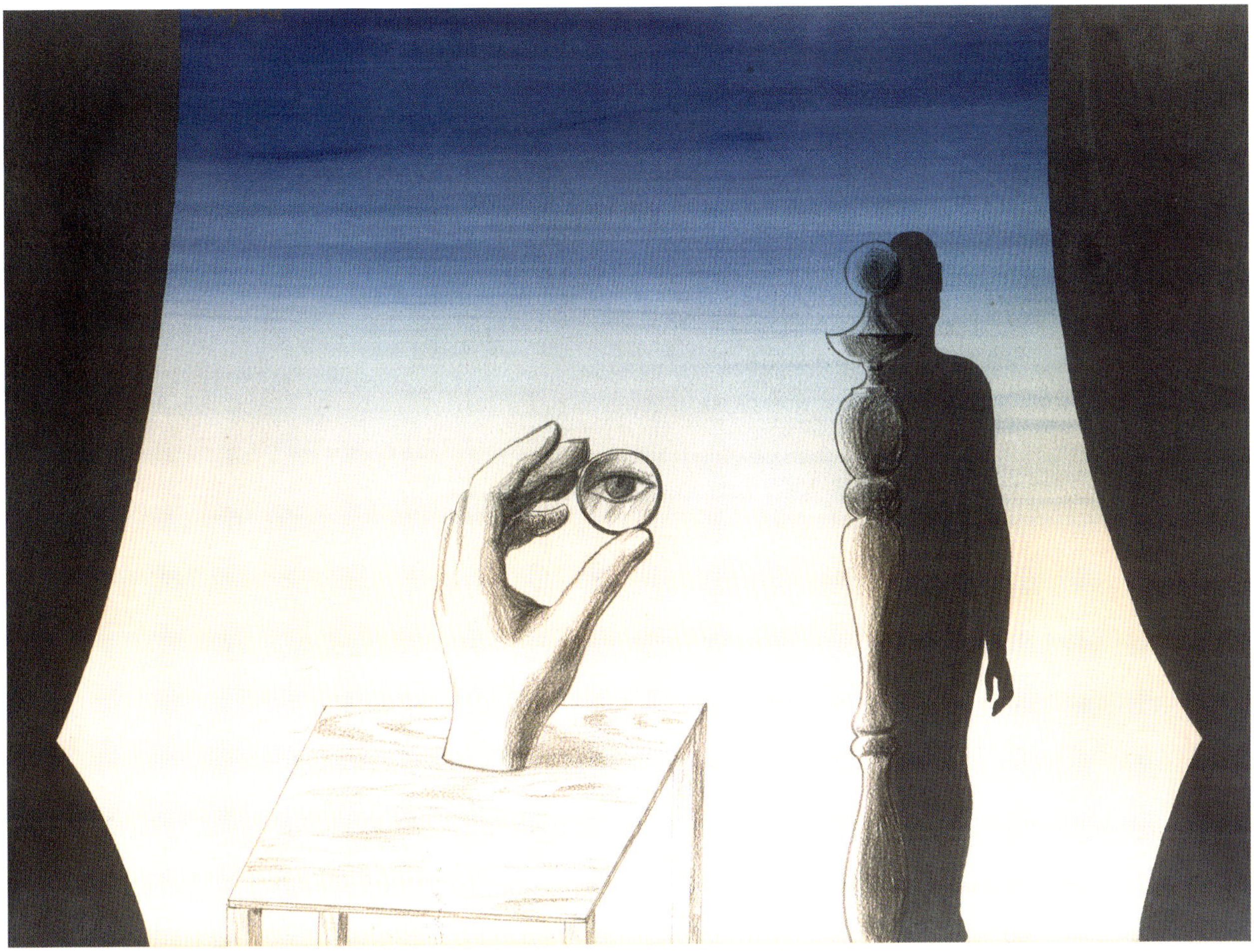

La Raison d'être (1928)

and hover close by in front of the three trees in the foreground. It is as though the Albertian perspective construction had been totally inverted and the viewpoint switched to the opposite end of the perspective pyramid. The impression given is that the whole scene is being viewed 'from behind'. Indeed, where the hypothetically reversed orthogonals approach their point of intersection and, hence where space diminishes and positional relations become indistinguishable, which is now the foreground, we see the table merging with the trees, in much the same way as objects at the horizon of a more conventional painting would fuse together in a hazy blur.

Yet another divergence from Alberti's system comes in the form of a challenge to the assumed position of the observer, a cornerstone of the perspective construct. A given for Alberti had been that 'both the beholder and the things he sees will appear to be on the same plane', in other words that everything is viewed from the front.[14] Magritte, however, set about perturbing even this elementary supposition. Going further than Erhard Schon's sixteenth century anamorphic

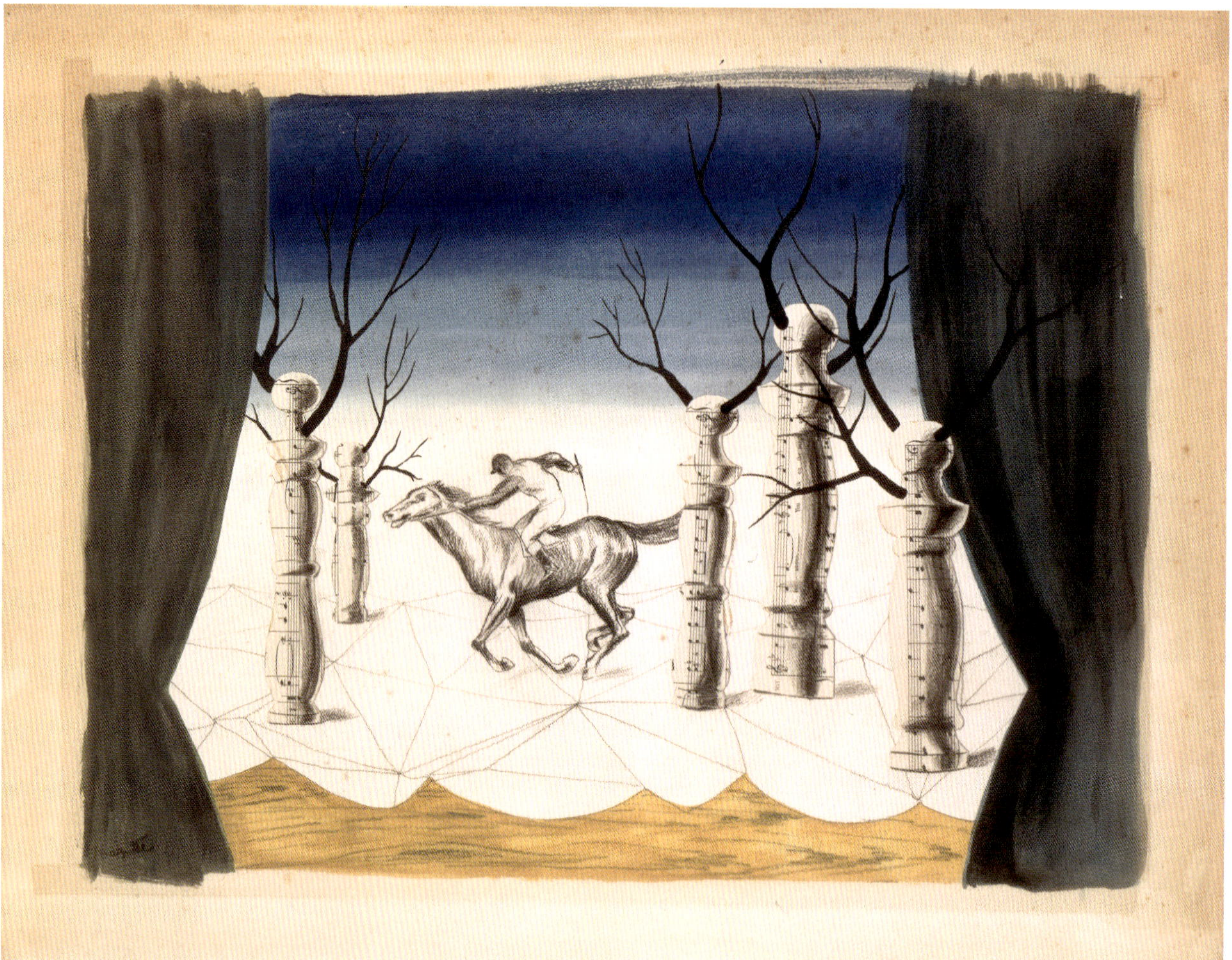

Le Jockey perdu (1926)

revisions of the frontality of the spectator's viewpoint, Magritte actually reversed the viewing point and, in some cases, dispensed with it altogether.[15] In *La Raison d'être* (1928) he depicted another table in Chinese perspective, but he also included a hand holding a monocle through which an eye is looking at the scene as though 'from behind'. The perspective cues make this the eye of the logical spectator, who would, consequently, be able to see the distorted table as corrected in true Albertian perspective. Magritte even positioned the viewing 'peephole' precisely where Alberti would have converged his orthogonals, at the exact centre of the horizon.

The assault on Alberti's canons continued with a breach of a further prescription in *Della Pittura*, the treatment of the pictorial pavement. Whereas for Alberti the intelligibility of the ground area was a prerequisite for correct composition – 'first I begin with the foundation' – the floor spaces in *La Fenêtre* and *L'Oasis*, as well as in *Cinéma bleu*, are incoherent and convey

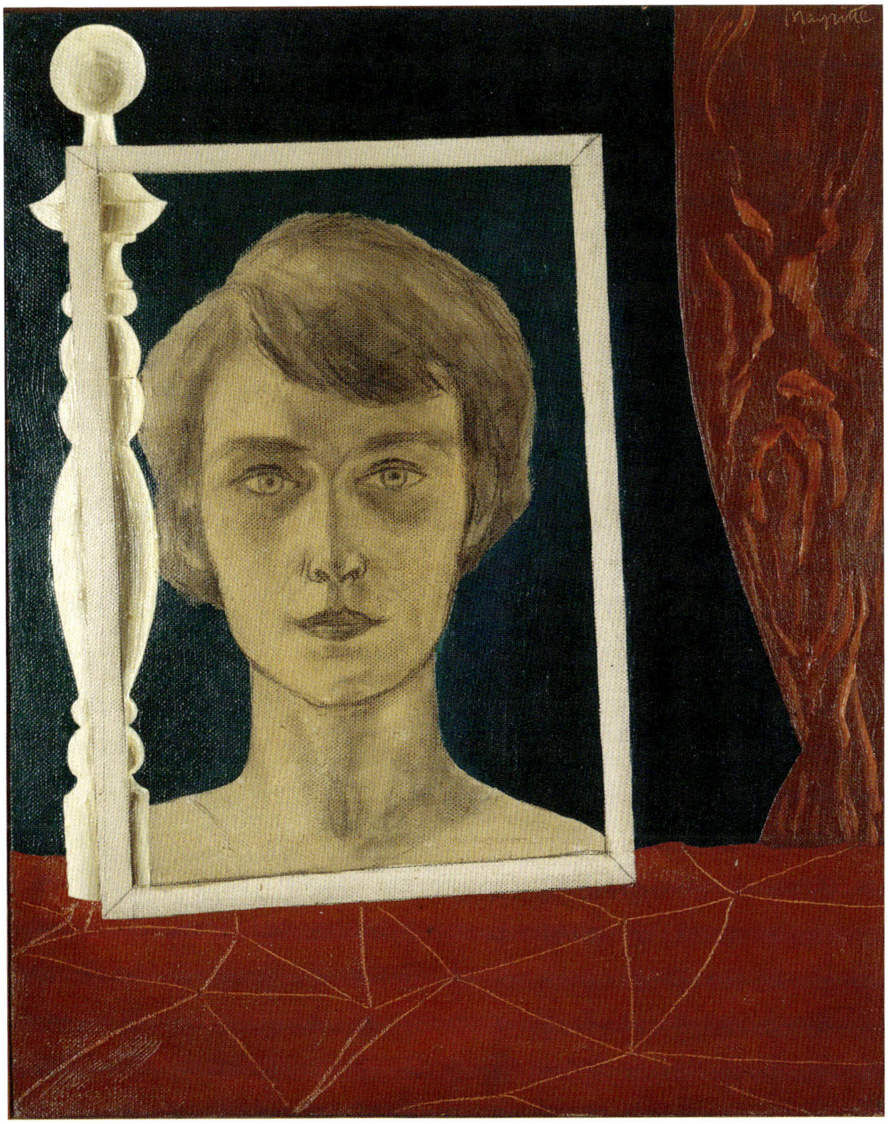

Georgette (1926)

only ambiguity.[16] Perspective cues are either inadequate or totally absent. In *Le Jockey perdu* (1926) and related works of the same year, however, the ground is criss-crossed with lines that force space to contradict itself.[17] Far from alluding to the 'converging tramlines' of perspective, these intersecting lines establish an irresolvable polyvalence of the lower horizontal plane. Although the incised lines in *Georgette* (1926) may appear to indicate a surface of shallow pyramids, it is, in fact, impossible to determine whether any of the individual delineated sections protrude or sink. Since there is no shading, each pyramid has two equally valid alternative readings and so the way in which it is perceived continually changes. This is because the visual data are inadequate and, thus,

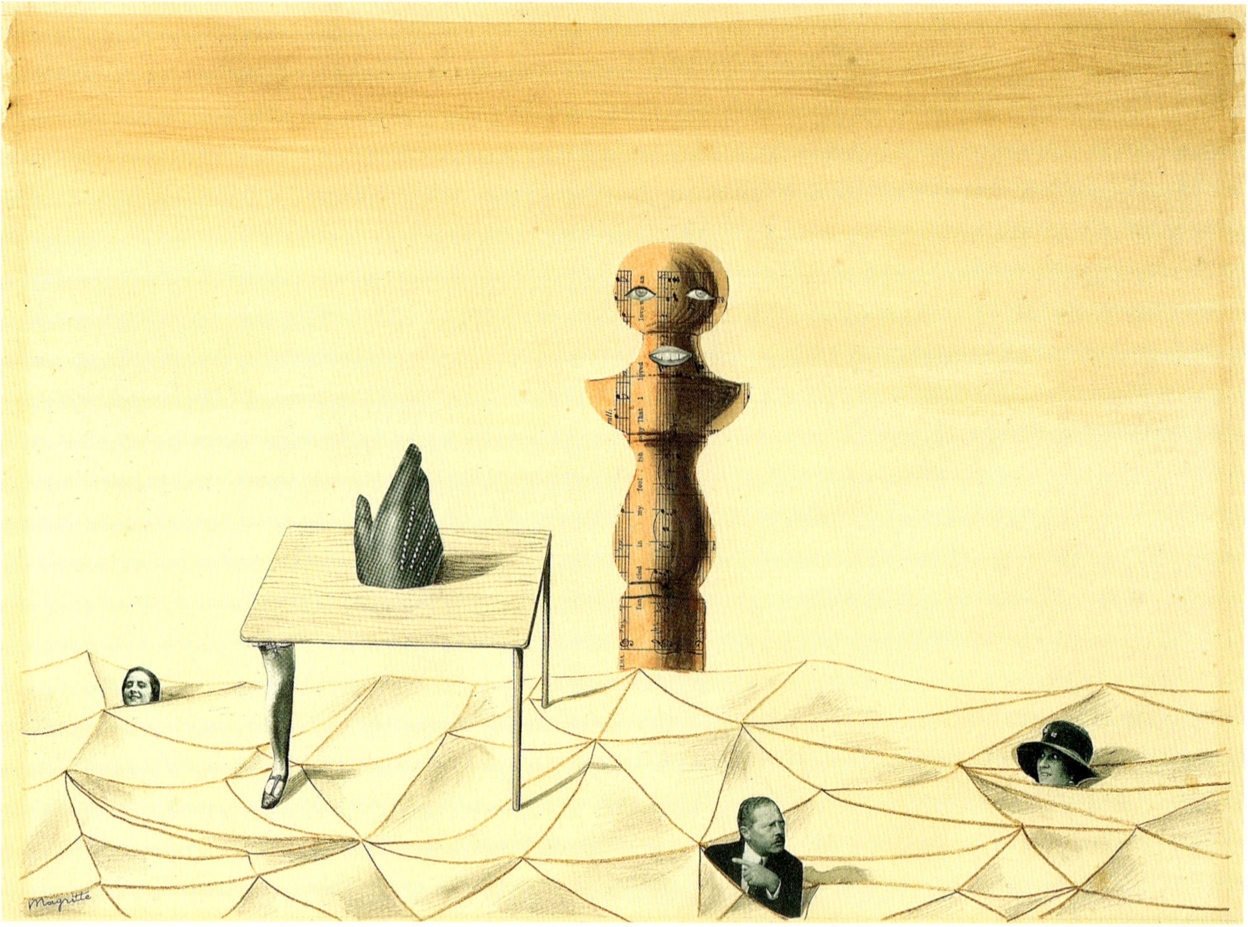

Untitled collage (1926)

the uppermost part of any one of the pyramids can also be interpreted as the base of another. Yet, when the overall sequence is considered, not even this already problematic bivalency becomes possible; whether a polygon is seen as concave or convex, the consequent interpretations of the adjoining forms produce an impossible spatial continuum.[18] If, for instance, the first pavement pyramid on the left in *Georgette* were a hollow, then the next one would have to have been perpendicular to it and so point directly at the spectator, making the ground vertical, as well as horizontal. As in another work executed in the same year, an untitled collage (1926) measuring 44 x 58 centimetres, there is a compounding of spatial inconsistency that, as Gombrich remarks of Cubism, 'den[ies] us the resolution of a coherent reading'.[19] As the visual cortex interprets the configuration of objects in terms of the orientation of angles and edges, Magritte's indecipherable polygonal pyramids, which comprise solely lines and angles, prevent us from formulating a fixed spatial hypothesis and we remain baffled at a rudimentary level of ocular perception.[20]

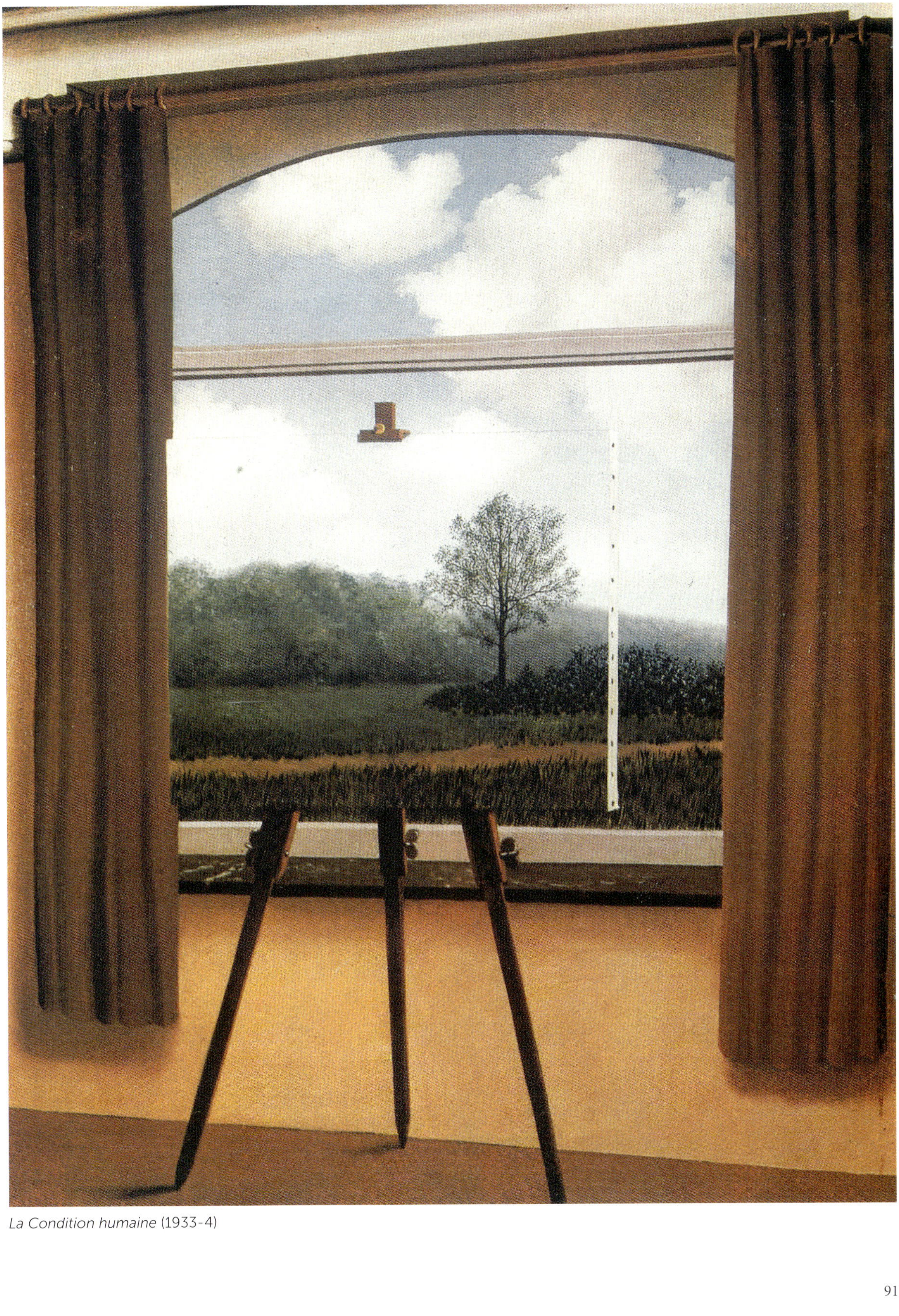

La Condition humaine (1933-4)

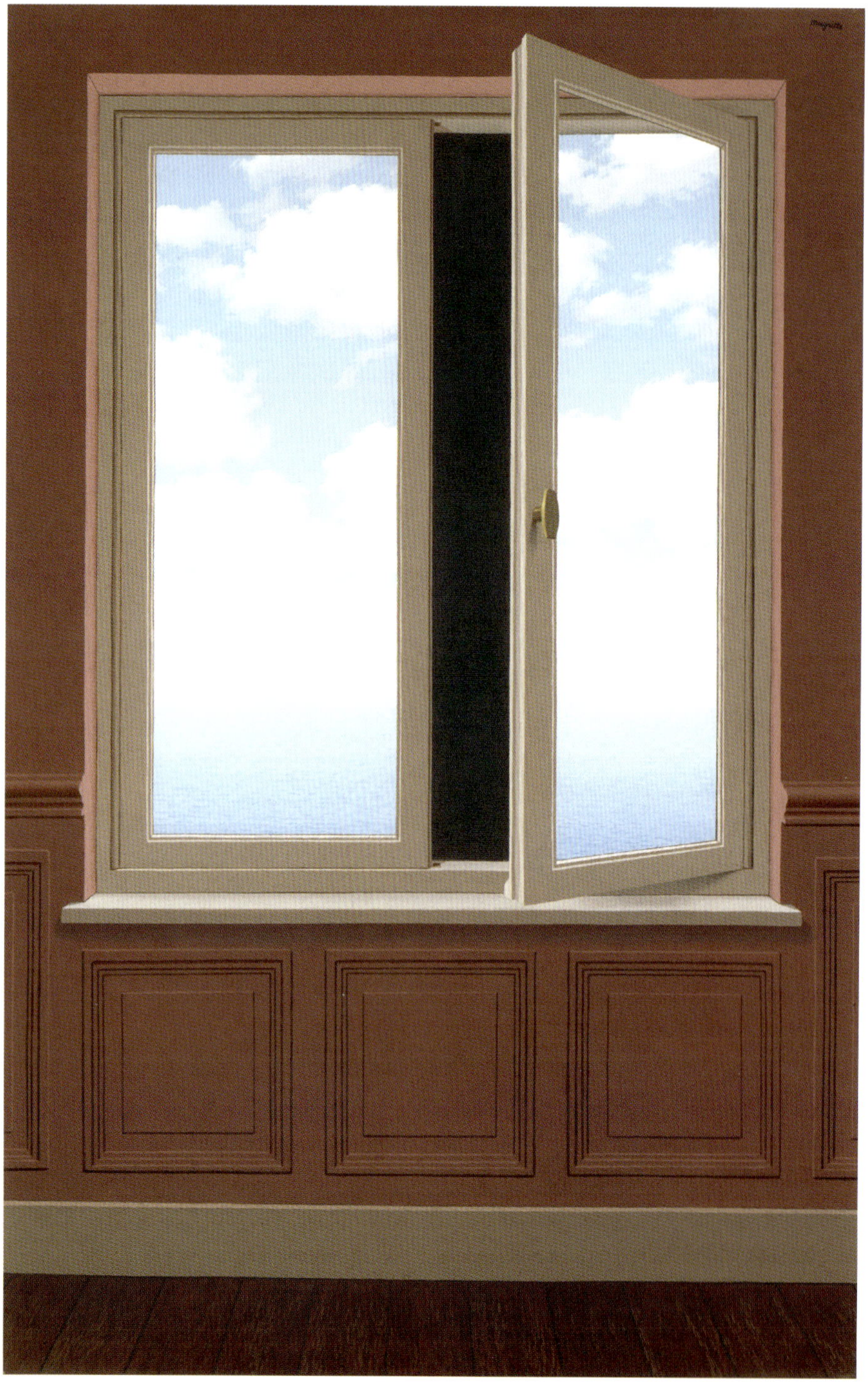

La Lunette d'approche (1963)

The discord in the pavement of *Georgette* is more than matched by the interrelational confusion between its objects. As had been the case in *Cinéma bleu*, spatial recession in *Georgette* is problematic. This is not so much due to the inconclusiveness of compositional ties, however, as to their incongruity. The skittle, for example, could be seen as being partially hidden by a framed picture of Georgette, which, as in the case of the canvas of the later *La Condition*

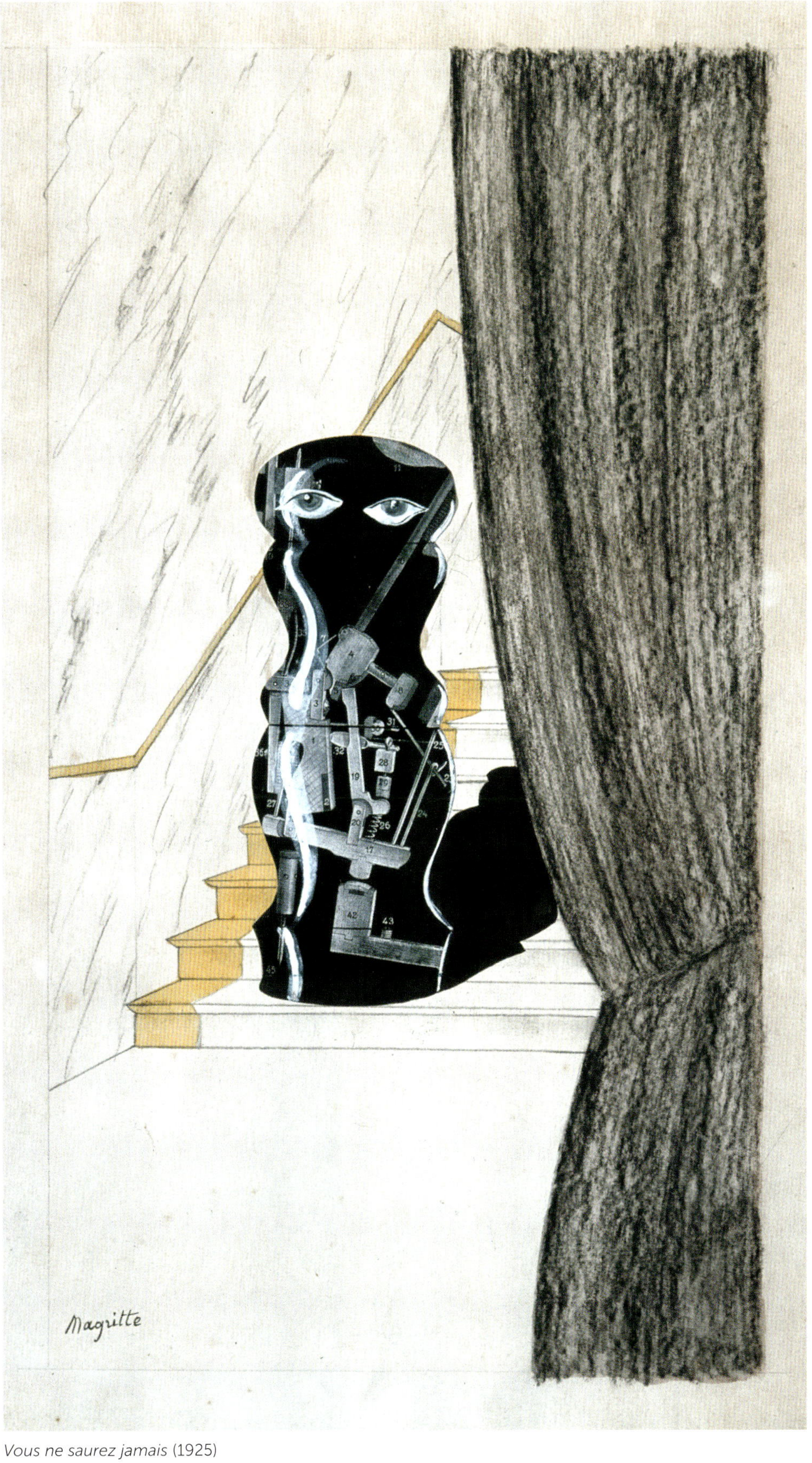

Vous ne saurez jamais (1925)

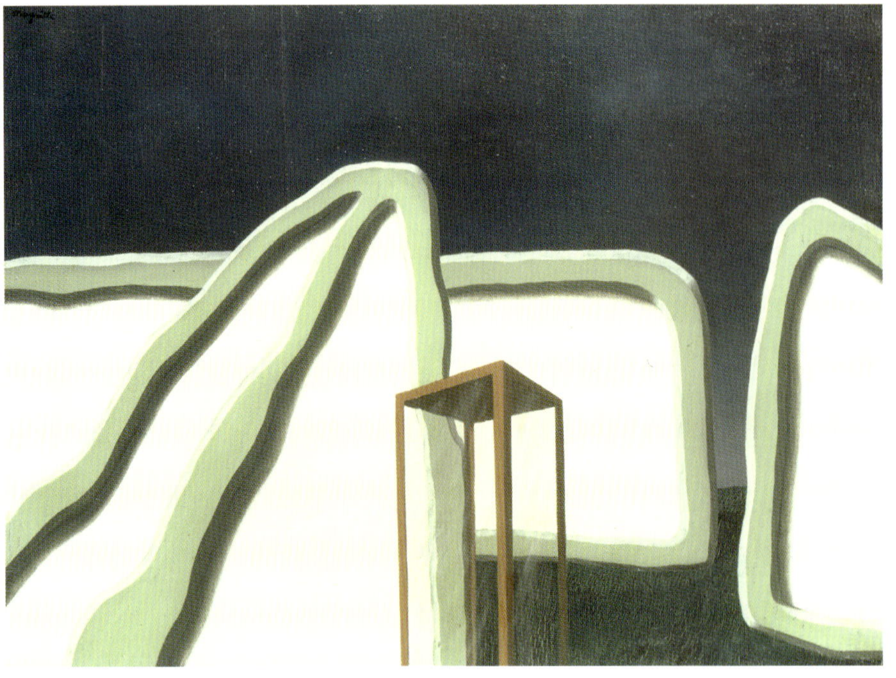

Le Prisonnier (1926)

humaine (1933-4), depicts precisely what it conceals. Nevertheless, this does not explain why the frame casts a shadow on the skittle. Alternatively, we could be looking at an empty frame through which the skittle and Georgette are visible. Seen in this way, however, Georgette would logically be positioned behind the red surface and so her shoulders would not overlap its far edge. Just as with the pyramids, both interpretations are flawed.[21] Pertinent to such a predicament is Judith Greene's observation that 'in a binary situation to affirm one possibility is the same as denying the other [...] a negative statement that one event is not the case amounts to an assertion that the other event is the case'.[22] In *Georgette*, however, neither alternative is plastically legitimate and the negation of one possibility is accompanied not by the affirmation of the other, but by a further negation. Magritte was to revisit this concept in 1963 with *La Lunette d'approche*, where the hypothesis suggested by the left pane, namely that the sky is being looked at through the glass, is contradicted by the black space to the right. The converse hypothesis, that a black space lies beyond and that the sky is painted on the panes, is also negated by the top corner of the right window. In just the same way, the arrangement of objects in *Georgette* does not so much result in an ambiguous scenario, where the alternatives would be equally probable, as in one in which the available interpretations are equally invalid.

Yet, by remaining to some extent within the bounds of what is conceivable, the painting cannot be classed as a true paradoxical illusion. Perhaps this was what Magritte meant when he wrote that his works 'aim, within what is possible, not

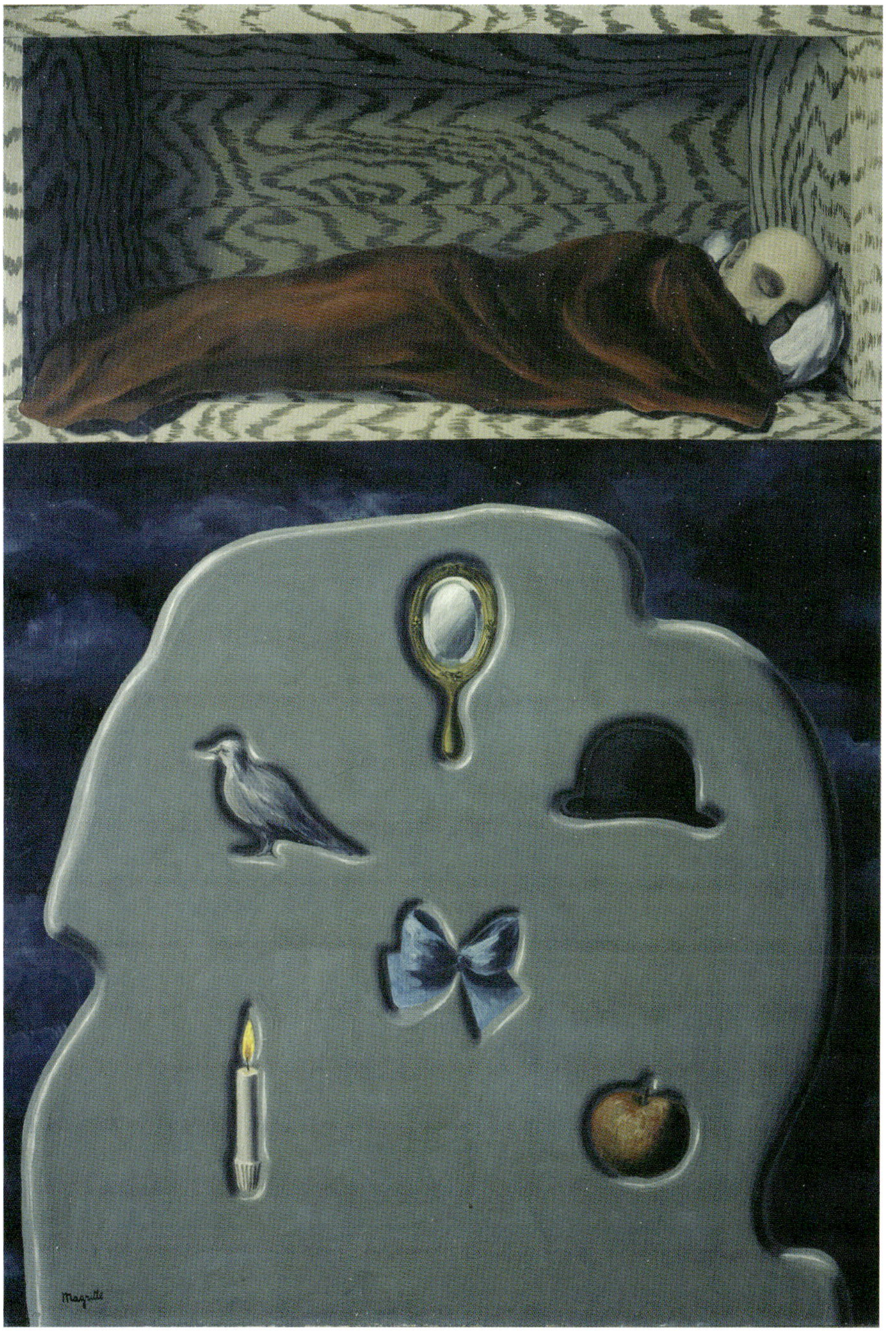

Le Dormeur téméraire (1927-28)

to be deprived of Meaning; that is to say not to be deprived of the impossible'.[23] Indeed, even the untitled collage of 1926 counterpoises the spatial absurdity of the floor with a regular recession of skittles that adhere to Alberti's rule that 'the feet of the farthest correspond to the knees of the nearest'. The idea of intertwining the possible with the impossible is one with which Magritte toyed in various works. In *Vous ne saurez jamais* (1925) inconsistent visual cues allow the minimal and insufficient space on the step of a staircase to accommodate a skittle that could not possibly fit the width of the tread. Similarly, the apparently

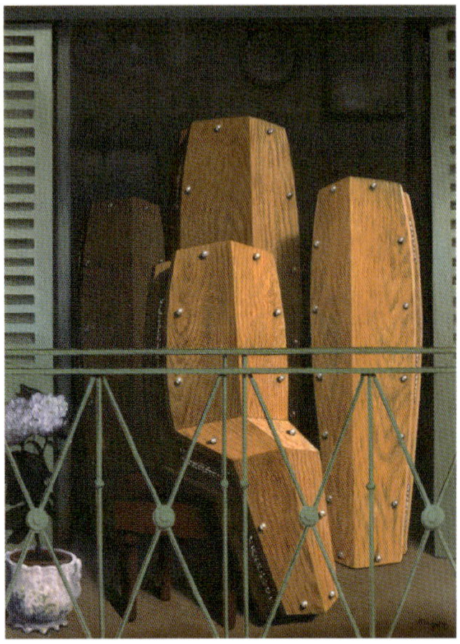

Perspective : le balcon de Manet (1949)

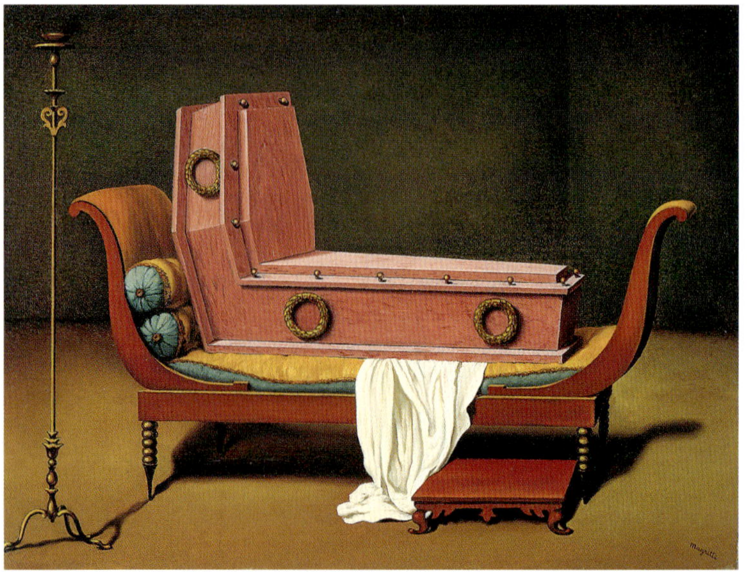

Perspective : Madame Récamier de David (1950)

solid polygons in the 1926 collage paradoxically give way under the weight of human figures, which are being swallowed up, whilst rigidly supporting the weight of a table. As far as Magritte was concerned, Alberti's compositional grammar, together with the consistency and comprehensibility that went with it, was there to be ridiculed.

✣ ✣ ✣

So far, Magritte's defiance of Albertian pictorial syntactics has been seen either to preclude the finite positioning of objects or to construct a paradoxical space for them. In a third twist to his derangement of pictorial context, Magritte proceeded to sever completely the links that hold the elements of a painting together. He simply isolated objects from one another. It became no longer a question of incomplete or polyvalent grammar, but of an outright pictorial agrammaticality. For the linguistic agrammatic, utterances become discontinuous and words are spoken in a staccato fashion because substantives are isolated from one another by silent pauses. In precisely this way, Magritte's agrammatic works are marked by representational pauses in the form of discontinuity between meaningful pictorial elements. To an extent, the objects in *Cinéma bleu* had been kept apart by the ill-defined spatial areas between them. In the more extreme grammatically dysfunctional works, however, the three-dimensional continuum is positively interrupted in a way that parallels the breaks in aphasic speech. Like the verbal caesuras of aphasia, the pictorial hiatuses in such paintings function as positive barriers and not just as omissions in the syntactic sequence. The individual object becomes

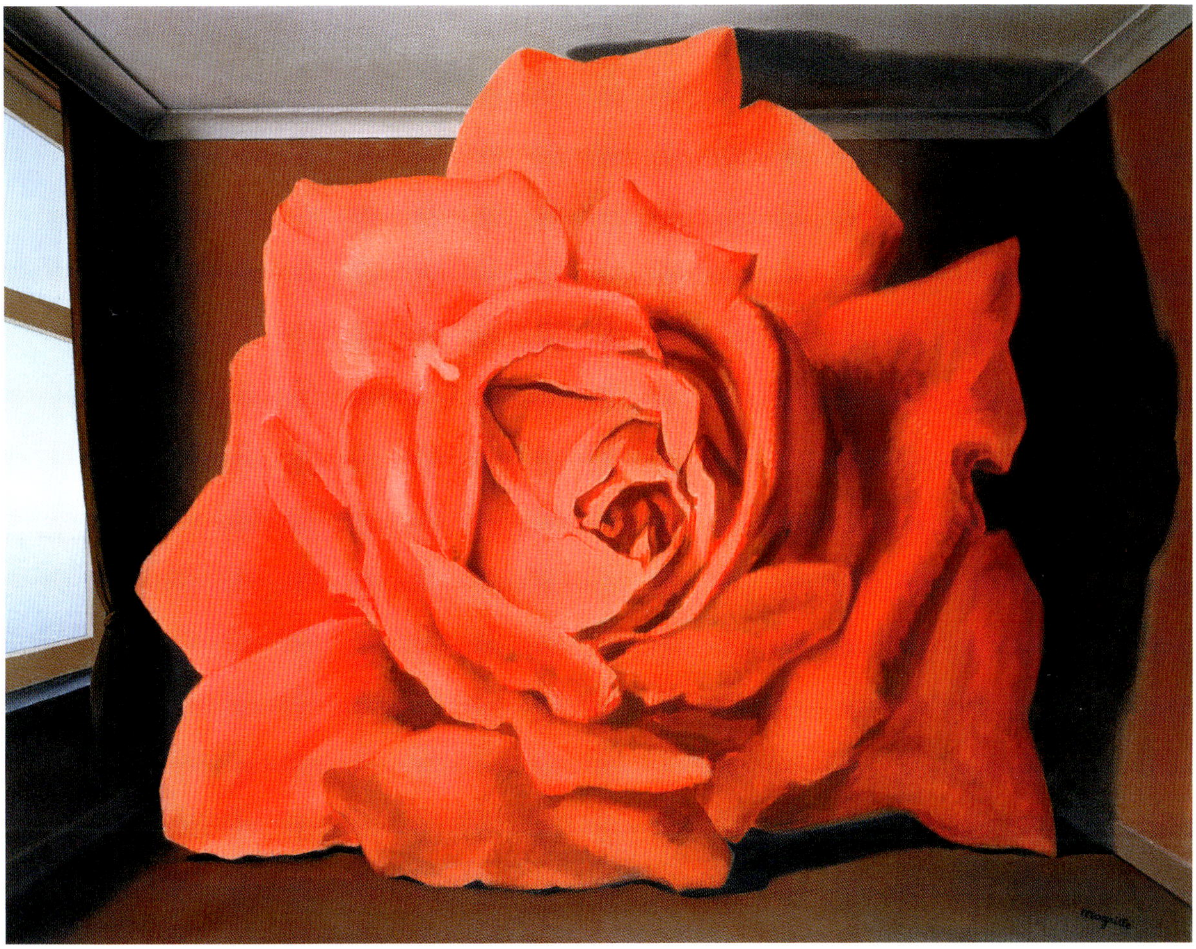

Le Tombeau des lutteurs (1960)

decontextualized not because it appears in a partially resolved space, as it had in *Cinéma bleu*, or in a self-contradictory space as in *Georgette*, but because it is confined within a compartmentalization of an explicit space. In his third form of agrammatism, Magritte cut objects off from one another in an overt way. As in agrammatic speech, the potential of an interrelation between semantic units exists, but, at the same time, it is frustrated. Alberti, of course, had gone to great lengths to construct a schema within which the parts of the painting would 'fit together'; Magritte, in his wilful contrariness, kept them apart.[24]

This heightened form of disjunction between semantic units first appeared in the aptly titled *Le Prisonnier* (1926), which depicts potential, but empty, receptacles. Within them space is clearly defined, but it remains vacant. The painting is a sign of things to come and formulates what could be seen as prototypes for the two forms of 'incarceration' to which objects would be subjected in due course. The upright, flat, irregular planes in the middle distance would eventually be moulded around objects so as to isolate and embed them within solid matter, as would occur two years later in *Le Repos de l'acrobate* (1928). The glass-panelled wooden box in the foreground, on the other hand, anticipates an alternative form of confinement based on encasement. The object has the appearance of a display case, but it is also cage-like and has the potential to entrap. The comparable compartments of the later *Le Musée d'une nuit* (1927) put objects on show, but also imprison them. In different ways, the two means of confinement create palpable impediments to the interrelation of pictorial elements.

Both types of pictorial isolation appear in *Le Dormeur téméraire* (1928), in which a sleeper is confined in a wooden box and six objects are embedded in a slab of set concrete or lead. In contrast to the swirling clouds in the background, the objects are frozen in their individual moulds. They appear as though pressed into tightly-fitting recesses outside of which they have no significance or pictorial impact; the mirror does not reflect its surroundings and the burning candle does not radiate its light. Circumscription ceases to be a point of transition between the object and its context and becomes more of a constraining circumvallation. The spaces between the objects are therefore not bridged by compositional concatenation, which would create relational ties; rather, each niche is a self-sufficient, insular space. Just like the cherubs, doves and crucifixes carved into the cemetery monuments amongst which Magritte had played as a child, the objects in *Le Dormeur téméraire* remain inert and cut off from any sort of outer context.[25] It is perhaps not incidental, therefore, that the upright grey slab in the painting should resemble a tombstone and that the sleeper should be asleep in a coffin, an object that Magritte was later to paint more literally in *Perspective : le balcon de Manet* (1949) and *Perspective : Madame Récamier de David* (1950).[26] Just like a corpse in a coffin, the recumbent sleeper is shown as encased and confined as the objects below him; his box is barely long enough to accommodate his extended body and within it he is again enveloped by a blanket.

The grammar of pictorial interrelation is disturbed on another level as well, that of perspective. The vanishing point is subtly placed slightly above the top edge of the canvas, with the result that the spectator's view point is misaligned with the entire content of the painting. Magritte therefore precludes any sort of correlation between the space of the observer and that of the painting and, as such, flies in the face of Alberti's condition that 'both the beholder and the painted things he sees will appear to be on the same plane'.[27] The painting as a whole ceases to be Alberti's 'open window', giving onto an illusory space that extends from the real space of the observer.[28] Not only are the objects in the painting separated from one another, but they are also separated from the spectator, who is excluded altogether. *Le Dormeur téméraire* offers only syntactic disjunction and spatial occlusion, a concept, incidentally, with which Magritte would continue to experiment in *Le Tombeau des lutteurs* (1960), where it is the object itself that swells to fill its enclosure. Whilst in *Cinéma bleu* the defiance of the grammar of painting had been brought about by an inconsistency of spatial relations, in *Le Dormeur téméraire* it arises from an interference with compositional ties. Pictorial elements are mutually alienated and locked in a rigid inertia that belies a seemingly plausible voluminous setting. Whether they have an irresolvable void between them or they are deprived of peripheral space, the objects in this phase of Magritte's experiments inhabit an indefinable expanse that is grammatically destabilized by ambiguity, paradox and discontinuity.

---

[1] Pierre Demarne, 'René Magritte', *Rhétorique*, 3 (Sept. 1961): n. pag.

[2] Leon Battista Alberti, *On Painting*, trans. John R. Spencer (London, 1956), p. 58.

[3] The comprehensibility of the floor area was central to Renaissance art. In Donatello's schiacciato predella of *St. George* (1415-7), the pattern on the floor meticulously defines a considerable penetration of depth.

[4] In the year of the painting, 1925, Magritte had in fact designed the stage set for a performance by the Groupe Libre, Brussels. André Blavier, in René Magritte, *Écrits complets* (Paris, 1979), p. 672.

[5] A drawing of the same year, 1925, by Magritte, in Marcel Lecomte's *Applications* (Louvain, 1925) shows the same confusion of the vertical and the horizontal. Whereas the represented girl's right foot is held vertically, with the toe pointing down, the foot is also a continuation of the edge of the horizontal carpet.

[6] According to André Blavier, in Magritte, *Écrits complets*, p. 25. Patrick Waldberg, *René Magritte* (Brussels, 1965), p. 212.

[7] His publicity design *La Festa* (1924), made for the Norine fashion house, features a similar figure, resembling an 'abstract' Art Déco mannequin. The *Exposition des arts décoratifs* took place in Paris in 1925 and included a section on fashion. According to Lester Gaba, the Art Déco mannequin was angular and had 'pointed toes', *The Art of Window Display* (London, 1952), p. 18.

[8] Alberti stressed that the painter must know well 'how each thing ought to be done and where located', and that in this respect there must be 'the greatest certainty', Alberti, *On Painting*, p. 96.

[9] It seems possible to perceive a sense of movement in a static representation: 'Perception will tend to run ahead of the evidence [...] Nobody thinks that the sailing boat is actually racing out of the frame, but there are experiments to suggest that if we understand its direction and speed we will anticipate its shift to some extent'. E. H. Gombrich, 'Illusion and Art', in R. L. Gregory and E. H. Gombrich (eds), *Illusion in Nature and Art* (London, 1973), p. 228.

[10] The technique first appeared in the misty hills of Verrocchio's *Baptism* (1470). The background of this painting and the angel on the left are usually ascribed to the young Leonardo da Vinci, who painted in the workshop of Verrocchio, Alberti, *On Painting*, p. 48.

[11] René Magritte, in José Vovelle, *Le Surréalisme en Belgique* (Brussels, 1972), p. 67. This confusion of relative distances is characteristic of Magritte's questioning of the way in which perception makes sense of the visible world: 'despite the complicated combinations of details and nuances of a real landscape, I could see it as though it were simply a curtain placed in front of my eyes. I became uncertain of the depth of the countryside, hardly persuaded of the far distance of the light blue of the horizon [...] I was in the same state of innocence as the child who thinks he can, from his cot, grab the bird flying in the sky', Magritte, *Écrits complets*, p. 106.

[12] Referring to Magritte's use of space, Michel Foucault remarked that 'the old perspective pyramid is no more than an old molehill about to collapse', *Ceci n'est pas une pipe* (Montpellier, 1973), p. 48.

[13] Alberti, *On Painting*, pp. 52 & 56. This also occurs in André Derain's *La Table* (1911).

[14] Alberti, *On Painting*, p. 56.

[15] Another example is the skull in Hans Holbein the Younger's *Jean de Dinteville and Georges de Selve. The Ambassadors* (1533).

[16] Alberti, *On Painting*, p. 70.

[17] *Georgette* (1926), *Roses de Picardie* (1925-6), *Le Jockey perdu* (1926, two versions), two untitled collages of 1926.

[18] The same is true of M. C. Escher's *Waterfall* (1961), where, although each part of the work is comprehensible, the overall sequence is impossible. Despite the correctness of each part of the composition, the manner in which these parts are linked is inconsistent with the modelling. It has been stated that: 'If we follow the various parts of this construction one by one we are unable to discover any mistake in it. Yet it is an impossible whole because changes suddenly occur in the interpretation of distance between our eye and the object', Anon., *The Graphic Works of M. C. Escher* (London, 1961), p.16.

[19] E. H. Gombrich, 'Illusion and Art', p. 238.

[20] Colin Blakemore, 'The Baffled Brain', in *Illusion in Nature and Art* (London, 1973), p. 29.

[21] The technique of simultaneously depicting opposing and conflicting situations was to become a major theme in Magritte's work post-1930.

[22] Judith Greene, *Psycholinguistics, Chomsky and Psychology* (Harmondsworth, 1972), pp. 123-4.

[23] Magritte, *Écrits complets*, p. 376.

[24] Alberti, *On Painting*, p. 70.

[25] Magritte, *Écrits complets*, p. 105.

[26] Magritte painted gravestones in *Le Sourire* (1943) and *La Fontaine de jouvance* (1957).

[27] Alberti, *On Painting*, p. 56.

[28] Alberti, *On Painting*, p. 56. Alberti further stated that the observer should feel involved in the painting: 'In an istoria, I like to see someone who admonishes and points out to us what is happening there; or beckons with his hand to see, or menaces with an angry face and with flashing eyes, so that no one should come near; or shows some danger or marvellous thing there', Alberti, *On Painting*, p. 78.

Shattering Anatomy

Magritte's affront on pictorial convention has so far been seen as a dismantling of the concatenation *between* objects. Quite systematically, he set about breaking every rule that his art school 'perspective' classes would have drilled into him, eventually doing away with all orthodox ways of interrelating the parts of a composition. Magritte's rebellion, however, did not stop there. As well as calling into question the ways in which figures in a painting can be interconnected, he also challenged the principles according to which they are individually assembled. Just as he had cocked a snook at his lessons on 'composition', he equally went on to defy what his 'anatomie' tutors had taught him. In an alternative type of pictorial disintegration, it is the unit form that is interrogated and the focus switches to a disintegration that is played out *within* objects. In ways that would have dismayed his figure-drawing teachers, Magritte left the anatomical body unfinished, fragmented, dismembered or simply ill-defined. For him, the academic analysis of form into its constituents not only provided a blueprint for consolidating the parts of a body, but also offered a ready-made scheme for disjointing them. Barely disguising his disdain for formal art training, Magritte cynically described his anatomy and perspective classes as 'all that a painter must know *a little bit* about'.[1]

According to Marcel Paquet, Magritte's treatment of the human body has, at its heart, a fundamental transformation of anatomy.[2] The interrelations of corporeal constituent parts, we are told, are reinvented and the human body is revised in a way that has nothing to do with anatomical laws. Like a puzzle made up of pieces that do not fit together, it becomes discordant, incoherent and disordered. It loses its integrity and inner cohesion to become a place of novel variations, leaving a sum of disparate parts that come together to form a fragmentary, shattered multiplicity. Paquet, however, also insists that this transformation of the human form is by no means arbitrary and adheres to some sort of implicit methodical formula.[3] Of course, a systematic approach to pictorial demolition has already been seen in Magritte's treatment of 'composition', which can be analysed in terms of aphasic linguistic degeneration. The same, as it turns out, can be said of his corruptions of 'anatomy', which, arguably, can also be rationalized within the aphasic model. From this perspective, Magritte's disassembly of the body emerges as a process that parallels the more acute forms of agrammatism, in which contiguity is impaired not only between words, that is on the level of syntax, but also within the construction of words themselves. In this type of aphasia 'the minimum free form' is no longer the word, and the utterance typically comprises no more than disjointed morphemes, phonemes and sometimes even isolated phonetic units.[4] Correspondingly, the second type of Magritte's deconstructive works reverts to the more elemental units of painting. *His* 'minimum free forms' become the members, planes and outlines that Alberti had considered as mere 'stages' of painting. The hitherto central question of the degree to which the 'parts fit together' is overshadowed by an alternative reductionism that evokes uncertainty about the very identity of what is depicted. In this phase, 'figures' gradually cease to be decipherable and increasingly lose their representational capacity. They shrink semantically to mere marks on the canvas and can be said to be the visual equivalent of the utterances of the anomic, whose words are replaced by unintelligible monosyllables or simply empty gaps in speech.[5]

In concert with the anomic, who is unable fully to articulate the substantives of language, Magritte degraded his 'pictorial nouns' to indefinite forms or even pictorial voids. He progressively broke down the unit form by contravening Alberti's stages of painting one by one and, in effect, reversed the academic formulae for constructing figures. This, however, was not the only process being played out in these 'anomic' works, which would otherwise have ended up depicting denuded forms in a meaningless amorphousness. What in fact occurs alongside the depletion of content is an accompanying intensification of compositional ties. As though compensating for a waning semanticity, Magritte augmented the relational ties between his diminished shapes. In this light, the parallel with aphasia is striking. The more a fluent aphasic's nouns are eroded, the more utterances become dominated by relational markers and, in the absence of meaningful words, verbal fluency can only take the form of a framework of grammatical colligation. Against this model, Magritte's semantically impoverished works are invariably underpinned by a well-articulated grammar of space. Anatomical dearth, in other words, is counterbalanced by compositional repleteness.

Equally in keeping with the aphasic model is that Magritte's deconstruction of 'anatomy' is marked by an inverse proportionality of grammaticality to semanticity: the lesser the semantic content of a painting, the greater the compositional ties between its elements, whilst, the greater the semantic content, the weaker the compositional ties. Put another way, the more the pictorial units become incomprehensible, the greater the concatenation between them. As in aphasia, it is either the contextual setting or the meaningful content that is brought to the fore. This accounts for the fact that the paradoxical, indefinite space of *Cinéma bleu* is inhabited by comprehensible objects; the young woman, the skittle, the curtain and the inscribed signpost are all clearly denoted. The converse mechanism operates in paintings in which shapes that are vague or incomprehensible are, nevertheless, unambiguously interconnected within a coherent space. In the 'anatomical' phase of his pictorial 'dissolution',

Magritte gradually reinstated the contextual matrix that had been absent in the 'agrammatic' paintings, and was thus able to denude the painted object, whilst remaining within the confines of a structured image.

Nevertheless, the recourse to aphasia as a model for Magritte's early paintings is, in one sense, problematic. Whilst the works of the 1920s can be mapped as successive stages of a linear process in which context and semanticity progressively increase or decrease in an inversely proportional manner, linguistic aphasia occurs as a rather more clear-cut dichotomy in which either grammar is mostly lost and meaning is pronounced, or meaning dissipates whilst concatenations predominate. What aphasia can certainly be said to model faithfully, therefore, are the structures operating at the extremities of Magritte's progressive spectrum. Beyond that, the parallel is less evident. Yet, it is also true that the two types of aphasia are not actually diverse conditions; they may be divergent, but they remain facets of the same generic communication deficiency. Concatenation may predominate at one end and identity at the other, but between these extremes there are shades of agrammatic and anomic language loss. Admittedly, these gradations cannot be said to be as nuanced as Magritte's own subtle mixes of pictorial concatenation and signification, but they do mark trajectories that are echoed in his work. Whilst aphasia may not be a model that provides a one-to-one correspondence, it does define a process and a broad taxonomy that rationalizes a phased pictorial deconstruction. Rather than adhering to the painterly method of fully determining pictorial space and its anatomical denizens, Magritte brought together the axes of semantic selection and grammatical combination as would an aphasic, in unequal portions and in varying degrees of resolution. Form and space are interwoven but, from work to work, each is left unresolved, hanging at a particular stage of visual development.

As this study has shown so far, the stages of compositional depletion amount to a relatively small number of variations in the way space is put together. But when it came to anatomical dissolution, Magritte made greater distinctions. The steps he took in this direction show a more graduated approach, which began with no more than a simple edging away from the finiteness of form. In its initial stage, the breakdown of form merely affects the 'stability' of the individual shape, whilst its fundamental integrity remains intact. In *Les Pipes amoureuses de la lune* (1928), for instance, the pipes in question are not veritably 'taken apart'. All that happens is that they are denied fixed form. It is as though a process of mollification were beginning and no more. The pipes may have been softened, but have by no means reached the point of melting away beyond recognition, even if their changing shapes suggest that this is inevitable. From right to left, the pipes become increasingly elastic, as though portraying different stages of a progressive dissolution. The implication is that, ultimately, the process will arrive at the state of liquid viscosity seen in *La Sortie de l'école*

(1927), where the object is reduced to an un-representational amorphousness. In *Les Pipes amoureuses de la lune*, though, the subject is far from effaced and the pictorial dissolution focuses more on the contextual setting, which, like that of the previously considered agrammatic paintings, remains vague. The pavement in particular has an indeterminate quality, since nothing actually rests on it and the pipes, like the 'Norine' figure in *Cinéma bleu*, are left ambiguously floating in mid-air. To add to the lack of articulation in the setting, the horizon line is blurred and only clumsily separates the ground area from the sky. In fact, in the absence of adequate orientation cues, the horizontal can barely be distinguished from the vertical and space in general has little cohesiveness. This, in turn, blurs the correlation of the foreground objects with the more remote areas and even the illusion of a sky, stretching beyond the immediate scene, is contradicted by the three broad horizontal strokes of dark colour below the moon, which remain outside the pictorial illusion.

Yet, neither is the setting totally lacking in logic. To a minor extent and bearing out the aphasic model's principle of inverse proportionality, the space of the painting does incorporate some measure of regulation. The tentative demise of the anatomical elements can be seen to be compensated by degrees of finiteness in the composition. The curtain on the right, for instance, may not itself be situated explicitly, but it allows us to gauge the position of other objects; the shadow of a mouthpiece places one of the pipes squarely *in front* of the curtain, whilst the dark stripe in the sky disappears *behind* the curtain. Of course, these are no more than suggestions of an increasing grammar but they do show that the abatement of anatomy does have a compositional foil. Only when Magritte went on to dismantle the composite form of the human body, however, did his dissolution emerge as a genuinely counterbalanced procedure.

The rules of anatomical construction with which Magritte would have been inculcated at the Academy and which he was to subvert would have been based on the treatises of Vitruvius, who had rationalized the human form by isolating and measuring its parts, and Alberti, whose *On Sculpture* is probably the most significant source of the formal analysis of the body.[6] According to the latter, the figure is to be viewed not only as a collection of delimitations in space, but also in mechanical terms, as extensions and movements. Alberti's 'dimensio' analyses the parts of the body in terms of their relative magnitude, each limb or portion being seen as a fraction of the whole and as corresponding to the other parts: 'dimensio', he wrote, 'is the accurate and constant recording of measurements, whereby the state and correspondence of the parts is observed and numerically represented, one in relation to another and each to the whole length of the body'.[7] Alternatively, 'finitio' limits the dynamic range of the parts and determines the extent to which a limb moves and the geometric confines within which that movement occurs: 'finitio is the means whereby we record

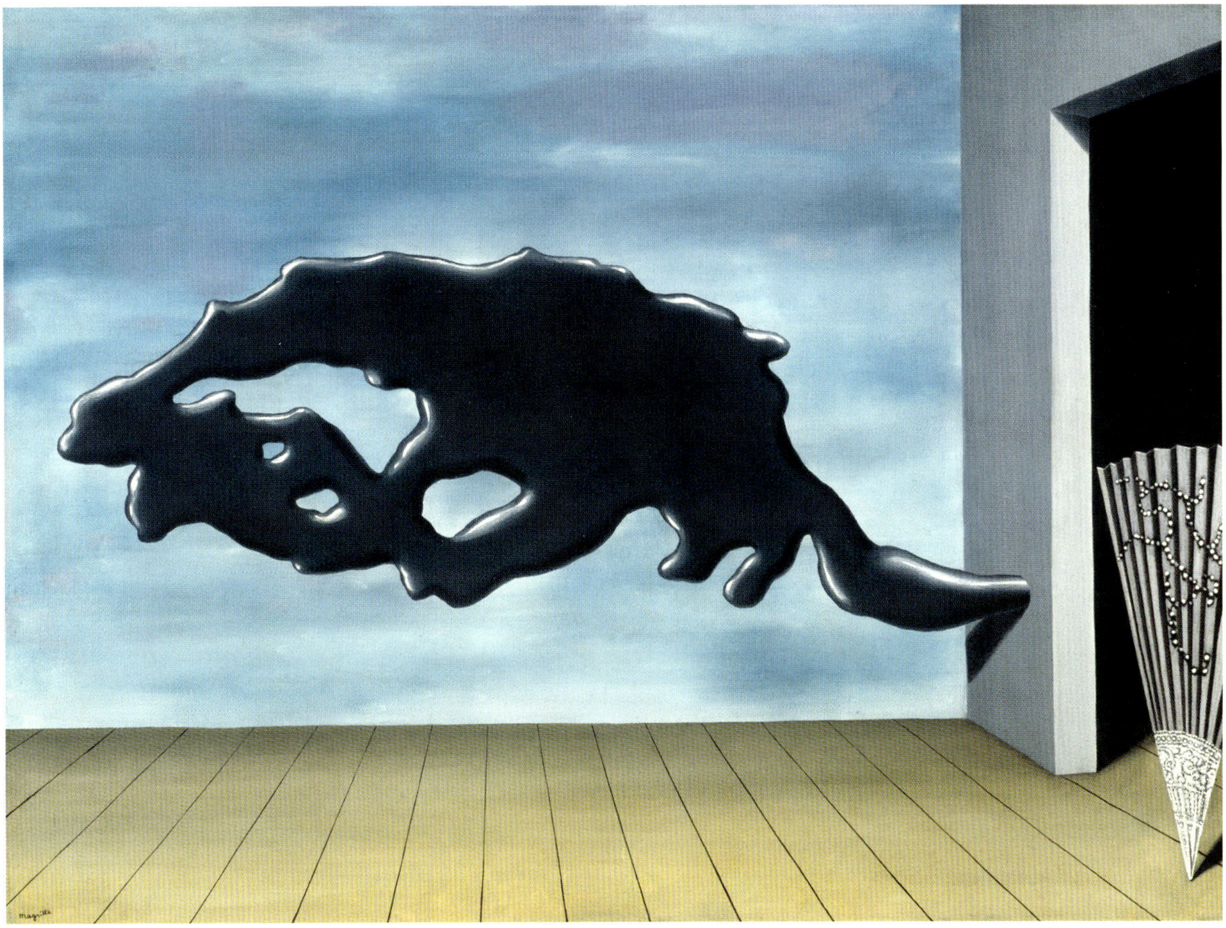

La Sortie de l'école (1927)

with sure and accurate method the extensions and curves of lines, and the size and shape and position of all angles, protuberances, and recesses'.[8]

Besides specifying two methods of measurement, *On Sculpture* goes on to elaborate two ways of subdividing the body. 'Anatomy', focuses on the different strata below the surface, 'the number of bones and the projections of muscles and sinews'.[9] Alternatively, 'anthropometry' divides the external form across its axis to create a series of comparable segments. As Alberti explained, 'it is [...] very important to understand how we observe the outlines of the body by sections'.[10] In this approach, the body is scanned linearly and measured as sections of the external form in order to establish its relative proportions. What results is a series of solid segments. There is a 'dissection' in the form of a fractionizing of the body. Significantly with regard to Magrittian deconstruction, the body is visualized as separate parts and therefore as an amalgam that is open both to disassembly, and to assembly. In one modern drawing manual the student is told to 'break down' and then 'rebuild' the human form.[11] In accordance with Alberti's conception of 'dimensio', modern art school drawing classes still subdivide the body into particular zones; as one twentieth century manual specifies, 'the trunk' is the 'top of the head to the fold of the buttock', the 'lower limb' stretches 'from the ground to the middle of the fold of the groin, level with the head of the femur' and the 'upper limb' extends 'from the acromion to the tip of the middle finger'.[12] In contrast, 'anatomy' deals with the way in which each layer of the body is structured. It starts by examining the arrangements of the bones and progresses to the more superficial layers, each stage of penetration being regarded in terms of its relational organization. In other words, anatomy details the *concatenations* within concurrent systems. '[A] thorough knowledge of anatomy', John Barrington observes, 'is to life-art what grammar is to language.'[13] At the primary level of the skeleton, for example, each bone is not only defined in its own terms, but also located in relation to the other bones and the rest of the figure. 'It would be useful', Alberti wrote, 'to isolate each bone [...] on this add its muscles, then clothe all of it with its flesh.'[14] Indeed, a typical modern art school exercise would be to 'draw the skeleton inside the figure'.[15] Students still examine each 'mechanism' and, with the aid of mounted skeletons, écorché displays and models, go on to build up the constituent layers of the body to arrive at the 'natural internal structure of the body'.[16] As opposed to the segmentation of anthropometry, the analysis is transversal.

Essentially, Alberti's scrutiny of the body amounts to a parsing. As he noted, his approach centred on the 'observation by sections of the body'.[17] But what remains important is the dependence of the parts to the whole. Unlike Magritte's fragmentations, there is never an observation of the sections in their own right. Although, ostensibly in concert with Magritte, Alberti advocated a way of seeing that reduced form into its primary factors, his aim was, ultimately, to achieve a precisely *assembled* integral form. Magritte, on the other hand, exploited such parsing to release form from the congruity of the whole. He drew on 'anatomie' and its analytical subdivision of the body to pervert academic norms, and contradict the rules of both 'dimensio' and 'finitio'.

---

1 René Magritte, *Écrits complets* (Paris, 1979), p. 624, italics my own. Magritte also wrote that: 'Painting limited to purely formal pictorial effects did not seem worth looking at', Magritte, *Écrits complets*, p. 552.

2 Marcel Paquet, *René Magritte, la pensée visible* (Cologne, 1993).

3 Paquet does not, however, explain what such a method might entail.

4 R. H. Robins in *General Linguistics: An Introductory Survey* (London, 1971), p. 185.

5 Anomia is also known as Wernike's aphasia.

6 Polykleitos had also tabulated the body as proportionate parts. Leon Battista Alberti, *On Painting, On Sculpture*, trans. Cecil Grayson (London, 1972).

[7] Alberti, *On Painting, On Sculpture*, p. 125.

[8] Alberti, *On Painting, On Sculpture*, p. 129.

[9] Alberti, *On Painting, On Sculpture*, p. 139.

[10] Alberti, *On Painting, On Sculpture*, p. 139.

[11] John S. Barrington, *Anthropometry and Anatomy* (London, 1963), p. 49.

[12] Barrington, *Anthropometry and Anatomy*, p. 42.

[13] Barrington, *Anthropometry and Anatomy*, p. 7.

[14] Alberti, *On Painting*, trans. John R. Spencer (London, 1956), p. 73.

[15] William A. Berry, *Drawing the Human Form: Methods/Sources/Concepts* (New York, 1977), p. 144.

[16] Barrington, *Anthropometry and Anatomy*, p. 7. Berry, *Drawing the Human Form*, p. 140.

[17] Alberti, *On Painting, On Sculpture*, p. 139.

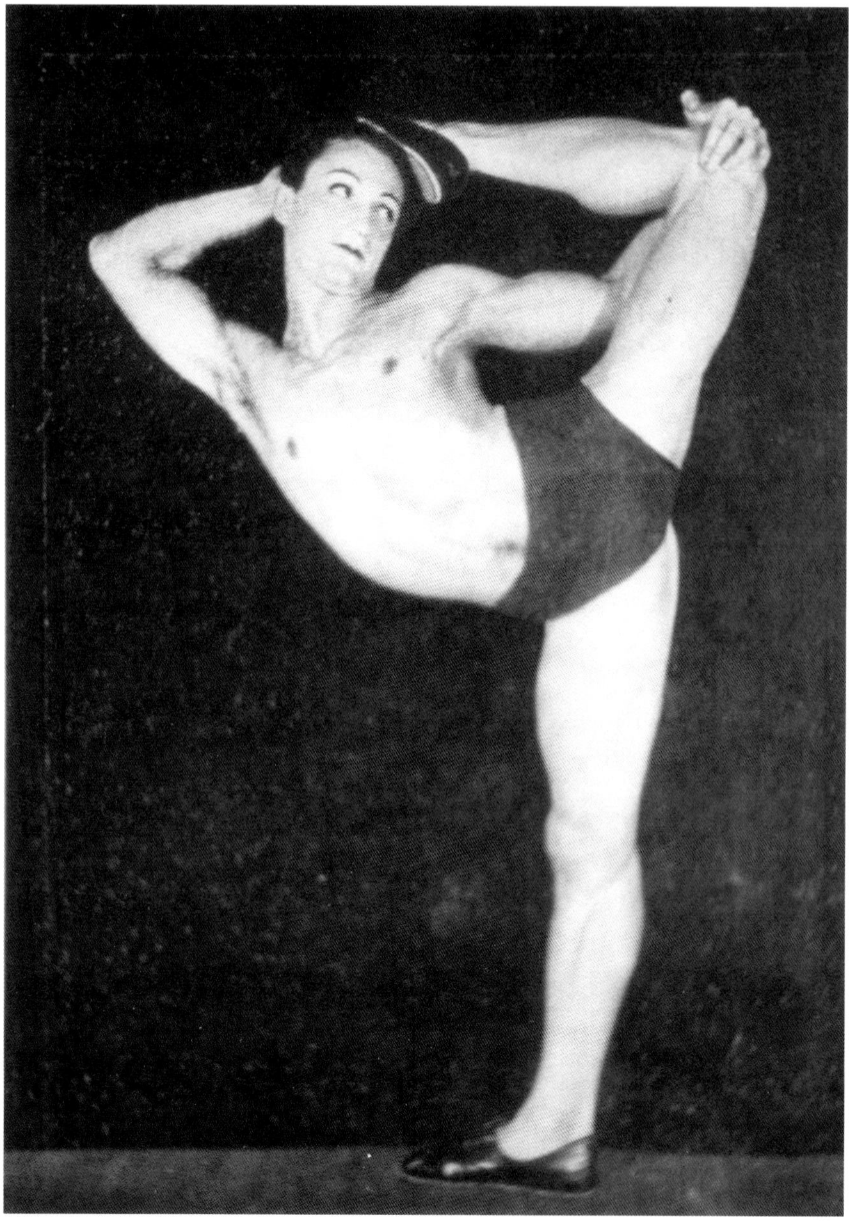

Atelier Robertson, *Le Danseur acrobatique*, in *Variétés*, 5 (1929)

Elastic Form

Before being systematically deconstructed, the human form undergoes what could be described as an anatomical assault course. It is depicted in extreme poses and situations that stretch it to breaking point. Figures teeter on the boundary between staying whole and disintegrating into bits.

One of Magritte's strategies for undermining the body was that of pushing it to the limits of its capability in what resemble physical trials. The gruelling gymnastics of *Les Impatients* (1928), for instance, puts muscular athletes through strenuous ordeals. One sportsman is straining to jump over an obstacle, possibly a hurdle just out of sight, whilst the other is shown in the opposing stance of stretching down, as though about to dive into a pool or perform a backward somersault. Both are flexing their limbs as far as humanly possible and, to an extent, beyond. The angle of the upward-pointing arm, for instance, is much too vertical to be plausible. Magritte pushes the elasticity of the body beyond credibility and his protagonists seem more like contortionists than gymnasts. They certainly echo the tortuous pose of a staggeringly lithe 'acrobatic dancer' featured in Paul-Gustave van Hecke's *Variétés*, which Magritte could well have seen pre-publication.[1] It may be telling that the reference to acrobacy in the magazine caption recurs in several of Magritte's titles at this time.

A painting that deforms and flexes the body still further is *Les Idées de l'acrobate* (1927-8). Unlike *Les Impatients*, it goes beyond the bounds of credibility. The human limbs and flesh are stretched, elongated and twisted as though they were pieces of dough. In every way, *Les Idées de l'acrobate* contravenes Alberti's caveat that the members should:

> accord well with one another [...] For, if in a picture the head is enormous, the chest puny, the hand very large, the foot swollen and the body distended, this composition will certainly be ugly to look at. So one must observe a certain conformity in regard to the size of the members.[2]

Not only are the members altered in size and shape by Magritte, but they are also disordered and, in places, incorrectly sequenced. In a deliberately non-compliant manner it would seem, the body is, in fact, 'distended' and deformed to become an ectopic jumble that would undoubtedly have perturbed Alberti. The painting, however, can also be seen as a test-bed for methods of deconstruction that Magritte would go on to exploit in other works. For instance, it shows a lateral shearing technique that severs a torso across its axis; in 1930, *L'Évidence éternelle* was to present the body as cut up horizontally into separate segments. *Les Idées de l'acrobate* effaces detail, including facial features, as occurs in *La Fin des contemplations* (1927). Further, there is a deformation of a figure's outline that eats away at pictorial meaning itself.

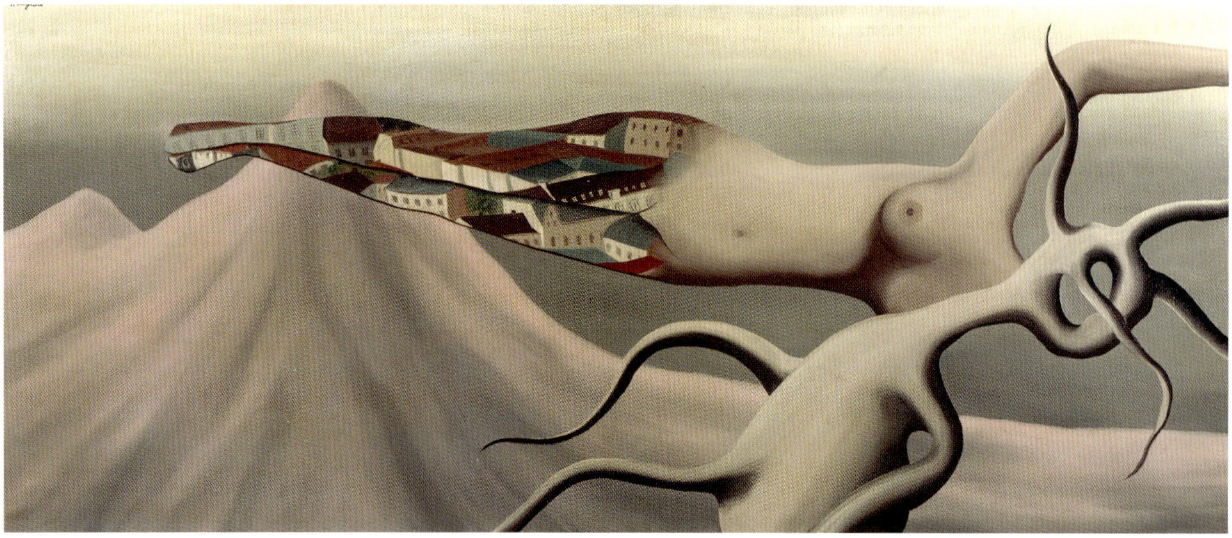

Les Grands Voyages (1926)

With its interconnected sequence of pictorial mutations, *Les Idées de l'acrobate* could be said to function as a flow-chart, mapping out the stages of a systematic disassembly of the body. It also signals a course set towards out-and-out pictorial dissolution, which had not been so much the case in earlier works, such as *Les Grands Voyages* (1926). As this particular work shows, modifications at that time were not focussed on a diminution of anatomy: the legs of the floating nude are distorted not so much by being lessened, as by being *augmented*, becoming a panorama of solid buildings. Rather than resulting in deconstruction, this alteration leads to an increase in substantiality. Only in the second, more flimsy tentaculoid figure is there a suggestion of impoverishment. But this is a mere hint of anatomical demise and *Les Grands Voyages*, as well as its contemporary *La Promenade du monstre* (1926-7) were still according as much emphasis to the construction of form as to its dissolution.

In paintings that challenge anatomy, even moderately, there are invariably tell-tale signs that the opposing axis of picture-making, 'composition', is being bolstered. In works such as *Les Idées de l'acrobate*, where figures are structurally disrupted and *internally* unstable, the space of the painting is constructed in a markedly coherent and even emphatic manner. The waning of the permanence of form in *Le Repos de l'acrobate* (1928), for instance, is counterbalanced by a decisively articulated context in the form of a rigid solid stone wall. In fact, Magritte overcompensates for the instability of the stretched and distorted corporeal parts by enveloping them in the contrasting stability of the sturdy masonry edifice that almost fills the painting.

Distension, however, was not the only form of abatement to which Magritte subjected the body at this stage of the anatomical dissolution. Experimenting

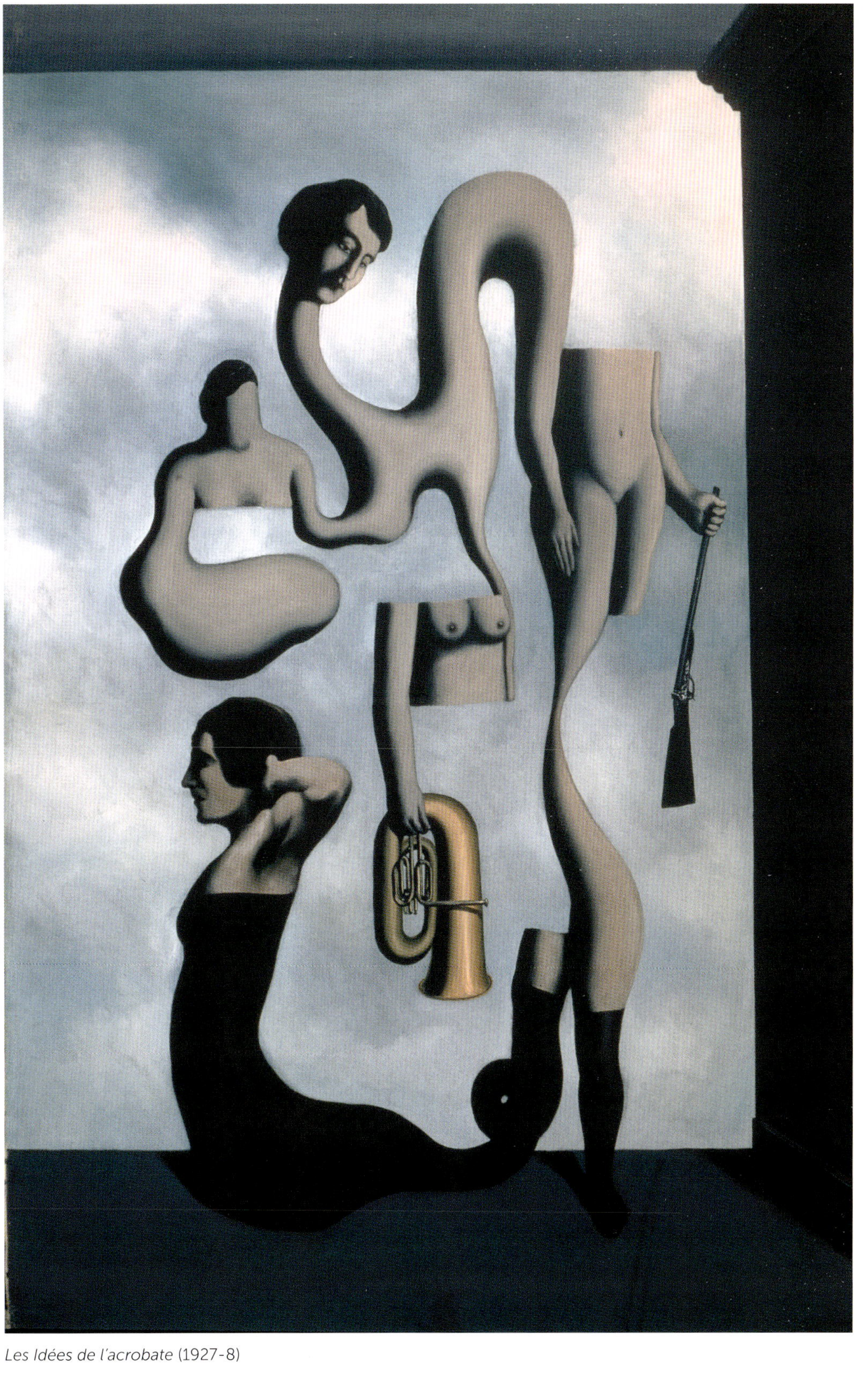

Les Idées de l'acrobate (1927-8)

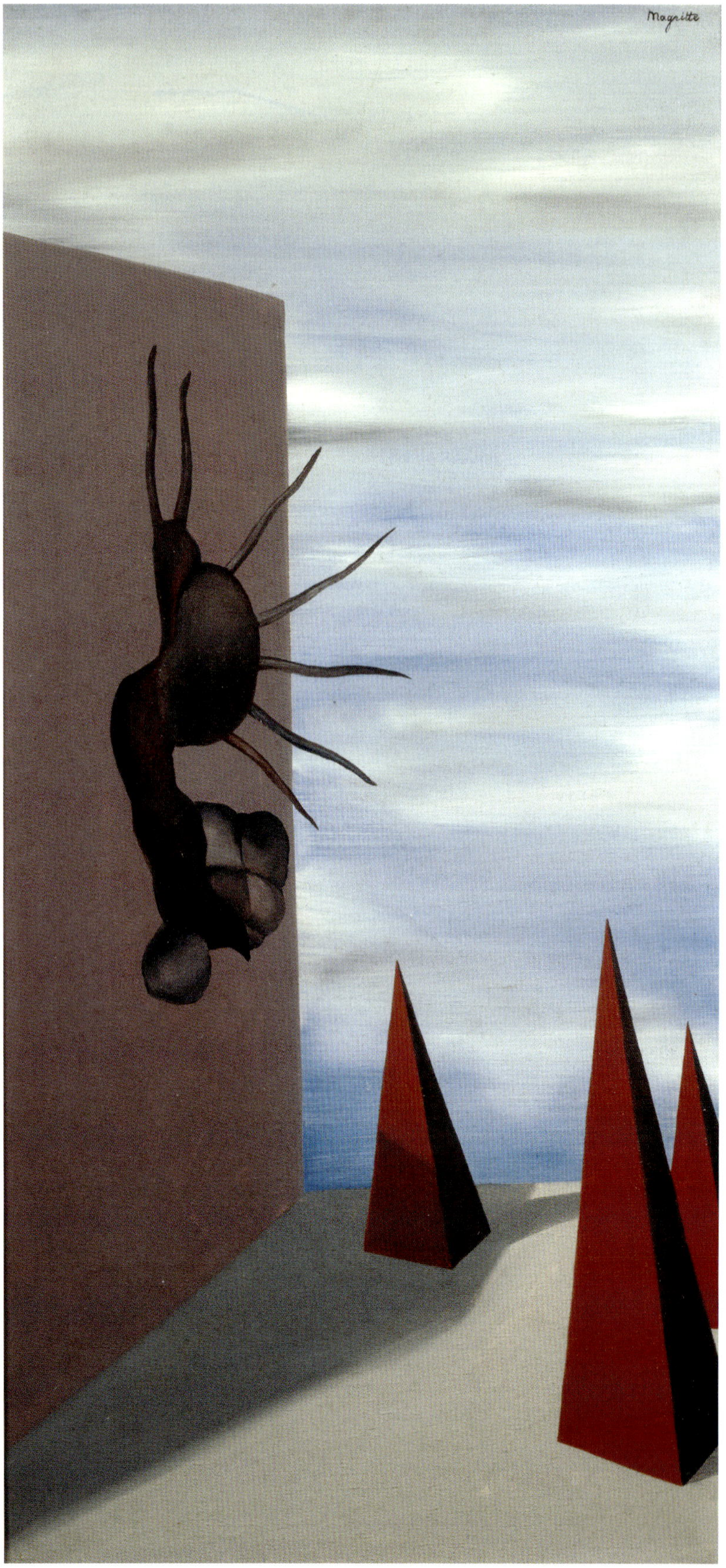

La Promenade du monstre (1926-7)

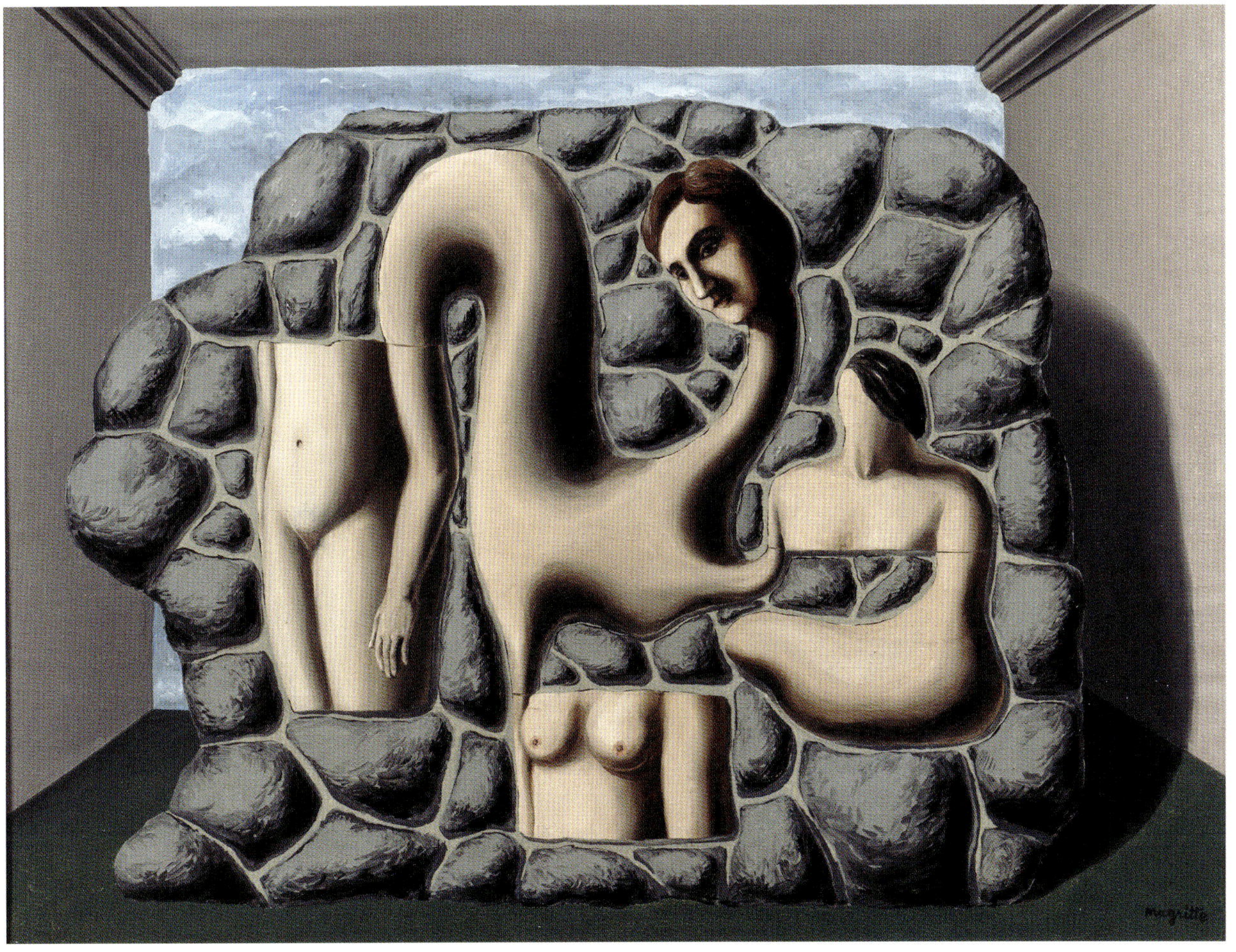

Le Repos de l'acrobate (1928)

with the converse approach, he put it through the ordeal of being compressed. Instead of extending pictorial elements beyond 'finitio', he constricted them to a space inside its boundaries. In *Les Chasseurs au bord de la nuit* (1928), for instance, two huntsmen fretfully struggle against the confines of a space which is closing in on them. The irony, of course, is that it is hunters, armed to the hilt and ready to entrap their prey, who are themselves ensnared. So limited is the available space that the protagonists are beginning to be swallowed up by the open-sided box in which they find themselves. One man has lost his head and is pushing against the wall as though to retrieve it, while the other looks down in horror at his right calf, which has disappeared almost as far as the knee. In opposition to the various forms of protraction seen in *Les Impatients*, here there is an overwhelming contraction. In many ways, the two paintings are mutually antithetical. The expressions of self-assured confidence of 'les impatients' contrast with the obscured faces of the panicking huntsmen. Equally, the claustrophobic closing-in of space in one painting, opposes the

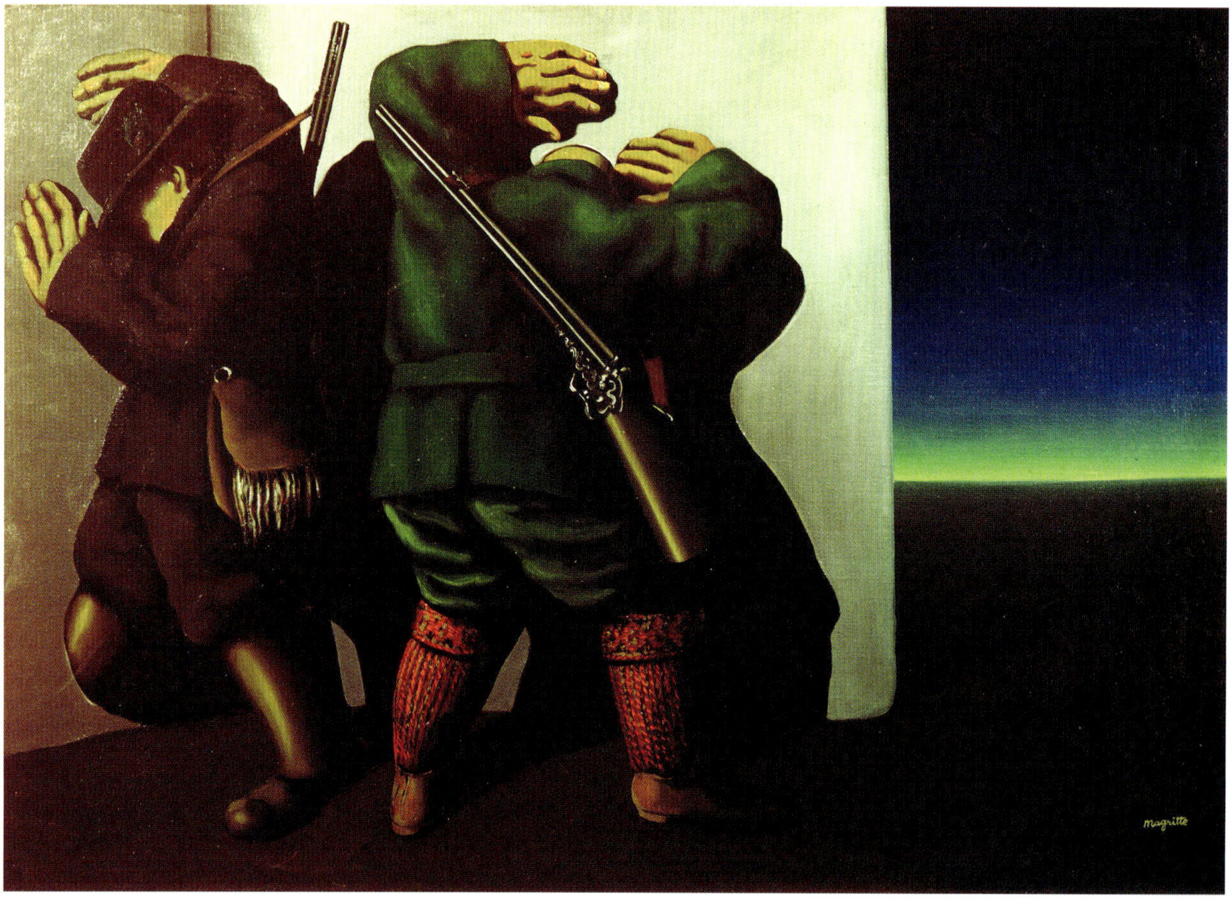

Les Chasseurs au bord de la nuit (1928)

emptiness around the unclad athletes of the other. Constriction contrasts with an absence of restraint. Above all, *Les Chasseurs au bord de la nuit* represents a privation of movement: it shows 'finitio' as inhibited in an extreme way. This idea of cramped impaction is taken even further in *Le Village mental* (1926), where a dismembered arm is being crushed between two walls. Not only is the force so irresistible that, like the huntsmen, the fingers and thumb have already penetrated solid matter, but the process appears to be ongoing and the space ever-diminishing.[3] Whilst *Le Repos de l'acrobate* had encased parts of the body, now they are being swallowed up. Entrapment becomes progressively enveloping, as it also does for a woman slowly sinking into the ground in *L'Odeur de la campagne les fait avancer* (1928). Despite her arduous swaying, she is glued to the spot and cannot take her next step. Like the walls in *Le Village mental*, the earth anchors and absorbs her. In the untitled collage (1926), measuring 40 x 55.5 cm, the figures have sunk even more and are almost completely submerged.

One thing that these particular methods of corporeal demise have in common is that they are enacted in an overt manner, in full view of the spectator. Magritte,

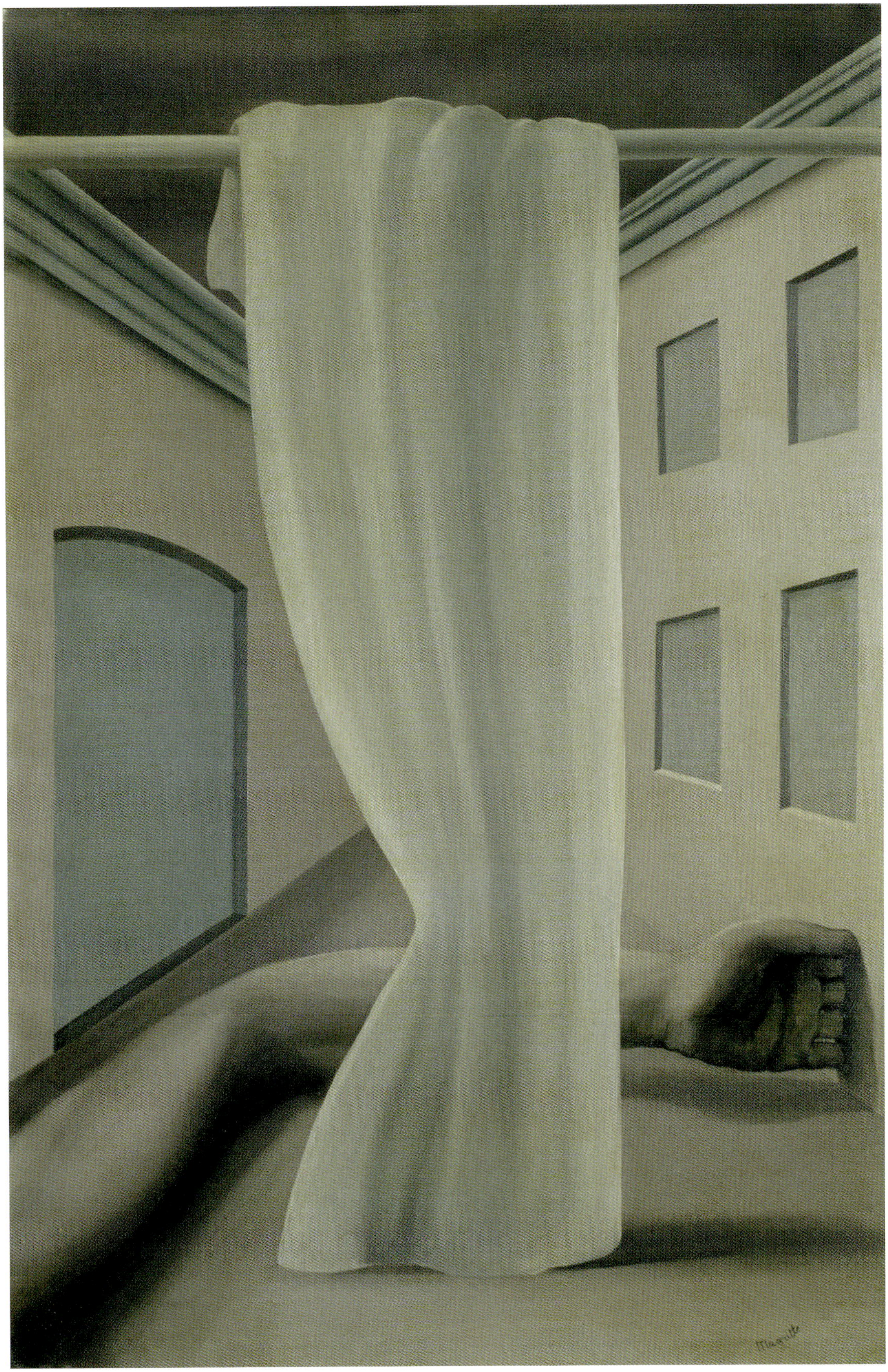

Le Village mental (1926)

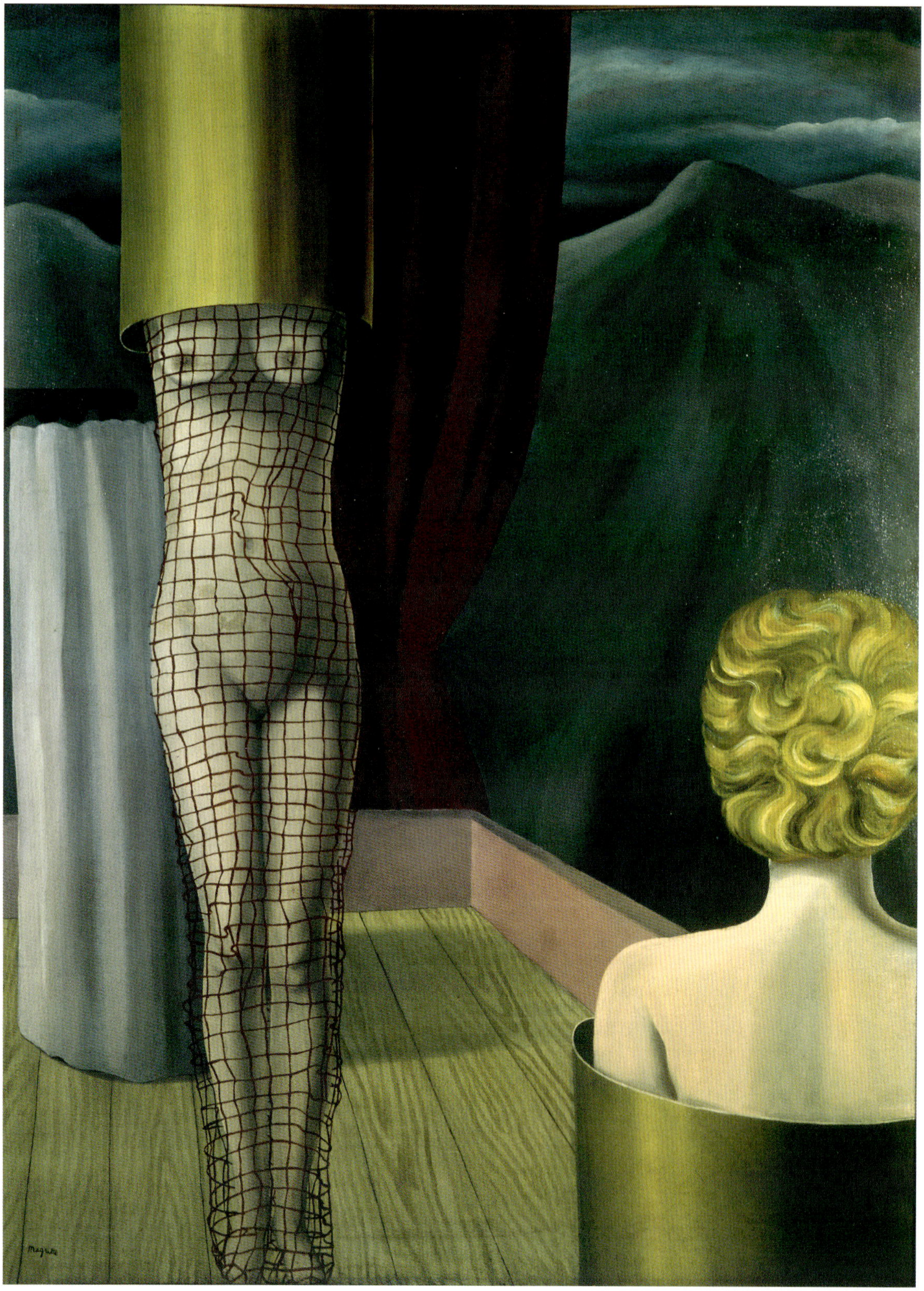

Les Complices du magicien (1926)

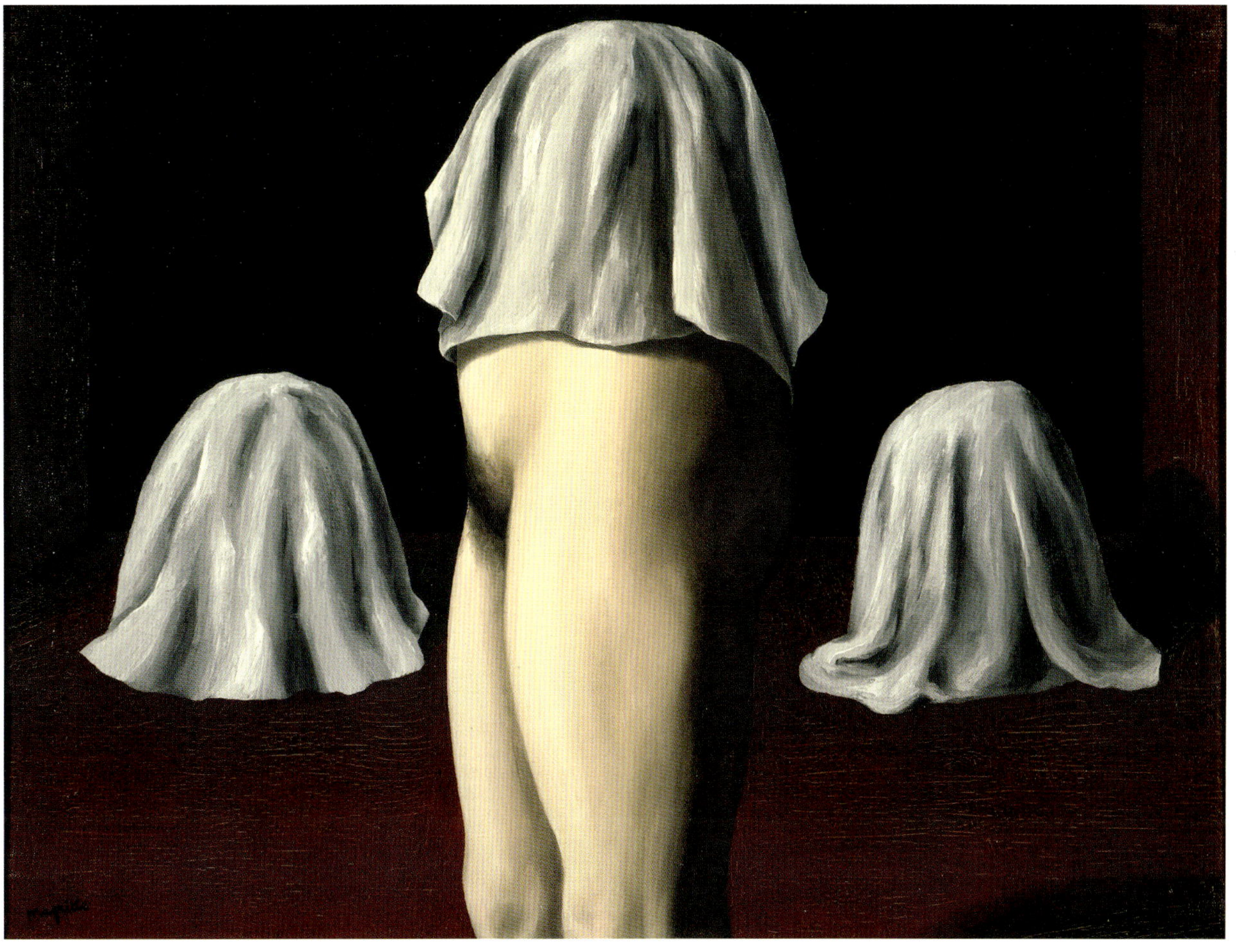

La Ruse symétrique (1928)

however, also employed a third, rather more hidden, way of interfering with the human form. In some works, his distortions are presented as covert machinations, hidden behind shrouds or inside boxes. Some sort of derangement is clearly taking place in these paintings, but its workings are never revealed. Cause and effect remain uncorrelated, just as in a magician's trick, a metaphor that Magritte occasionally evoked directly, as, for example, in *Les Complices du magicien* (1926), which depicts a prestidigitator's performance. The 'trick' involves sliding an assistant through a tightly-fitting tube into a pocket of hanging netting. What is inexplicable is how the assistants are able to enter the tubes with their arms pointing down, as the foreground example shows, and emerge with arms raised. The tortuous switch, as is customary, takes place out of sight and we can never know. Concealment is central to another 'trick' in the aptly-named *La Ruse symétrique* (1928). This time, a shroud thrown over a figure causes the upper body to disappear down to the waist or, in the case of the background forms, to disappear almost completely. At this stage, Magritte has

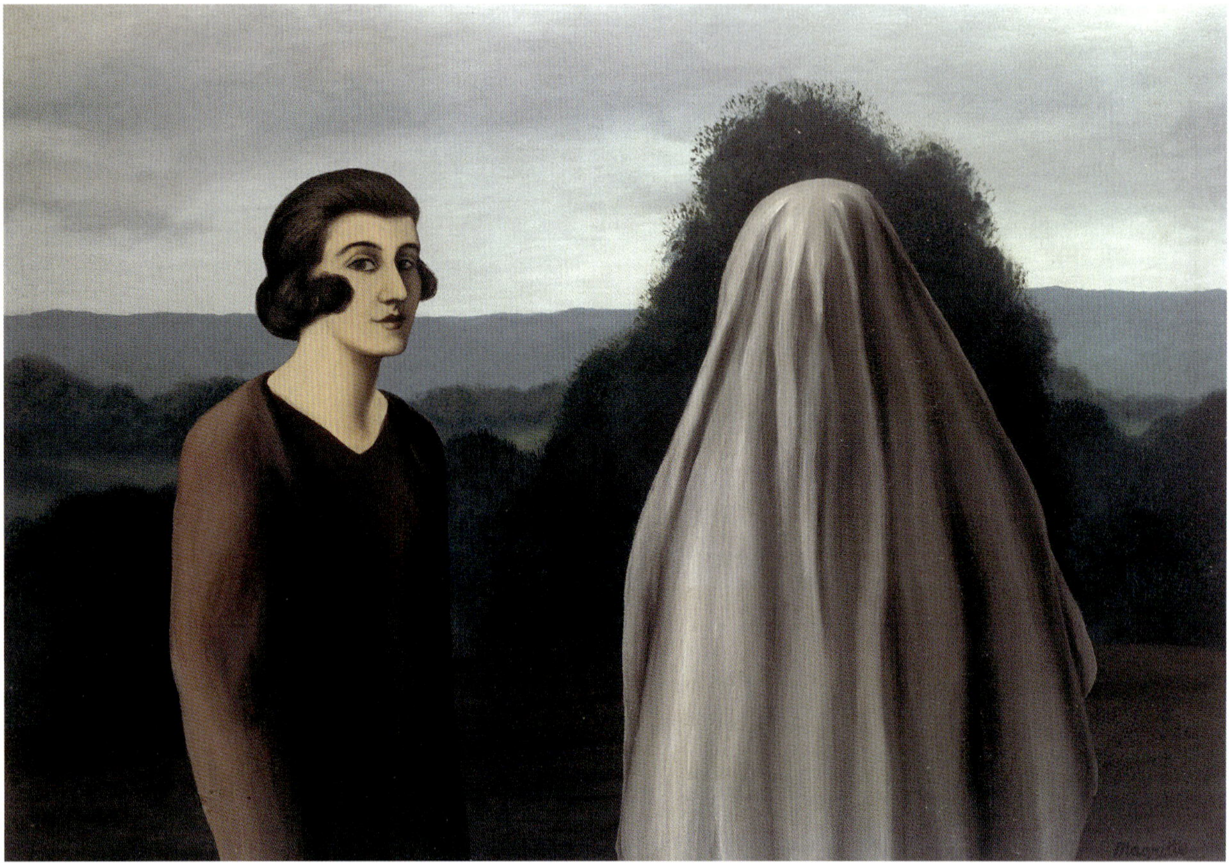

L'Invention de la vie (1928)

not performed the finale of lifting the cloth to reveal thin air. As *L'Invention de la vie* (1928) and *La Gravitation universelle* (1943) suggest, he carries on playing a game of peek-a-boo that hides, enwraps, swallows up and shrinks the body.

---

1 *Variétés*, 2ème année, 5 (15 Sept. 1929): unnumbered plate on the fifth of six pages of illustrations inserted between pages 322 and 323. This post-dates *Les Impatients*, but, given that Magritte was acquainted with the magazine's editor and that he had been a contributor, he may well have had access to the material at the time of the painting. In 'Portraits de Magritte', David Sylvester makes the point that Magritte drew on printed pictures (exhibition catalogue *Rétrospective Magritte*, Palais des Beaux-Arts, Brussels, 1978), pp. 47-76.

2 Leon Battista Alberti, *On Painting, On Sculpture*, trans. Cecil Grayson (London, 1972), pp. 73-5.

3 The idea of pictorially restricting the space a figure can occupy was later exploited by Marcel Mariën in his 'rétrécissements'. He 'shrank' photographs of figures by cutting away parts of the image. The figure is thus forced into a smaller space and acquires new, distorted contours.

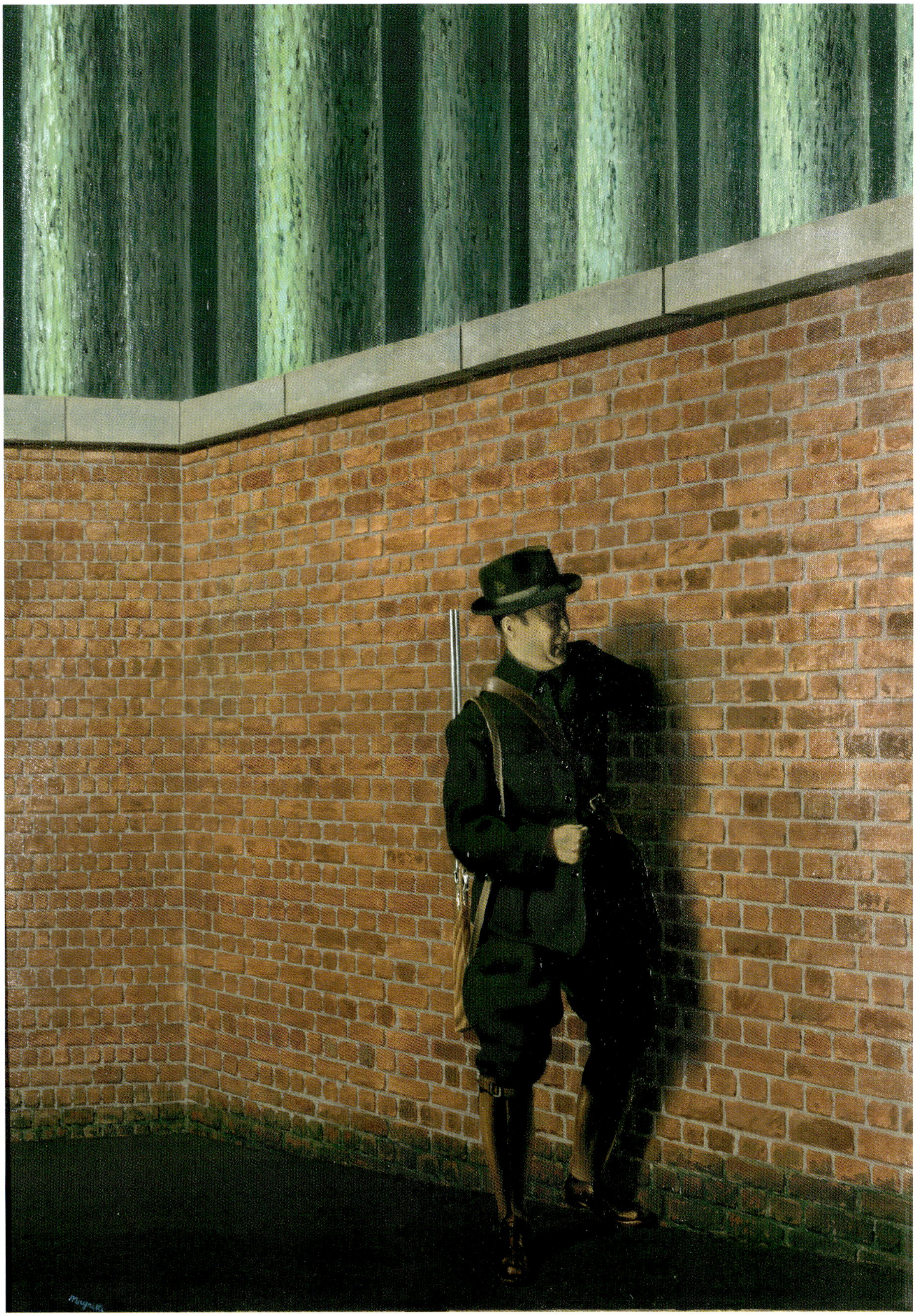

La Gravitation universelle (1943)

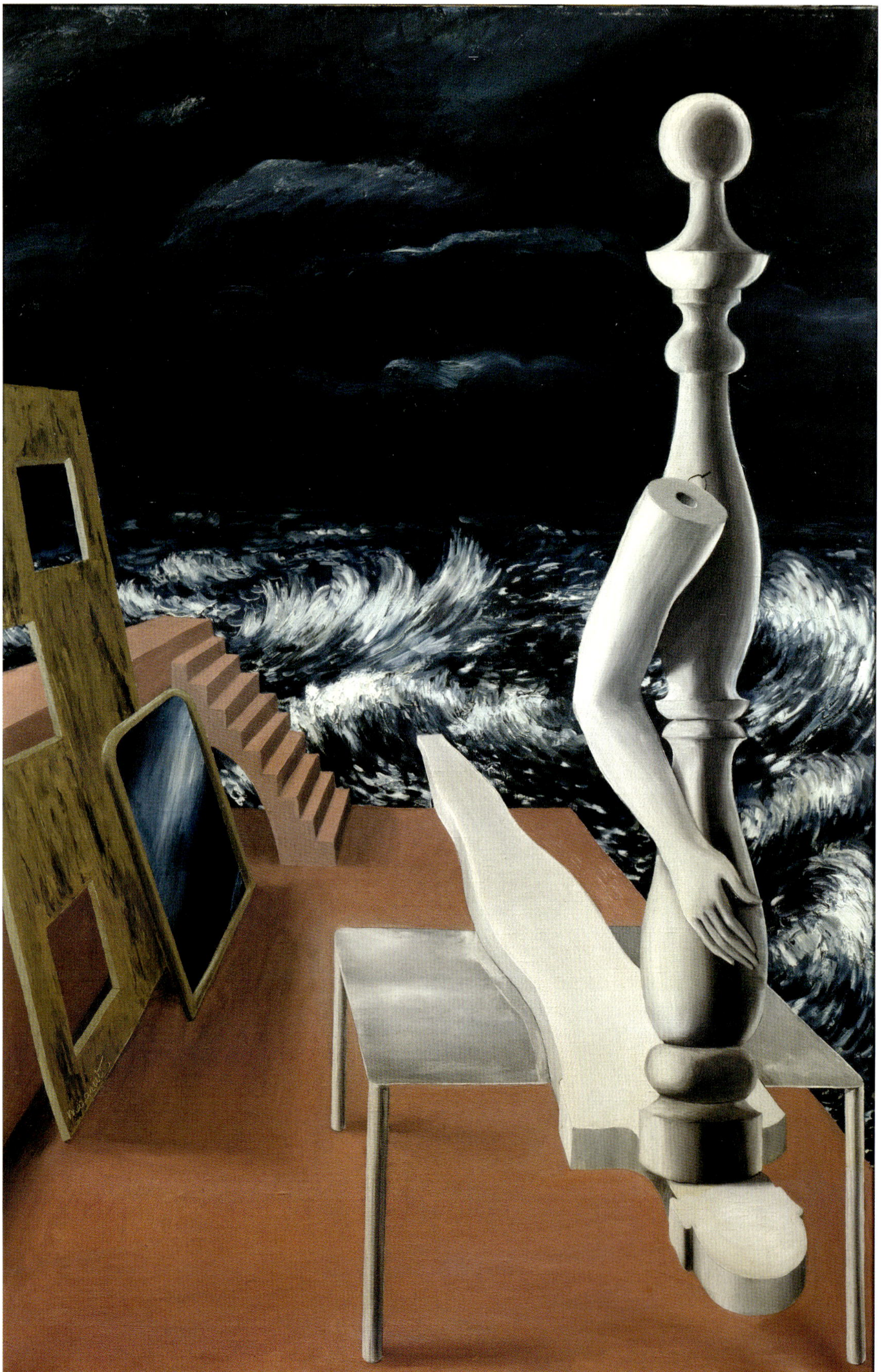

La Naissance de l'idole (1926)

Fragmentation

Having bent, stretched, squashed and concealed the body, Magritte went on to take it to bits. The approach he adopted to this further twist to the dissolution, the *fragmentation* of the human form, was twofold. Firstly, he sectioned it into separate parts and treated the object as a solid entity that could be dismantled, subdivided and broken up. Alternatively, he deconstructed the formal constituents of representation, such as reception of light and circumscription.

In both lines of attack, the focus remains squarely on the female body, which, according to Robert Lebel, lends itself to being 'cut up into pieces'.[1] Indeed, Magritte repeatedly reduced it to its primary components by slicing it up or detaching its limbs. For him, female anatomy became a sum of independent and removable parts. Just like the then novel *assembled* mannequins, with which his commissions for the furrier Samuel had made him familiar, the representational body comes across as a fluid entity, capable of being subdivided.[2] As he would have discovered, the display dummies that he sketched, together with Samuel's fashionable furs, were assemblies of numerous elements: 'an upper half, consisting of the head and waist-length torso [...] a lower half, consisting of the hips and legs [...] two detachable, swivel-jointed arms that hook into the armholes of the bust [...] two detachable, swivel-jointed hands that hook into the wrist holes of the arms [...] a wig made of horsehair'.[3] In other words, mannequins define a sequencing of the body and so, logically, offer a ready-made formula for its *dis*assembly, a fact that had not been lost on Magritte. In a suite of works tellingly executed at the time of his association with Samuel, he started to treat the human form precisely as though it were a dummy and dismembered it accordingly. Time and time again, he harked back to fashion dummies and the ways in which they came apart. *La Naissance de l'idole* (1926), for instance, shows an artificial disjointed arm, complete with the socket hole that would connect into a mannequin's bust. It also depicts a giant skittle balanced on a plank, a motif that had featured in Magritte's contemporaneous fashion illustration for Samuel's 'Matinal' fur coat. Further borrowings from the display dummy turn up in the form of a detached hand in *La Traversée difficile* (1926), a severed head in *La Salle d'armes* (1925-6) and a pair of abandoned wigs in *Le Mariage de minuit*. In every case, Magritte makes the point that these parts have been dismantled, as those of a dummy might be, from a more complete body. Whenever the opportunity arises in his 'mannequin series', Magritte shows the prongs, hooks and sockets that would have linked in with other parts. These interconnections, however, are also shown to be redundant. The rods protruding from a torso in *Le Supplice de la*

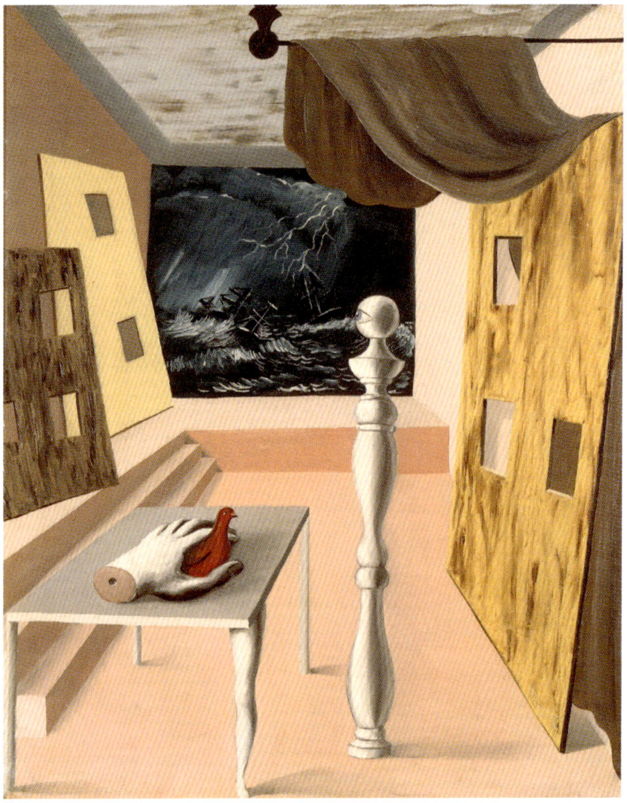

La Traversée difficile (1926)

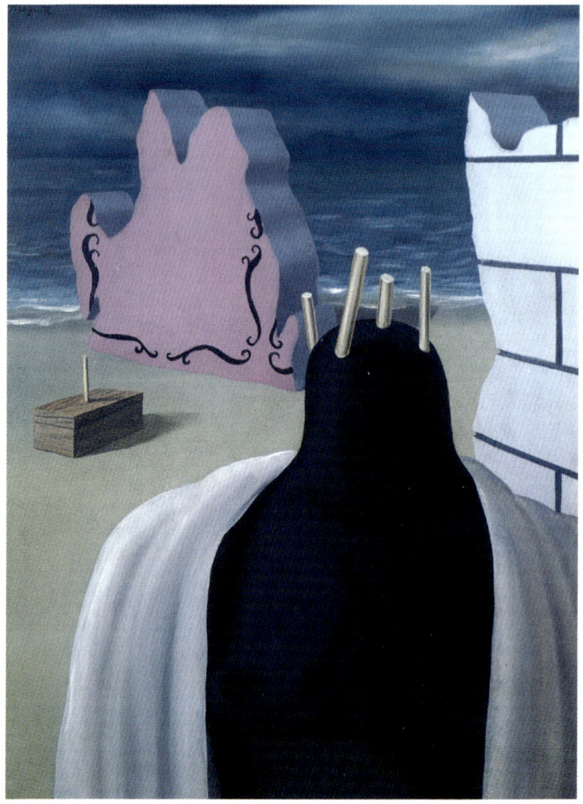

Le Supplice de la vestale (1926-7)

vestale (1926-7), for example, are clearly designed to fix into a head, but this is nowhere to be seen. Similarly, the clumsily inappropriate way in which the arm in *La Naissance de l'idole* hangs on the skittle emphasizes that the limb has been separated from its long-lost torso. Again and again body parts are left starkly disconnected.

As the parts belong to hollow mannequins as opposed to veritable bodies, the dismantling process can only be *anthropometric*. By probing what is no more than an outer shell of the human form, Magritte was obliged to implement his subdivisions longitudinally, along surface contours. Only where there are substrata of flesh and bones can a dissection be truly transversally *anatomical*. *La Lumière du pole* (1927) clearly shows that when the mannequin-figure breaks open there is nothing at all beneath the carapace; internal stratification is, unsurprisingly, wholly absent. Thus, the only path to disassembly open to Magritte was that of segmentation. Indeed, by choosing lifeless dummies as his protagonists he made precisely this point. All that concerned him at this juncture in his anti-academic mission was not so much the defiance of anatomy as a whole, as the sub-discipline of 'dimensio', Alberti's most basic method of analysis. With his irreverent treatment of mannequins, Magritte derided the drawing classes in which the body

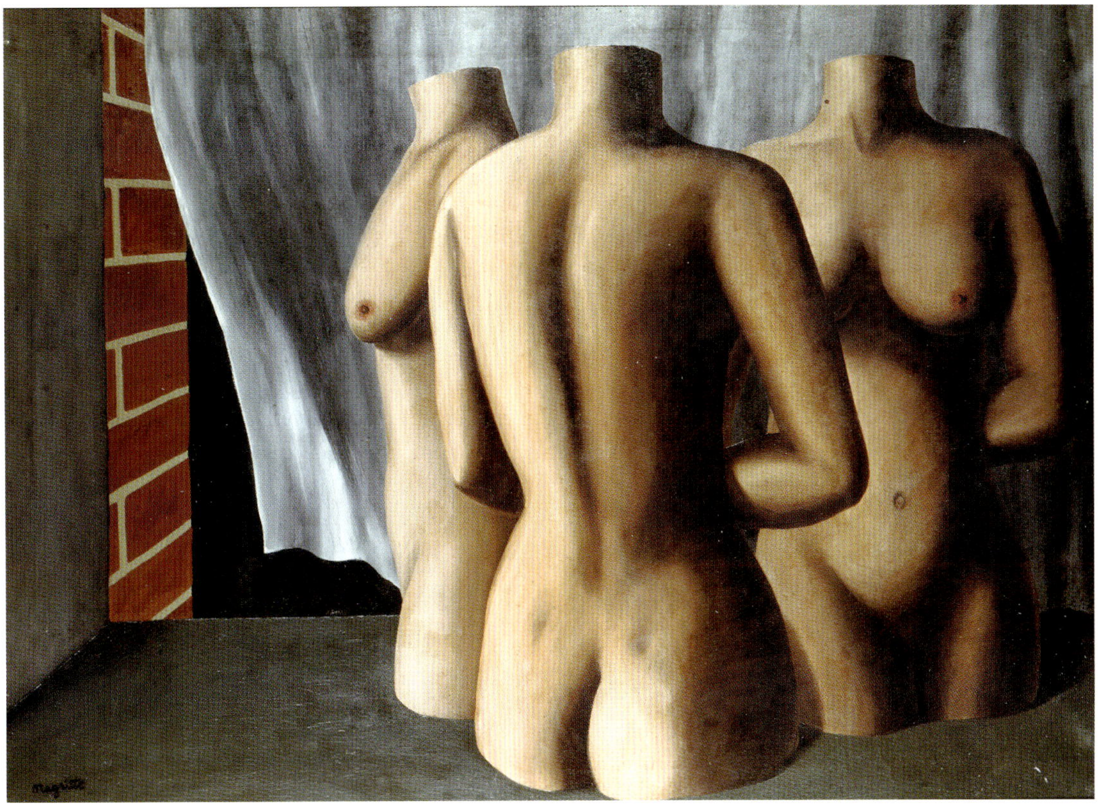

Dialogue dénoué par le vent (1928)

had been measured up and apportioned into prescribed segments, no doubt in accordance with Alberti's explanatory diagrams, which had fastidiously mapped the body to separate zones and stipulated the permitted relationships between them. Indeed, Alberti had insisted not only on the 'observation by sections of the body', but also on a specific 'correspondence of the parts'.[4] Echoes of the exacting discipline endured by Magritte are still felt in the present-day drawing class, which teaches the punctilious distinctions between these same parts.[5] That Magritte's dissolution homed in on this academic segmentation of the body is evident in *Dialogue dénoué par le vent* (1928), in which three torsos are sliced up precisely in accordance with Alberti's prescribed subdivision of the body. Respecting orthodox anthropometry, Magritte sectioned the figures at the measurement points 270 and 520 in Alberti's schema, making cleavages at the bottom of the chin and at the fold of the buttock. It is as though Magritte were re-enacting one of his formal life-sketching classes, albeit mischievously. He even dutifully depicts his model from the three textbook viewpoints, frontal, posterior and lateral, as he might well have been instructed to do at the Academy. Indeed, every aspect of the staging in this painting – the positioning of the subjects in the tightly-knit formation, the implied raised platform that

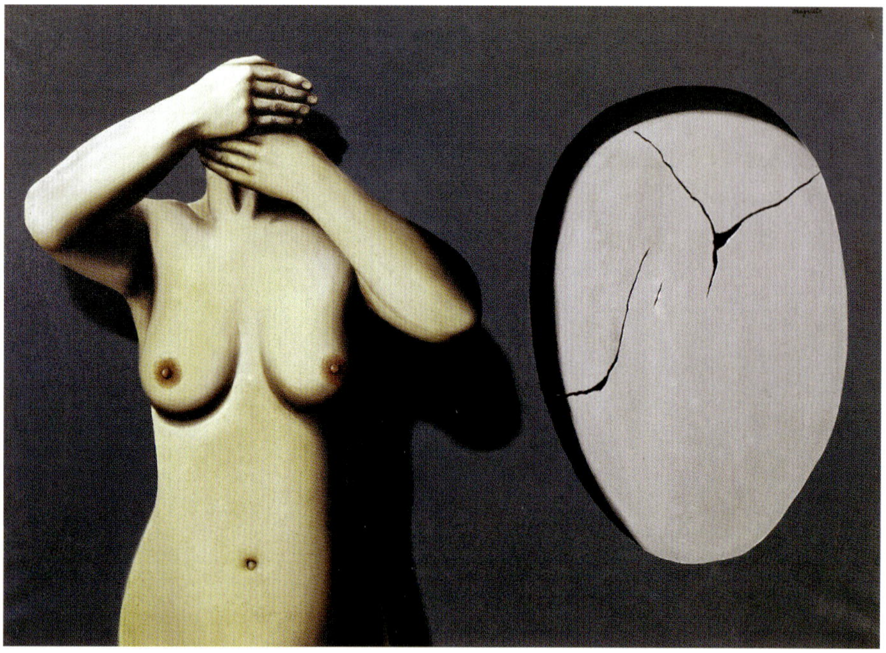

Le Genre nocturne (1928)

puts the figures at eye level, the directional lighting, the plain backdrop – suggests the pedagogical still-life class. But this is not the sole implication of this overly exacting compositional setting. Arguably, it also functions as a pictorial 'control' against which the remainder of the painting's content can be gauged. Given that compositional space is so fully resolved and integral, it acts as a foil to the contrastingly fractured objects contained within it. The finite spatial context, the intelligible pavement, the clearly perpendicular surfaces, the strong shadows, the clarity of distances between objects, the over-simplified, single-point perspective all emphasize just how far anatomical form has been depleted. Had space and relative distance been expressed imprecisely, as in *Les Pipes amoureuses de la lune*, the disassembly of the figures would not have been so marked. It is not so much that space inhibits the human presences, as in *Les Chasseurs au bord de la nuit*, where figures are swallowed up or crushed, but that anatomy is seen to fragment in its own right and not in response to a compositional constraint.

In some cases, this *anatomical* breaking up of the body is in some way concealed from the spectator and only conveyed indirectly. We know that the head of the figure in *Le Genre nocturne* (1928) is absent not because we can see that it is but, given that it is hidden from view, as a result of a series of deductions; only by making a judgement can we conclude that the two hands purporting to mask a head completely do nothing of the sort and that the standing nude is, in fact, headless. More typically, Magritte would use the motif of the wall or the door to divide up the body by means of concealment. The solitary head in *La*

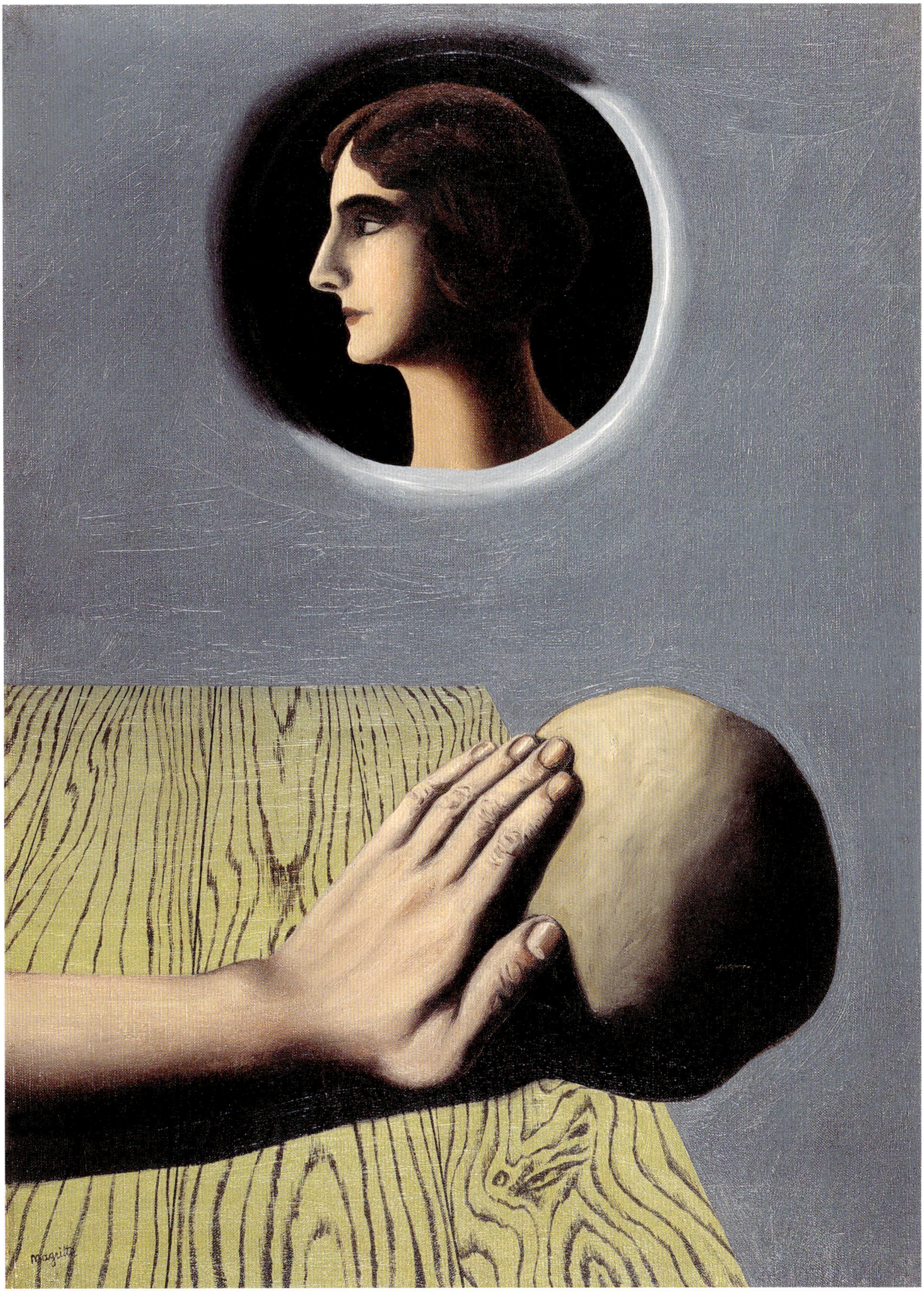

La Promesse salutaire (1927)

Promesse salutaire (1927), for instance, is visible through a hole in a wall that effectively separates it from the displaced hand in the foreground. Similarly, a bodiless head levitates in mid-air behind the barrier of a closed door in *L'Espion* (1927-8). Parts of the body are not only concealed from the spectator by such obstructions, but they are also fenced off from one another. Whereas in paintings like *Les Chasseurs au bord de la nuit* encroaching walls had imposed restrictions on the body's interaction with external space, now they serve as interrupters of its *internal* continuity. They physically apportion members into separate spaces. As *La Confidence capitale* (1928) shows, a wooden partition can act as a disjunction between a torso and its head. The physical obstacle creates two distinct spatial areas, one in front and one behind, that accentuate the segmentation. Even more emphatically than Alberti, who apportioned the drawn figure into zones with horizontal lines, Magritte subdivides and separates his protagonists' body parts into discrete pictorial zones that are delineated by solid palisades.

As well as disjointing a torso at the shoulders and neck, *La Confidence capitale* also erases its features: there are no breasts, waist or umbilicus. More than severing a body, Magritte obliterates its nuances. The torso is present as a mass that occupies space, but it is also devoid of pictorial finiteness. As such, the depleted form acquires an ambivalence that leaves it open to interpretation and allows it to drift from its original semanticity. The female body is diminished here not just by being physically minimized, but also by being diverted towards alternative pictorial meanings. In the later *L'Invention collective* (1935) Magritte was to use this very configuration to dispense with human anatomy altogether and, instead, piece together a neological fish-woman. Even a *partial* fragmentation of the body can, as Magritte shows, fundamentally compromise anatomy. The ambiguous shape in *La Confidence capitale* can just as easily be resolved into a fish as into a human torso. Anatomical segmentation reaches a point, therefore, at which identity itself is compromised. The dismantling of objects, it would appear, goes hand in hand with an attenuation of finite pictorial meaning since it severs the one-to-one relation between symbolic form and what it signifies. 'Everything leads us to think', Magritte stated, 'that there is little relation between an object and what it represents.'[6]

La Confidence capitale, however, expresses a potential rather than a realized semantic deflection. Despite being divested of its innate meaning, the 'torso' is not assigned an alternative role. It is only in *Entracte* (1927-8) that Magritte took this further step in his disruption of the pictorial object. As in *La Confidence capitale* and *Dialogue dénoué par le vent*, he depicts isolated body parts, but this time these have alternative functions. 'Limbs', according to Roger Manvell, 'become entities of their own, or thighs combine with arms in their own living choreography.'[7] As opposed to simply being segregated,

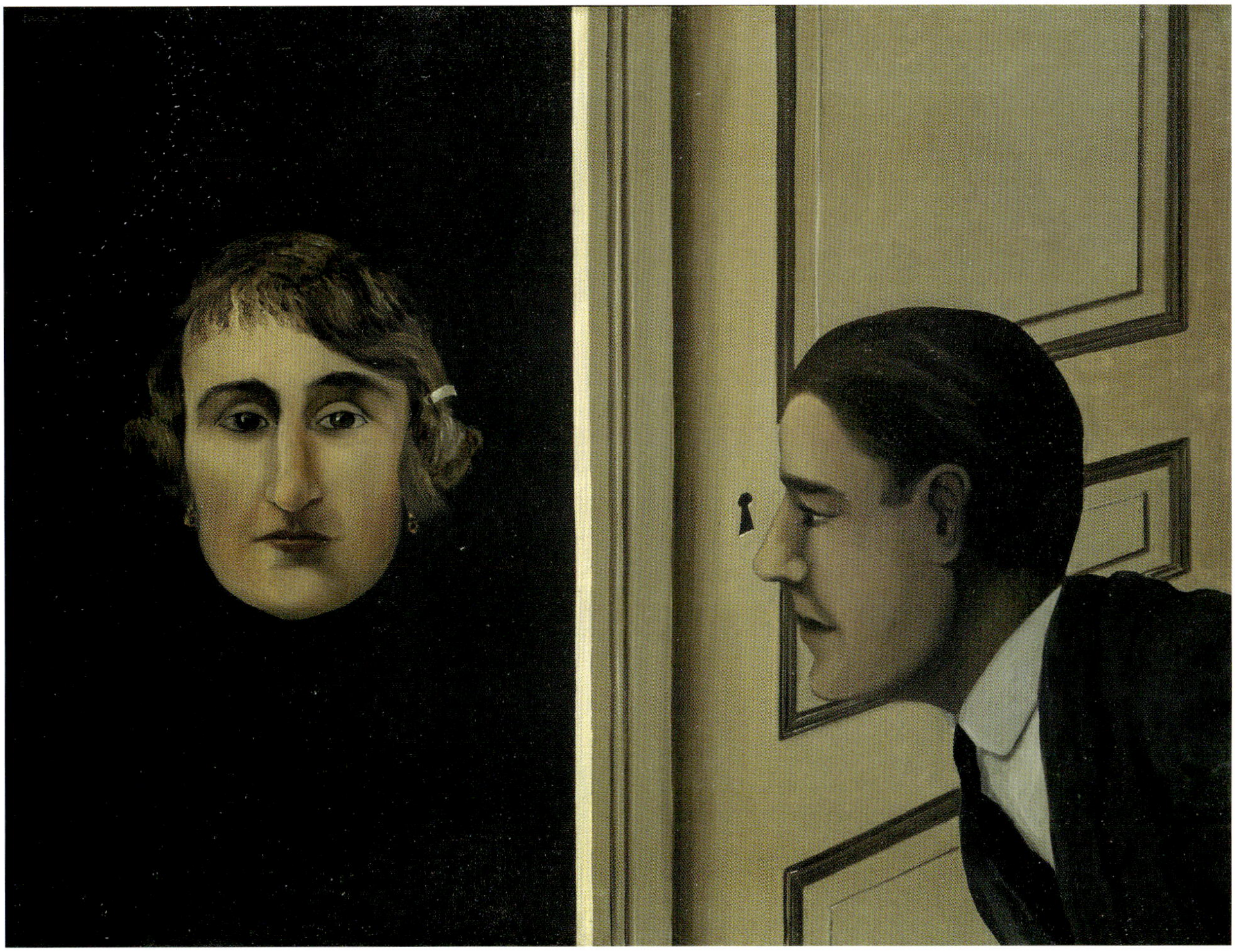

L'Espion (1927-8)

arms and legs are reutilized in novel corporeal arrangements. What Magritte does here is to delete the section of the body between Alberti's measurements 270 and 440 and fuse the remaining members, with the result that knee joints operate as waists, legs take on the role of rudimentary torsos and an arm is joined to a thigh, which simultaneously acts as shoulder and buttock. Magritte instigates an endless game of displacement, which, incidentally, was later to be taken up by Hans Bellmer, who saw the process as 'the synthesis of two images simultaneously revised'.[8] For Bellmer, as for Magritte, it was a question of reallocating meaning:

> The 'sex-armpit' analogy is established, the two images intermingle their content by superimposing themselves on each other, the sex on the armpit, the leg naturally on the arm, the foot on the hand, the toes on the fingers. What results is a bizarre fusion of the 'real' and of the 'virtual', of the 'permitted' and of the 'forbidden', composites in which one vaguely acquires presence in proportion to what the other gives up.

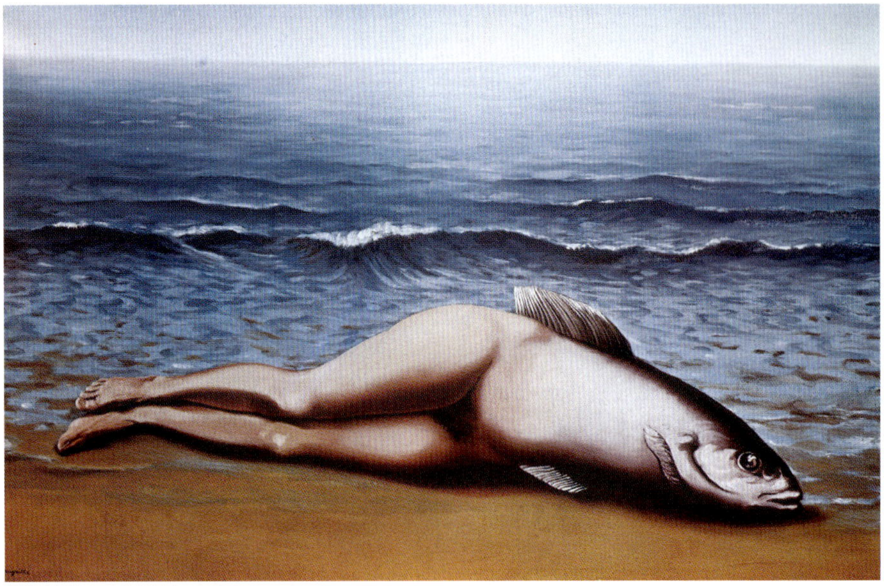

L'Invention collective (1935)

It is precisely this notion of bringing together and superimposing spatially separate parts of the body that operates in *Entracte*, as well as in the later *Le Viol* (1934), which enacts 'the oppositional affinity [...] of the mouth and the sex' that Bellmer would describe. Such pictorial simultaneity brings about semantic duality. Just like words, unbridled anatomical members acquire an interpretative fluctuation that leads to semantic flux. As Bellmer continues in terms that parallel Alberti's insistence on the comparability of the elements of representation and those of language, 'the body can be compared to a sentence which invites us to disarticulate it so that it can recompose itself, by means of an endless series of anagrams'. Once the unit form is fragmented in Magritte's paintings, fixed pictorial meaning is lost and replaced only by unstable signification.

✣ ✣ ✣

Besides analyzing the body in terms of its external components, Alberti had also remarked that 'it would [...] be extremely valuable to know the number of bones and the projections of muscles and sinews'.[9] This alternative approach, which centres on anatomy in its stricter sense, as opposed to anthropometry, is the basis of Magritte's second method of shattering the body. At times, he would depart from treating the object as a series of outer contours and superficial features, which he had already successfully cut up or effaced, as in *La Confidence capitale*, in order to turn his attention to *internal* composition. He would delve below surface form to show that objects had concurrent structural

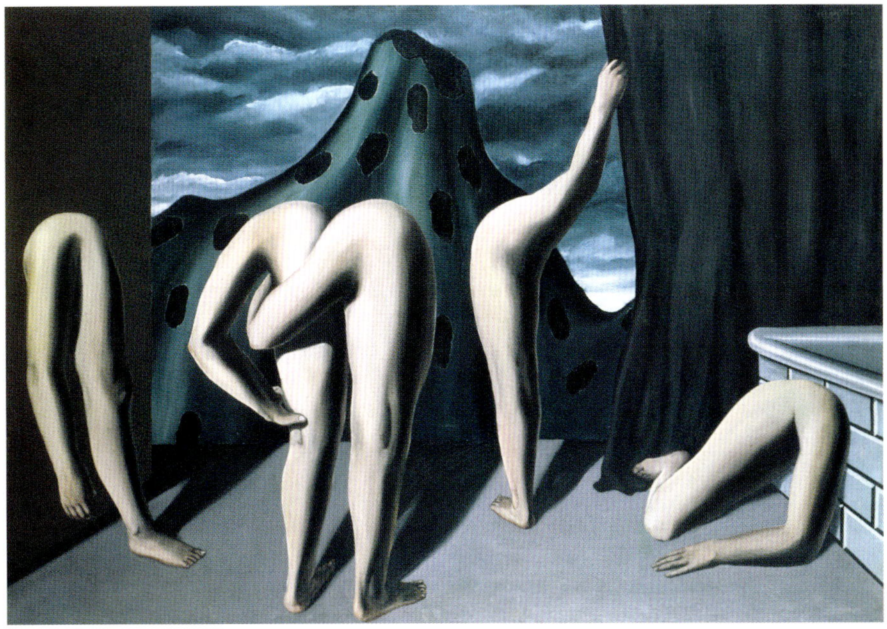

Entracte (1927-8)

layers that could be penetrated and manipulated. As Passeron puts it, 'it is not so much that the painting is made in layers as the fact that the pictorial image is stratified'.[10] The course of Magritte's fragmentation therefore progressed from an essentially linear breaking up of the body to what could be described as a transversal subdivision. What now emerges, to use Foucault's words, is 'the internal relationship of subordination or of organization [...] that traverses the thickness of the body'. The breakdown of form, in other words, begins to operate on the substrata of anatomy.[11]

The transition from a dissolution that targets the *concatenation* between anatomical members to one in which the body is disassembled into concurrent *layers* occurs most strikingly in *L'Importance des merveilles* (1927). This work contains both segmentation and stratification. The female body is, once again, sliced horizontally, with divisions made at the groin, the waist, the neck and the shoulders, very much in line with Alberti's prescribed apportionment. Rather than being dispersed into autonomous units, however, the parts are retained within their original sequencing and distanced solely through differences in scale. They become smaller in stages and appear to fit into one another so that the groin section contains the abdomen, the abdomen houses the thorax and the thorax accommodates the head and arms. What this means is that a purely sectional division, by virtue of being accompanied by a series of progressive modifications in size, has also resulted in the creation of interdependent strata. As with a Russian doll, there are divisions along the cross-section, but also there are structural tiers enveloped within one another that give a sense of *interiority*.

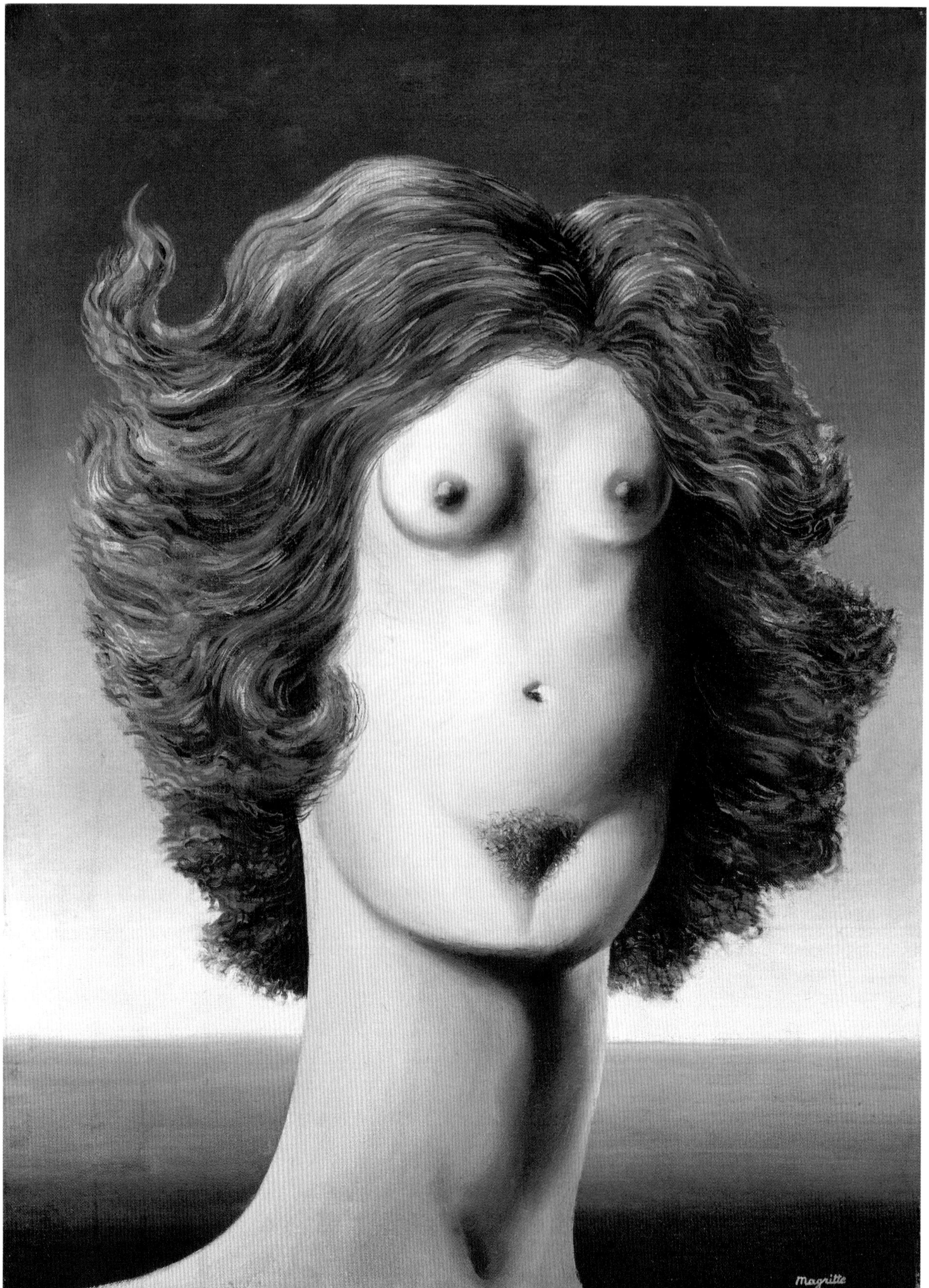

Le Viol (1934)

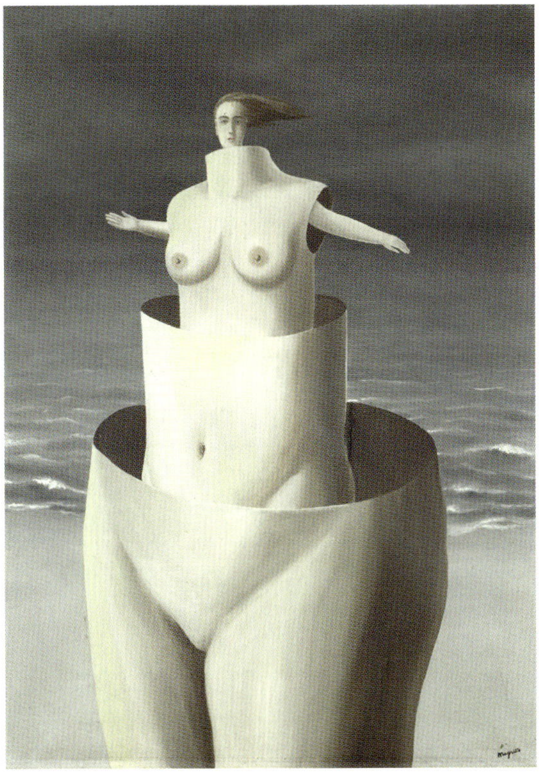

L'Importance des merveilles (1927)

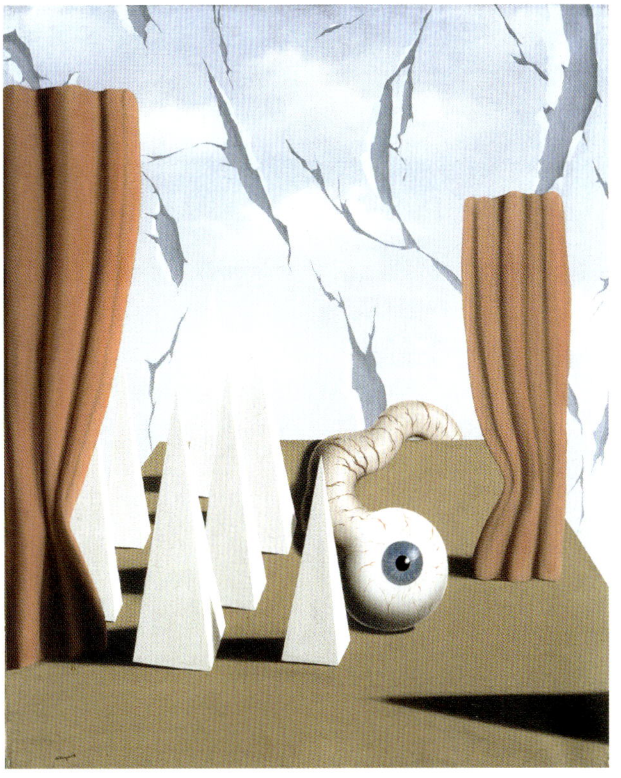

Le Monde poétique (1926)

The former, strictly linear, notion of sub-divisibility is extended to incorporate differentiation between overlapping or overlaid gradations. Thus, whilst being firmly rooted in segmentation and in no way depicting the interior construction of the body, the painting does point Magritte's fragmentation in the direction of *stratification*.

A painting that does commit to this idea of *penetration* of the layers of the body is *Le Sang du monde*. Whilst the three partially visible bodies it depicts are not 'segmented' sensu stricto and retain their normal external contours, Magritte does take them apart in a different way, by removing their epidermal layer. The fleshy tones he had used in *Dialogue dénoué par le vent* are replaced here by the starkness of skinned forms that expose the network of blood vessels and arteries under the surface. As in de Chirico's *The Scholar's Playthings*, we are presented with écorché representations of the human form. As though to emphasize that he is taking us into an interior world, Magritte depicts an entire complex of magnified blood vessels, lymph cells and deep tissue. He delves beyond what is superficial and immediately visible into the inner fabric and substrata of the body.

In *Le Monde poétique* (1926) the concept of corporeal ingress is presented in a more targeted manner; the body, it would appear, has been penetrated at a single point, the eye socket, to reveal a disembodied eye, complete with a worm-like, distended optic nerve. Whether or not there is allusion to a cerebral

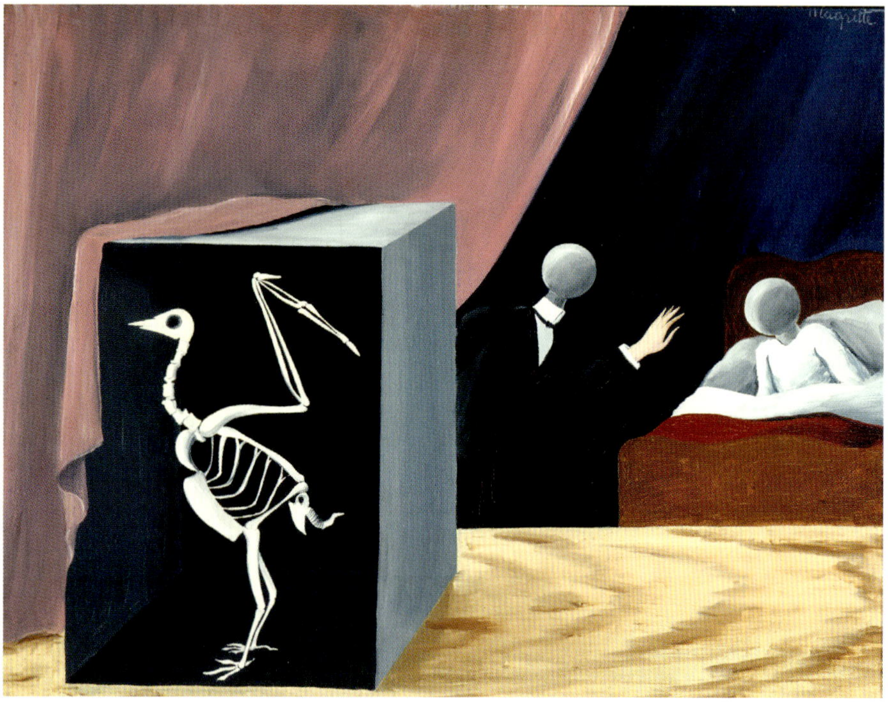

La Grande Nouvelle (1926)

cross-section drawn from inside the skull is open to debate, but certainly the painting implies a fathoming of the body, just as in *Le Double Secret* (1927), where it is prized open or *La Grande Nouvelle* (1926), in which the skeleton is laid bare. As Scutenaire put it, Magritte went 'under the crust of objects'.[12] In a general sense too, the idea of penetrating depth is echoed by the overall composition of *Le Monde poétique*, which incorporates a sharp perspective reinforced by rows of pyramids receding along the orthogonals. Even the horizon does not cut short this sense of permeation, since the distant sky cracks open to reveal an impossible dimension beyond. It is as though matter itself were being burrowed into.

✣ ✣ ✣

Implicit throughout the process of fragmentation is that the body is analyzed through an itemization of its parts. As though inventorying a set of inanimate components, Magritte isolated portions of the human form, which, like Picabia, he treated as the removable and interchangeable parts of a machine.[13] In a recurrent sexual-mechanical analogy, Picabia derided human anatomy, equating corporeal functions with the workings of machines. As in Magritte's work, the body became an assemblage of distinct parts that were shown as capable of

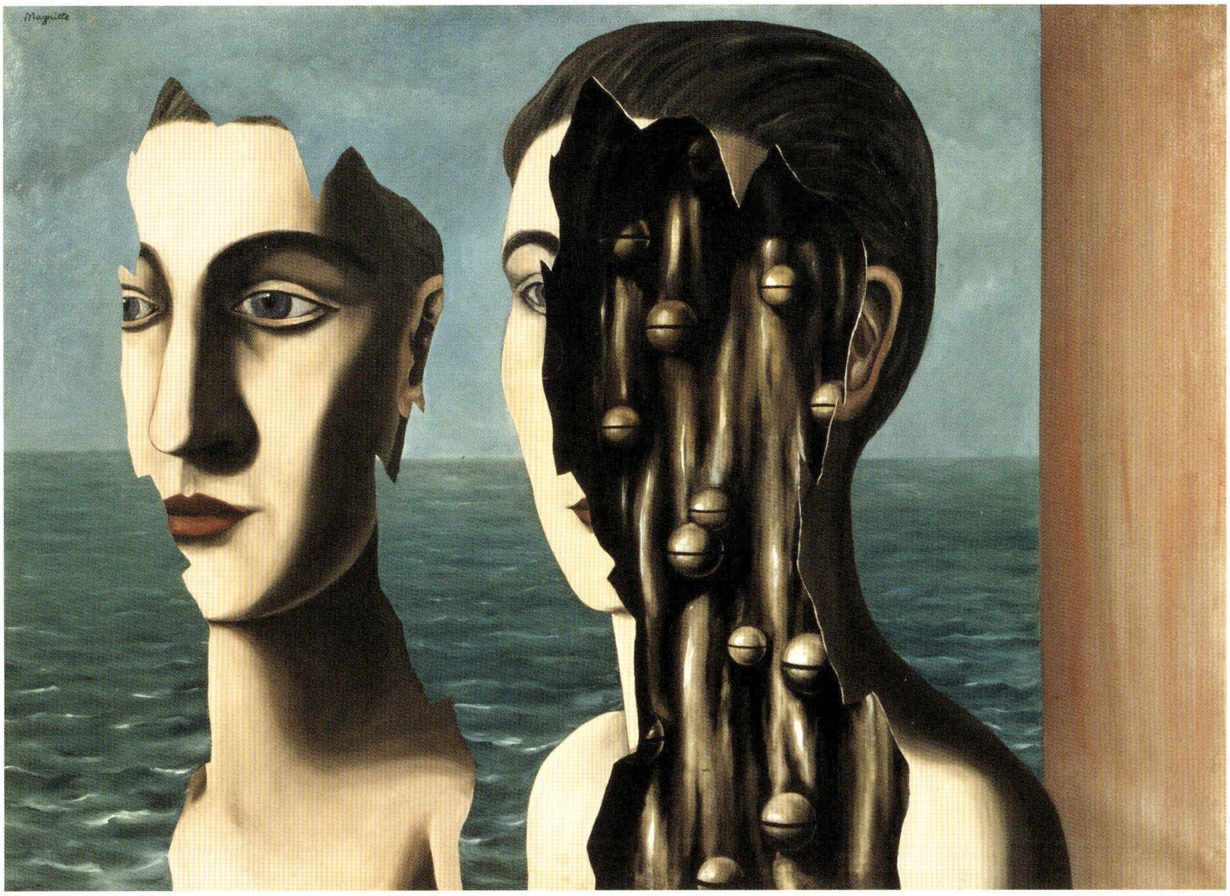

Le Double Secret (1927)

being *dismantled*. Picabia's *Parade amoureuse* (1917), for instance, shows the body-machine as comprising separated and separable components; the depicted fork-like shape could, clearly, be seen as detachable from the two cylinders into which it is inserted. Picabia was also at pains to show how the components of his pseudo-machine 'fitted together'; he painted the screw heads, nuts, rivets, hinges and screw threads that showed not only how the parts of his assemblages could be secured together, but also how they could be *taken apart*.

That Magritte went on to adopt his fellow Dadaist's conceit is apparent in *Vous ne saurez jamais*, in which an anthropomorphic skittle is shown to contain an array of internal pistons and levers that, just like the mechanical parts in *Parade amoureuse*, are interlinked by pivots, springs and screws. Indeed, Passeron commented that it was 'with Picabia's machines [that] he discovers this sense of mechanical interconnectedness'.[14] The body-machine analogy is even more explicit in *L'Âge des merveilles* (1926), where it is a human figure, as opposed to an allusion to it, that is seen to be animated by internal machine parts. In the manner of a 'cut-away' anatomical model, the lower abdomen of a nude is opened up to show the wheels and pistons that turn beneath its outer shell. Similarly, each of its legs is shown to be internally attached to the trunk by solid rods geared to a series of wheels and cogs. What is implied is that the body is merely mechanistic.

That is not to say, however, that Magritte's 'mechanized' bodies do not work. On the contrary, his contraptions stand in sharp contrast to Picabia's inoperable machinery. The latter's title page illustration for number 4/5 of *Dada* (1919) was composed of the parts of a *broken* watch and *Parade amoureuse* was not so much a real machine as an awkward amalgam of unrelated and un-relatable mechanical fragments. Conversely, the wheels and cogs depicted by Magritte in *L'Âge des merveilles* do propose a remotely conceivable form of functioning operability. Unlike those of Picabia, these particular clockwork components *do* interlock to form a coherent arrangement of turning wheels and moving rods and the female figure, could, by a stretch of the imagination, be regarded as an operable mechanism. Similarly, in *Vous ne saurez jamais* there is an implication of a plausible sequential interaction between the various parts, which, being numbered, suggest an underlying rationale. What distinguishes Magritte and Picabia's portrayal of the machine is that, whilst the former preserves a sense of functionality, the latter is at pains to negate the notion of a credible mechanism. Picabia's mechanisms simply do not work. His analogy between the body and the machine is a contradiction in terms. It is a negation. By being likened to his brand of 'machine', the body is depreciated and effaced. Magritte, on the other hand, painted quasi-credible mechanisms and when he used the machine analogy it was to emphasise the *workable* concatenations and interdependencies within the body. For Magritte, the body was like a machine in that it was a complex of interconnected and coherently organized constituent parts. Therefore, when he went on to disassemble it he did so in a way that acknowledged its inherent structures, both in terms of anatomy and pictorial construction. Far from being arbitrary or capricious, Magritte's step-by-step fragmentation of the human form was a direct riposte to the logic with which it had been rationalised.

---

1 Robert Lebel, 'Avant et après Magritte', *L'Œil*, 159 (Mar. 1968): 34.
2 Photographs of this type of mannequin appeared in *Variétés*, 8 (15 Dec. 1929): 670, 722.
3 Lester Gaba, *The Art of Window Display* (New York & London, 1952), p. 50.
4 Leon Battista Alberti, *On Painting, On Sculpture*, trans. Cecil Grayson (London, 1972), p. 137.
5 John Barrington, *Anthropometry and Anatomy* (London, 1963), p. 42.
6 René Magritte, *Écrits complets* (Paris, 1979), p. 60.
7 Roger Manvell, 'Magritte and the Surrealist Image', *Humanist*, 84 (June 1969): 179.
8 Hans Bellmer, *Petite Anatomie de l'inconscient physique ou l'anatomie de l'image* (Paris, 1957), n. pag. Subsequent references to Bellmer relate to this text.

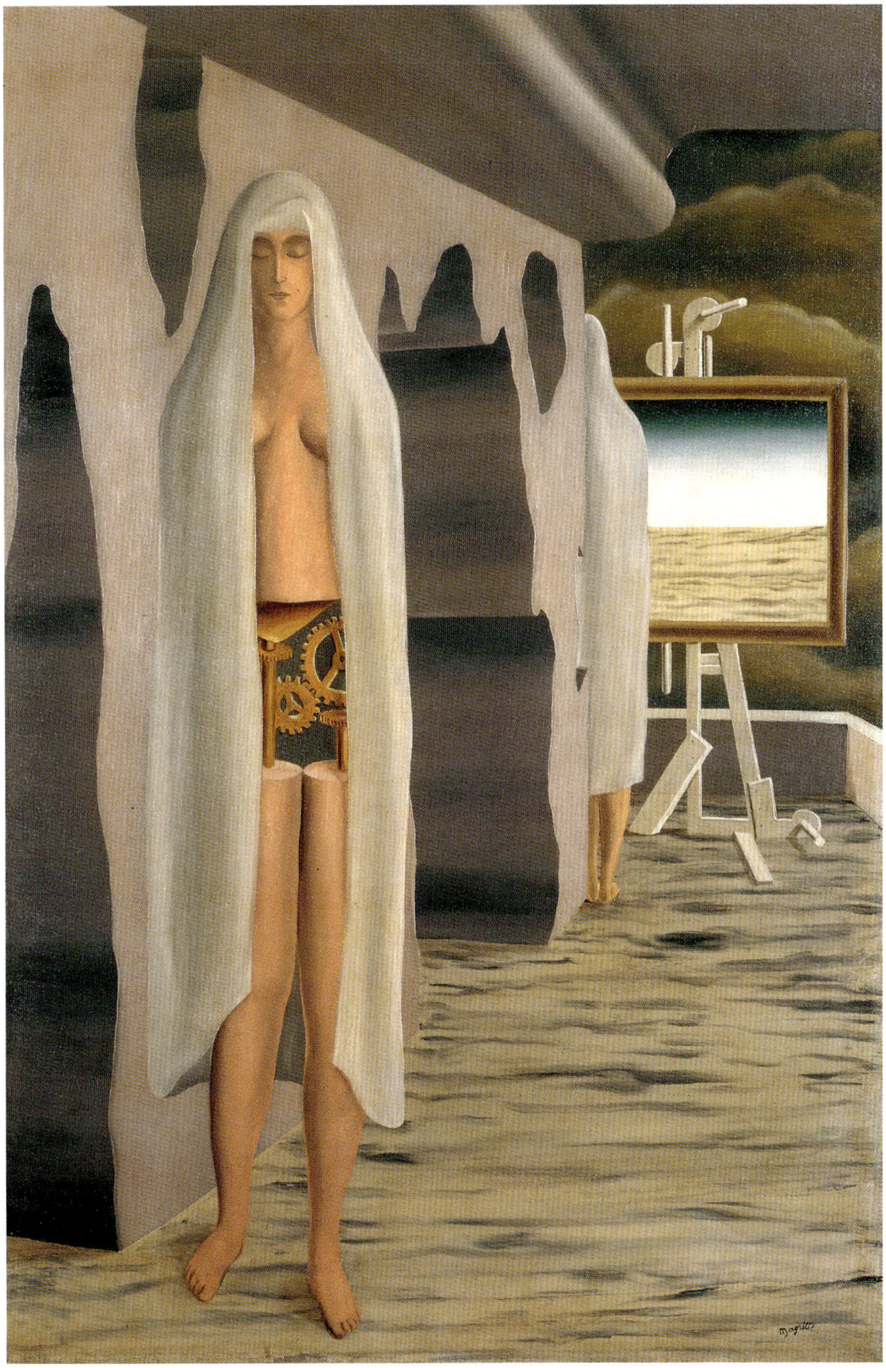

L'Âge des merveilles (1926)

[9] Alberti, *On Painting, On Sculpture*, p. 139.
[10] René Passeron, *René Magritte* (Paris, 1972), p. 74.
[11] Michel Foucault, *Les Mots et les choses* (Paris, 1966), p. 149.
[12] Louis Scutenaire, *Avec Magritte* (Brussels, 1977), p. 139.
[13] According to Pierre-Louis Flouquet in his article 'Servranckx, cet inconnu', the machine form was the central feature of Servranckx's art: 'He had formed a specific vision in which mechanical movements and vast coloured surfaces combined in an original way', *Fantasmagie*, 22 (Mar. 1966): 22.
[14] Passeron, *René Magritte*, p. 37.

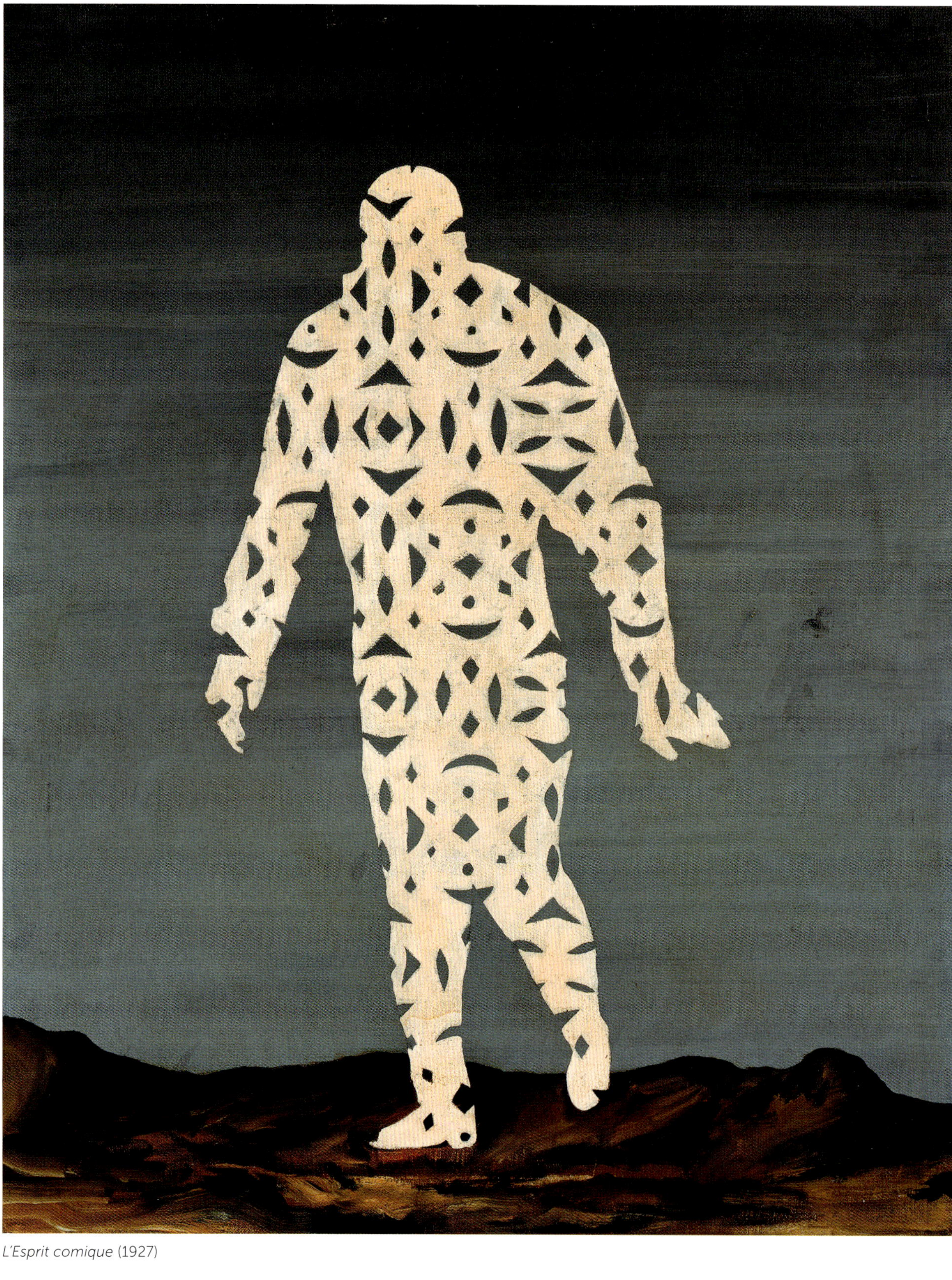

L'Esprit comique (1927)

Pictorial Primaries

With his assaults on anthropometry and anatomy Magritte effectively reduces the pictorial unit of the body into its constituent members. According to Alberti, however, the members themselves are composed of still smaller elements that he called 'planes'. These purely formal aspects of representation are precisely what the next development of Magritte's anti-painting proceeded to confront. He moved from representing dismantled objects to dismantling the methods of depiction themselves. As Mariën put it, there is a 'reduction of the means of expression'.[1] In a more radical diminution of the portrayal of the object, Magritte now leaves behind the concept of solid form and pares down anatomy through a systematic effacement of its formalistic rudiments. The technical 'stages' that Alberti had set out as essential for the attainment of a faithfully represented figure were not just contravened by Magritte; they were progressively reversed and, eventually, deactivated.

The process begins where Alberti had ended, at the concluding stage of the pictorial construction of the figure, the 'reception of light'. This phase of Magritte's deconstruction counters light and shade, colour and surface form. Essentially, it reduces the three-dimensional to the two-dimensional, the solid to the planar. The figure in *Le Chevalier du couchant*, for instance, is deprived of volume and ends up 'flattened'. We see a featureless head, the details of which have been squashed into a uniform plane surface. All that remain are the peripheral forms, delineating the cranium, the jaws and the ears. The representational content of this 'member' is thus reduced to two dimensions; Magritte regresses the figure to the constructional stage that precedes the 'reception of light', before three dimensions are defined. Whilst form is present as surface, surface nuance is absent.

This reduction of the corporeal form to the planar is more emphatic in *La Naissance de l'idole*, where it is not only the head but the body in its entirety that is deprived of volume. What is more evident here is that the recession to this stage entails a wholesale denudation of the pictorial unit, in which almost every detail of the body disappears; what is left is an armless trunk, a waist that is only hinted at, and lower limbs in the form of a single elongated stump. The form is little more than a flat plank and, as though to make this very point, it functions as a quasi-diving board, on which another figure stands. With his tenuous suggestion of a body, Magritte winds back the clock to an incipient stage of the representational procedure. As he would have been well aware, he was reverting to a more elementary stage in a process that he himself had described in terms of a progression:

> The linear representation made by the caveman was followed by an equivalent and increasingly perfected representation that set out to fill the silhouette of a body with the voluminous appearance of this body.[2]

What occurs in *La Naissance de l'idole* is the converse; far from advancing towards a 'perfected' depiction, Magritte purges the body of its 'voluminous appearance', taking it back to its more elementary 'linear' pictorial status.

Yet, even though forms may be divested of their surface features, they still retain a sense of palpable substantiality. They remain tangible and ponderous. Magritte's regression to 'the silhouette of a body', by which his representations were to forfeit all reference to voluminosity, was not to occur until the year after *La Naissance de l'idole* and *Le Chevalier du couchant*. It was in 1927 that Magritte was to make the transition from the 'solid' plane to one that was, to all effects, insubstantial. What marked this momentous conceptual shift was the unexpected appearance of the device of the 'paper cut-out' in Magritte's work. Compositional figures, situated within unexceptional but, nevertheless, coherent spatial settings, would incongruously and inexplicably be depicted as shapes made from perforated, paper-thin sheets. Magritte described these as 'masked paper'. As he explained, his innovative figures were 'made of paper in which differing geometric shapes have been cut in a regular pattern'.[3] More significant, however, is that this departure from customary pictorial methodology not only goes against Alberti's anatomical construct, but also reverses it. The figure in the oil version of *L'Esprit comique*, for instance, is presented in such a way that it contradicts its own semantic properties; a flimsy blank sheet of paper punched with holes across its entire surface could not be more incompatible with the broad-shouldered hulk of a man implied by the contours of the form. The figure stands as an unambiguous and dominant form within the structure of the painting, casting a strong shadow on the ground and unequivocally assuming the role of subject of the work. Yet, the very substance from which this stalwart silhouette is crafted remains, in effect, the epitome of fragility; it is devoid of thickness, rigidity and weight. It is as though the figure had been 'emptied' of its pictorial resolution by an erasure of the 'stages' by which a painted figure achieves form and substance. There is a regression towards the blank sheet of paper from which the figure would have emerged. Magritte did not stop there, however, and carried on with his erosion of the pictorial figure by depleting the paper support itself through his incisions.

The incompatibility between the pictorial narrative and the physical materiality of its protagonists is particularly marked in the gouache of *L'Esprit comique*, painted in the same year as the version in oil. Again, the figures are rendered in the same 'thin and transparent' sheeting, but the drama in which they are involved in this case makes the notion of anatomical enfeeblement all the more paradoxical.[4] As the paper cut-outs are not just shown in static poses

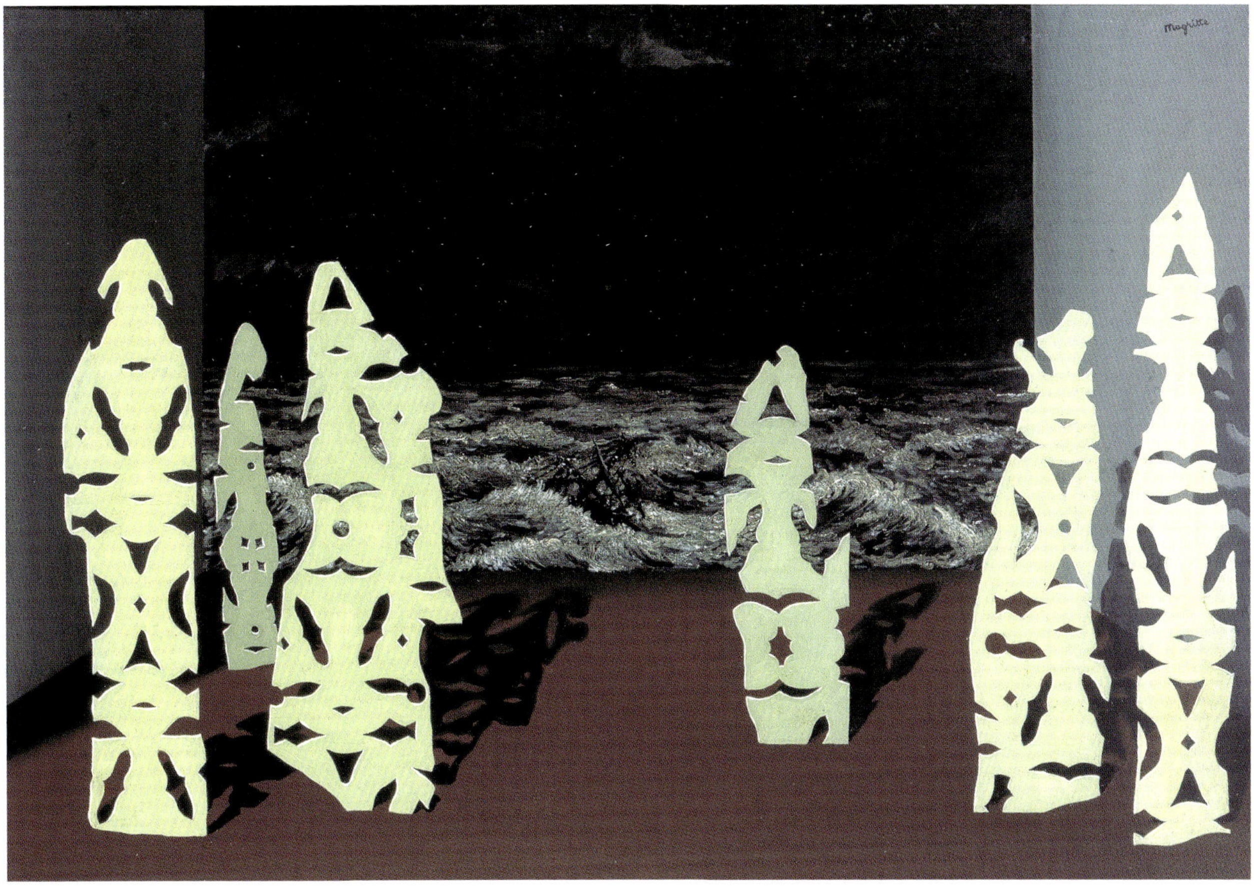

La Parure de l'orage (1928)

but, rather, as part of a dynamic and, indeed, violent drama, the insubstantiality of their make-up strikes us as contradictory. Whilst we are shown a juvenile who has picked up a heavy stone with which to strike a sleeping man, the idea that a delicate piece of paper could support the weight of stone, let alone deal a blow with it, is a nonsense. What this paradox shows is the extent to which Magritte had, by this stage in his dissolution, eroded and invalidated pictorial semanticity. Forms may still be vaguely recognizable, but they have become representationally redundant and inoperative.

The erosion of signification is carried still further, however, when even this last vestige of identity is effaced. In *La Parure de l'orage* (1928) a counterbalancing intensification of pictorial grammar accompanies the loss of the scant meaningful traces that had remained in the contours of the silhouettes in *L'Esprit comique*. In a further progression of the dissolution, the minimalistic outline of the human form is itself lost and all that is left behind are quasi-figures whose only corporeal attribute is uprightness. The pictorial subjects are depleted in the extreme and all that can be read in this painting is a complex of interconnectedness. There are no protagonists, but simply differentiated 'roles'; half a dozen non-referential paper cut-outs simply occupy various positions on a flat ground,

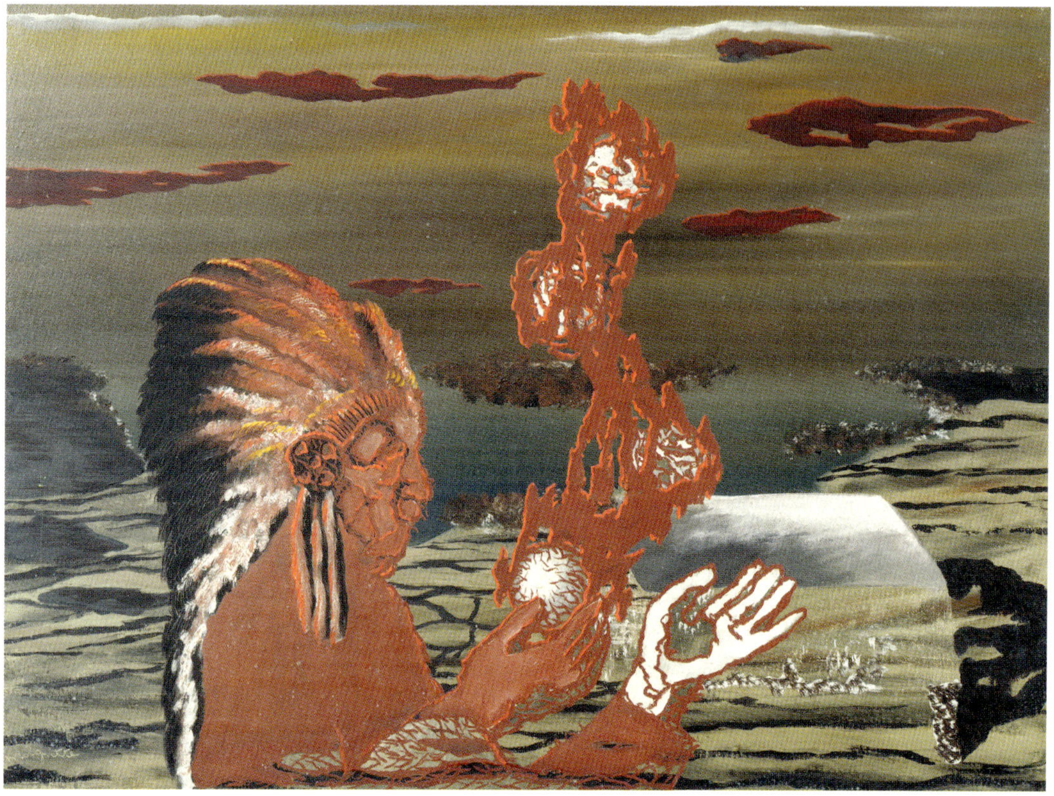

L'Âge du feu (1927)

like actors on a stage, engaged in some sort of complex performance. Some are slightly inclined, as though beckoning for attention or addressing an audience. Others are gestureless and passive. One figure lurks in the background near the wings, waiting to make an entrance, whilst another hovers in the middle distance with an air of indecision or stupefaction. Magritte stages a whole drama, but in so doing he only too clearly emphasizes that his performers have been semantically expunged. It is as though he were painting pure composition, uncluttered by anatomy. As he demonstrates, the more his flat phantoms tend towards insubstantiality, the more finite and cogent the compositional framework can become. Flying in the face of the Albertian construct, Magritte mischievously conjures up an *inverse* relationship between content and context. By intensifying the compositional ties within the painting he is able to construct a coherent work, populated by no more than the 'planes' that Alberti had described.

Notwithstanding, the progressive dismantling of the pictorial object has yet more levels to which it can be taken. The very first 'element' that Alberti had defined was the 'line' itself and it is on this incipient stage of representational methodology that Magritte's dissolution eventually set its sights. This level of the 'pictorial linear' is precisely what is focused upon in *L'Âge du feu* (1927), where lines themselves begin to disintegrate. The work as a whole is something of a compendium of the diverse stages of Magritte's 'technical' dissolution and shows that the demise of the line is the logical conclusion of a process. The division into planes is implied in the face of the figure depicted, which is not presented as a continuous, contoured surface but as a collection of individual and distinct flat facets. The cheek, in particular, has become split into several planes. The same is true of the ground area extending across the middle distance as far as the background, which is marked out into separate divisions of flat space. In the torso of the figure, surface nuance appears obliterated and reduced to the flatness and homogeneity of the plane. What we see is a uniform, uninterrupted surface that extends from the neck down to the lower extremity of the canvas. As in *L'Esprit comique*, all sense of detail vanishes into surface flatness. Yet, the abatement continues here towards an even greater reduction in pictorial definition. The treatment of the figure's hands, for instance, shows not only a negation of voluminosity, but also the elimination of surface integrality. The fingers and palms are conveyed by just rudimentary outlines, executed in a crude, rough and ready manner. Magritte presents no more than sketchy, unrevised forms that give the impression of incompleteness and which leave us in no doubt that he has taken us to an inchoate level of pictorial construction that precedes voluminous relief or even the basic continuity of flatness.

Another work that demonstrates this 'linear' phase of the dissolution is *Le Problème de l'espace* (1928), which depicts a brick wall daubed with a line drawing of a man who illogically appears to be smoking a pipe in *trompe l'œil*. As its title suggests, the work ponders the paradox of conveying space and volume within a two-dimensional medium. Being flat and literally impenetrable, the brick wall can accommodate neither protrusion nor recession; it is pure *surface* and depth is irrelevant to it. Indeed, by demonstrably representing his protagonist in terms of a veneer of paint applied to a façade, Magritte makes the point that line is limited to the domain of the planar. Any suggestion of solid modelling, therefore, is pure illusion. What is emphasized here is that line belongs to the periphery of three-dimensional modelling. Unlike the forms in *L'Esprit comique*, however, the linear figure of *Le Problème de l'espace* cannot even exist *as* a surface. Rather, it is inscribed *on* a plane, which clearly shows through it and continues beyond its circumscription. The figure is, in fact, less than a plane. It may define the extremities of a plane, but it is otherwise depleted of substance.

---

[1] Marcel Mariën, *Magritte* (Brussels, 1943), p. 12.

[2] René Magritte, *Écrits complets* (Paris, 1979), p. 275.

[3] René Magritte, in Harry Torczyner, *René Magritte, signes et images* (Paris, 1977), p. 165.

[4] A. M. Hammacher, *Magritte* (London, 1974), p. 92.

Mon cher ami,

Je regrette un peu de vous avoir écrit ma dernière carte, ce que j'ai pu dire du petit texte que vous m'aviez envoyé est peu de chose. Je pense que je m'expliquerais mieux avec ce fragment d'un texte que j'écris. (ce n'est encore que le projet)

— Un écrit, sans l'usage de l'analyse ni de la synthèse. Il ne serait pas une explication ni un plaisir. Mais avec des images, (qui seraient dans le texte pour désigner un état ou un objet quand son nom le désigne trop généralement) obtenir un effet qui secouerait violemment le lecteur.

Je crois avoir fait une découverte, dans la peinture, tout a fait saisissante: J'ai employé jusqu'à présent des objets composés, ou bien la situation d'un objet suffisait parfois à le rendre mystérieux. Mais à la suite des recherches que j'ai faites ici, j'ai trouvé une possibilité nouvelle qu'avaient les choses: c'est de devenir graduellement autre chose, un objet se fond dans un objet autre que lui même. Par exemple le ciel à certains endroits laisse apparaître du bois. C'est me semble til bien autre chose qu'un objet composé, puisqu'il n'y a pas de rupture entre les deux matières, ni de limite.

J'obtiens par ce moyen des tableaux où le regard "doit penser" d'une toute autre façon que d'habitude, les choses sont tangibles et pourtant quelques planches de bon bois deviennent insensiblement transparentes a certains endroits; ou bien une femme nue, a des parties qui deviennent aussi d'une matière différente. J'ai trouvé cela a la suite d'un tableau comme ceci:

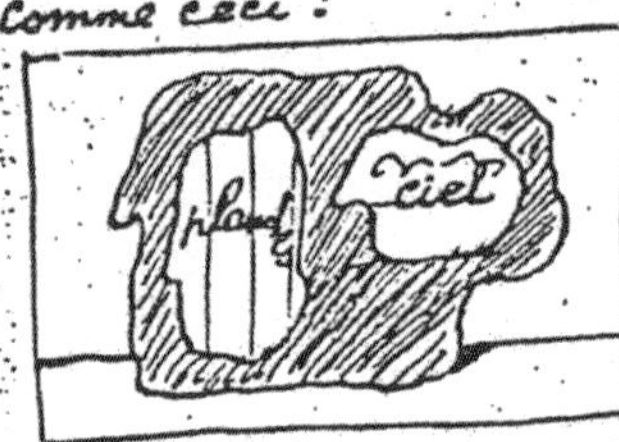

Il suffisait comme vous voyez de supprimer la forme qui sépare les planches du ciel

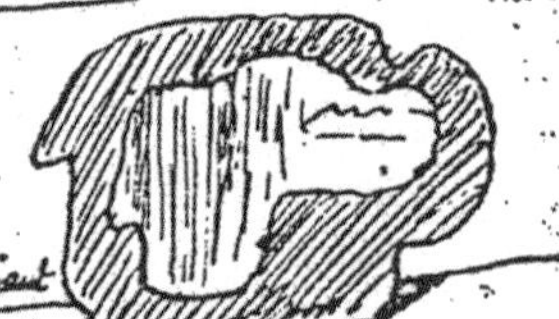

et de fondre l'une dans l'autre les choses qui se trouvaient séparées plus haut.

J'appelle ces dernières choses: L'illusion modèle, Le centre de la nature, La base du silence, L'expérience du miracle, L'avenir des voix, La fin du temps, La réclote des nuages, La maladie des planchers, Les embarras de la peinture etc.. Bien amicalement votre

Magritte

Manuscript (*circa* 1927)

Vague Things

As well as regressing the pictorial construct to the level of the line, *L'Âge du feu* introduces a further stage in the demise of anatomical representation. The line may carry only scant meaning, but it is still denotative in some way, leading towards fuller significance through its suggestive qualities. As in *L'Âge du feu*, however, the mark on the canvas can also cease to carry any meaning at all. The vague, indeterminate forms being tossed in the air by the figure in the painting are, to all intents and purposes, semantically vacuous. These are simply blobs of matter that are unrecognizable and wholly devoid of referential value.

How Magritte arrived at this notion of representational non-signification can be gleaned from a 1927 manuscript in which he had announced 'I think I've made a totally striking discovery in painting'.[1] Until that moment, he explained, he had been thinking in terms of finite objects and had either modified their context ('the situation') or had questioned the relation of their parts ('composed objects'). His novel approach was concerned with modifying not so much the external relations that an object might have, as its internal structure. Illustrating his argument with a sketch of *La Saison des voyages* (1927), which depicts the often-repeated format of a solid slab enclosing individual articles, he suggests that the layout of his 'encased' pictorial elements could be altered in such a way that the divisions between the compartments disappear so as to allow the otherwise isolated forms to merge freely.[2] In this way, the explanation continues, one thing could be melted into another and so gradually become something else. This hypothesis is illustrated by a second sketch in which the substances in question, sky and planks, blend together at their point of contact. As Magritte saw it, this permeation of one thing into another distorts the representation to such an extent that it becomes difficult to interpret. Because the intermingled plastic forms lose their finiteness and become ambiguous, he feels that the spectator's expectations would be disrupted: 'one has to look in a manner that is completely different from the usual'. What is missing here are 'the visible contours of objects', which he would specifically put into question a couple of years later.[3] As Magritte says, he removes the 'limit' of materials. In other words, he does away with the elementary pictorial marker of 'finitio' and, in so doing, throws pictorial finiteness into disarray. What results are the 'vague things' that he maintains images are capable of designating.[4]

With this concept, Magritte took a further significant step in his overall anatomical dissolution. Of course, *La Saison des voyages*, with which he illustrated his argument is already a progression from the earlier phase that had simply reduced anatomy into planes. The work differs from comparable

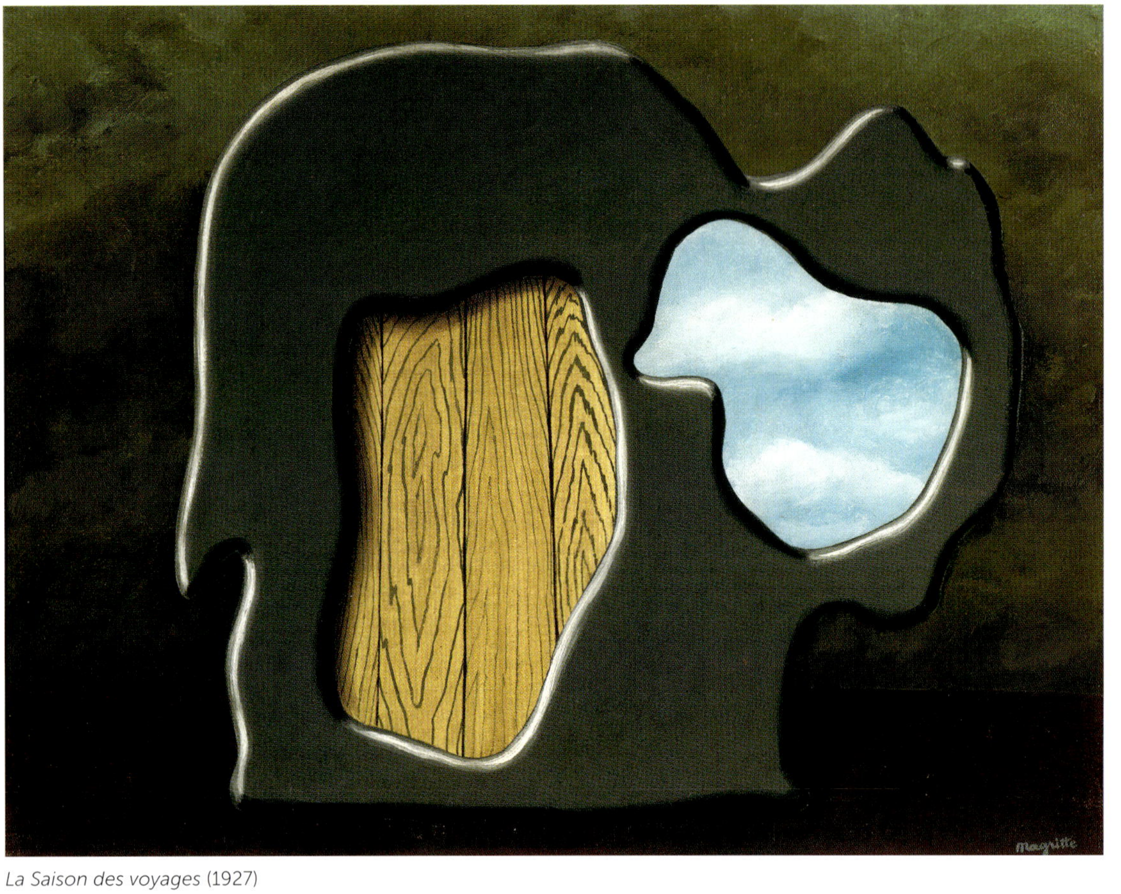

La Saison des voyages (1927)

'encasing' works, such as *Le Dormeur téméraire*, in that it deranges the *internal* integrity of the pictorial element. In *Le Dormeur téméraire* individual objects had been isolated from one another and denied pictorial interrelation, as well as being removed from any sort of 'composition'; however, within their respective circumscriptions, they maintained their anatomical totality, their form remained unaltered and their meaning persisted. To the contrary, when, as in *La Saison des voyages*, the same principle of encasement is applied, not to single objects but to 'materials', anatomical unity is at once compromised. If the items restrained within the grey slab are 'substances', such as sky, which is an unlimited three-dimensional space, or interlocked planks, which comprise a continuous surface and have no definite contours, then the function of the grey solid changes from that of *wrapping around* a form to that of *invading* it. The question is no longer one of compromised 'composition' but, rather, of interference with the internal make-up of an object. Clearly, whereas an object can be confined to its own outline, something which has no fixed delimitations is inevitably partially erased by confinement. It is anatomy itself, therefore, that is vitiated. This is more obvious in *Le Démon de la perversité* (1927), where

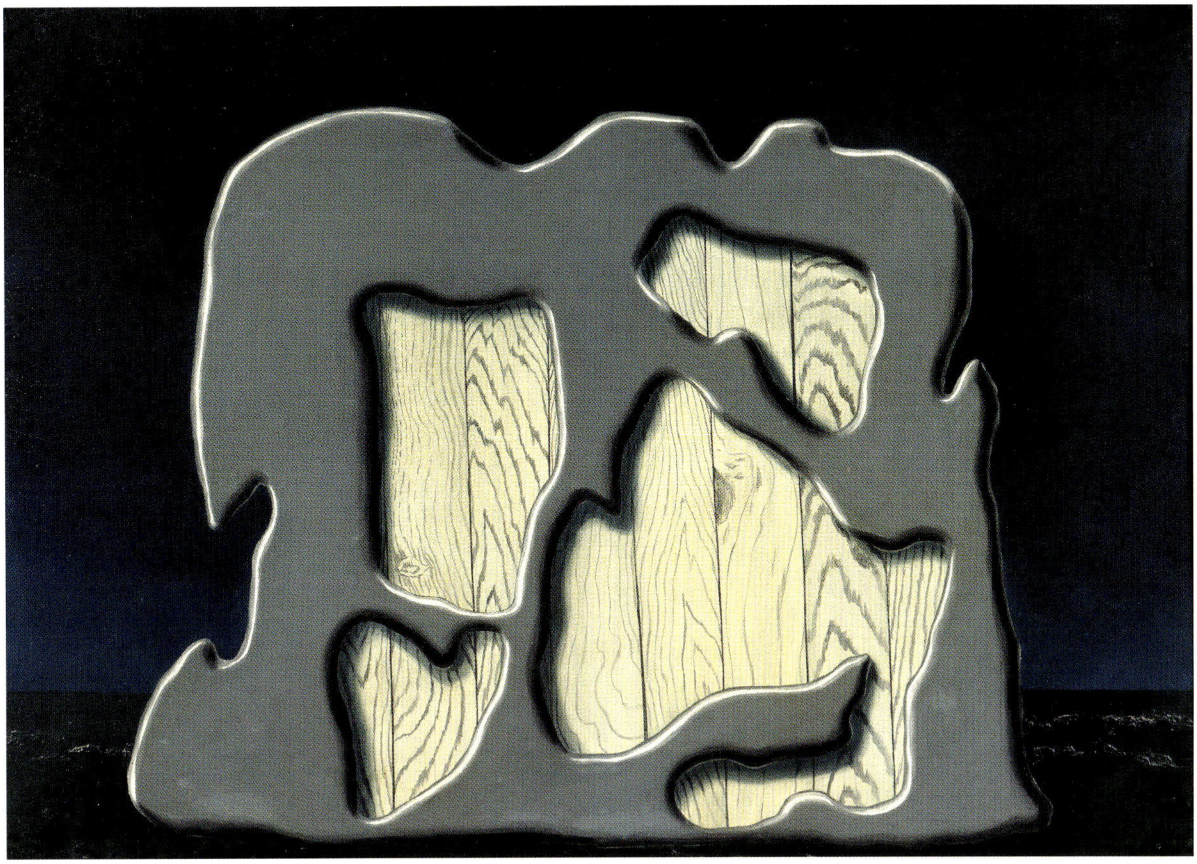

Le Démon de la perversité (1927)

the flowing grey form acts as an *interruption* of what is a continuous surface, whereas the planks in *La Saison des voyages* had merely been intruded upon. In the case of the sky, however, the impoverishment is unmitigated. With its inherently expansive qualities, this 'substance' is depleted in a drastic manner. In fact, its entrapment in a shallow niche is no less than a direct negation of its very definition of limitless voluminosity. Constriction in this case amounts to contradiction. For both substances all that remain are tokens of their representation. They are invalidated and rendered semantically inert.

Yet, Magritte proceeded to propose a further reduction. 'I have found', he wrote, 'a new possibility that was inherent in things [...] it is that of gradually becoming something else.' The next decrement of anatomy, it would seem, challenges the very identity of the pictorial unit. Magritte now begins to see individual objects as capable of being neither discrete nor differentiated. So, when he proposes that sky be mixed with wood and wood with sky – 'in certain places the sky allows wood to show through [...] some planks of solid imperceptibly become transparent in certain places' – he is laying pictorial intelligibility on the line. His removal of the partition between the sky and the planks does more than

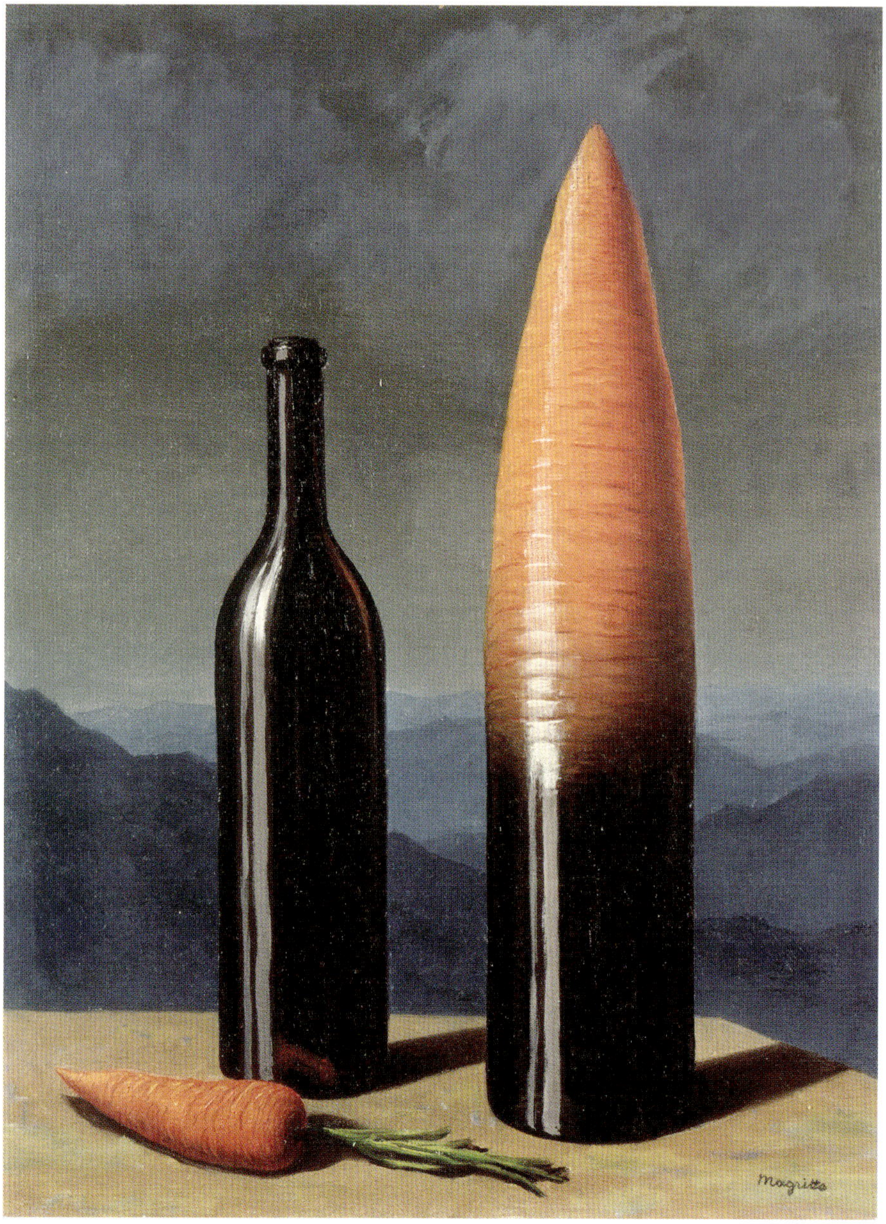

L'Explication (1952)

efface the circumscription of an object or the demarcation of the space occupied by each substance; it triggers ambiguity and indistinctness. As the sky and the planks 'melt' together, there is no point at which one ends and the other begins. All that can be identified are the extremities of a continuum that starts as planks and ends as sky. There is not even a point of juncture since, as Magritte says, he is not dealing with 'composed objects'. The heart of the sky/plank conglomeration is more of a locus of pictorial irresolution. It evokes what could be thought of as an incipient level of representation, at which meaning has yet to be instilled into

Le Bon Sens (1945-6)

visible traces. The 'new possibility', therefore, signals a transition from a stage at which a substance is engulfed by neutral, *meaningless* matter, more often than not in the guise of a grey, viscous, curd-like substance, to a further stage at which it is permeated by extraneous and discordant, but *meaningful*, matter. The upshot of this process is an attenuation or total erasure of pictorial anatomy. What starts off as clear pictorial denotation ends up as vague imprecision.

It is by creating this vague region of fusion and confusion that Magritte neared the end of his anatomical dissolution. By overlapping and superimposing materials, he challenged conventional pictorial monovalency. It is not so much a question of two alternative pictorial significations here – either sky is becoming wood or wood is becoming sky – as that of an equal presence of sky and wood. But, such a simultaneity inevitably triggers a cancelling out of each term by virtue of the presence of its opposite; what is being signified is neither sky nor planks since, if both exist concurrently, neither can exist autonomously. In the end, all that can be said is that Magritte creates irresolvable contradiction that results in representational amorphousness. The 1927 manuscript therefore begins with the notion of minimal pictorial signification, as it is seen in *La Saison des voyages*, and leads the argument towards the elimination of visual meaningfulness.

Yet, the fact that a painting can present manifest plastic presence that is, nevertheless, devoid of representational significance or that, as Magritte put it,

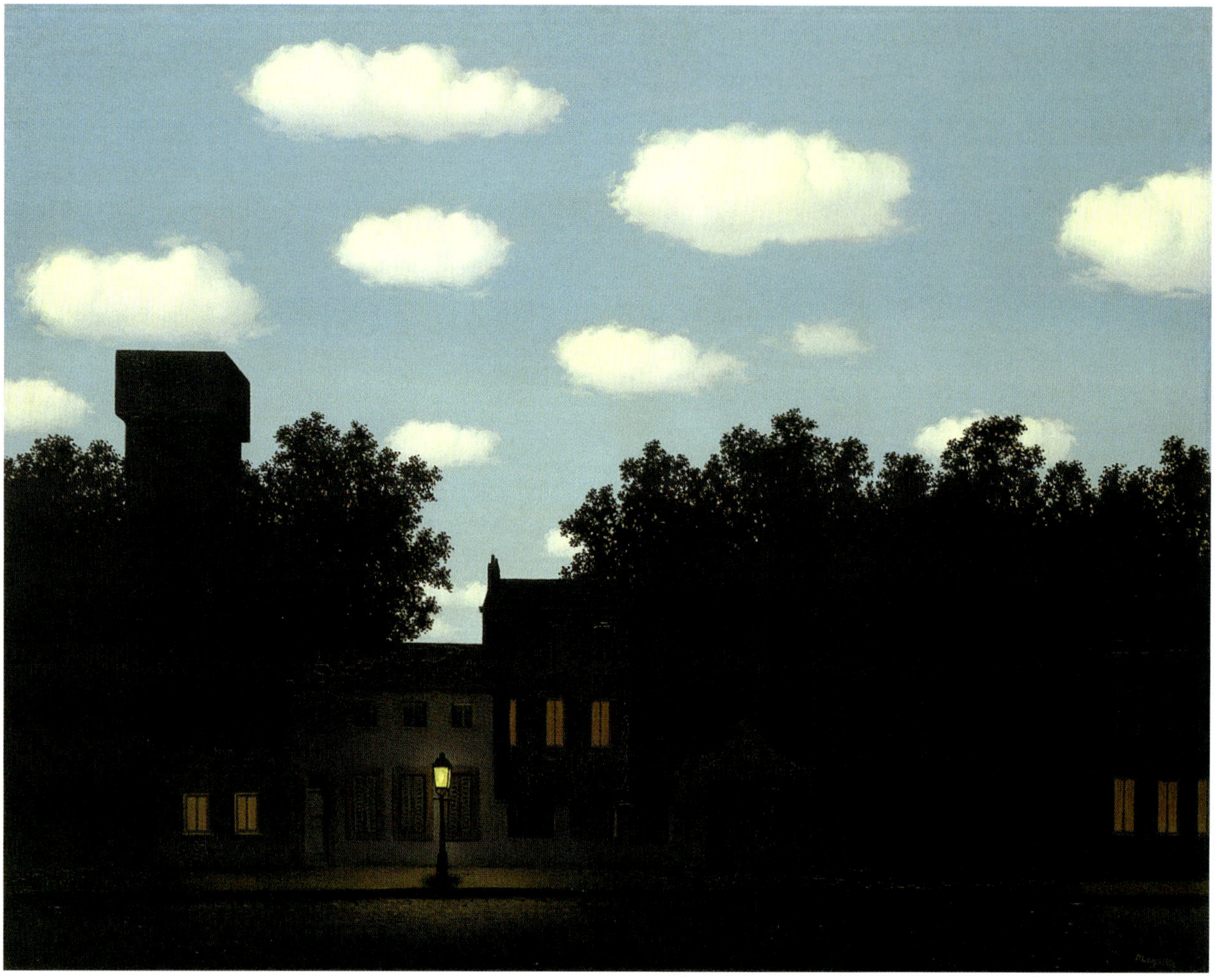

L'Empire des lumières II (1950)

'images sometimes designate vague things', is not directly addressed in the 1927 manuscript.[5] His preoccupation at this point was still with the precursory concept of plastic *contradiction*, which, according to Vincent Bounoure, was to pervade Magritte's work for decades.[6] For Bounoure, the various mechanisms employed by Magritte, such as 'isolation', 'modification', 'hybridization', 'incongruity', 'chance encounters', 'double images', 'paradox' and 'conceptual bipolarity', are all subsumed within 'one and only intellectual operation'.[7] Contradiction, Bounoure continues, amounts to 'the essential drive of his undertaking, the motive force of his thinking, the core of his sensibility'.[8] But when the argument goes on to make a distinction between 'an intellectual contrariness' and 'a plastic contrariness', it becomes clear that in 1927 Magritte had not yet delved into all aspects of the notion. Whilst the first kind of contradiction accounts for paintings such as *La Condition humaine*, which places the representation in conflict with the reality to which it refers, it is only the second kind, which entails the juxtaposition

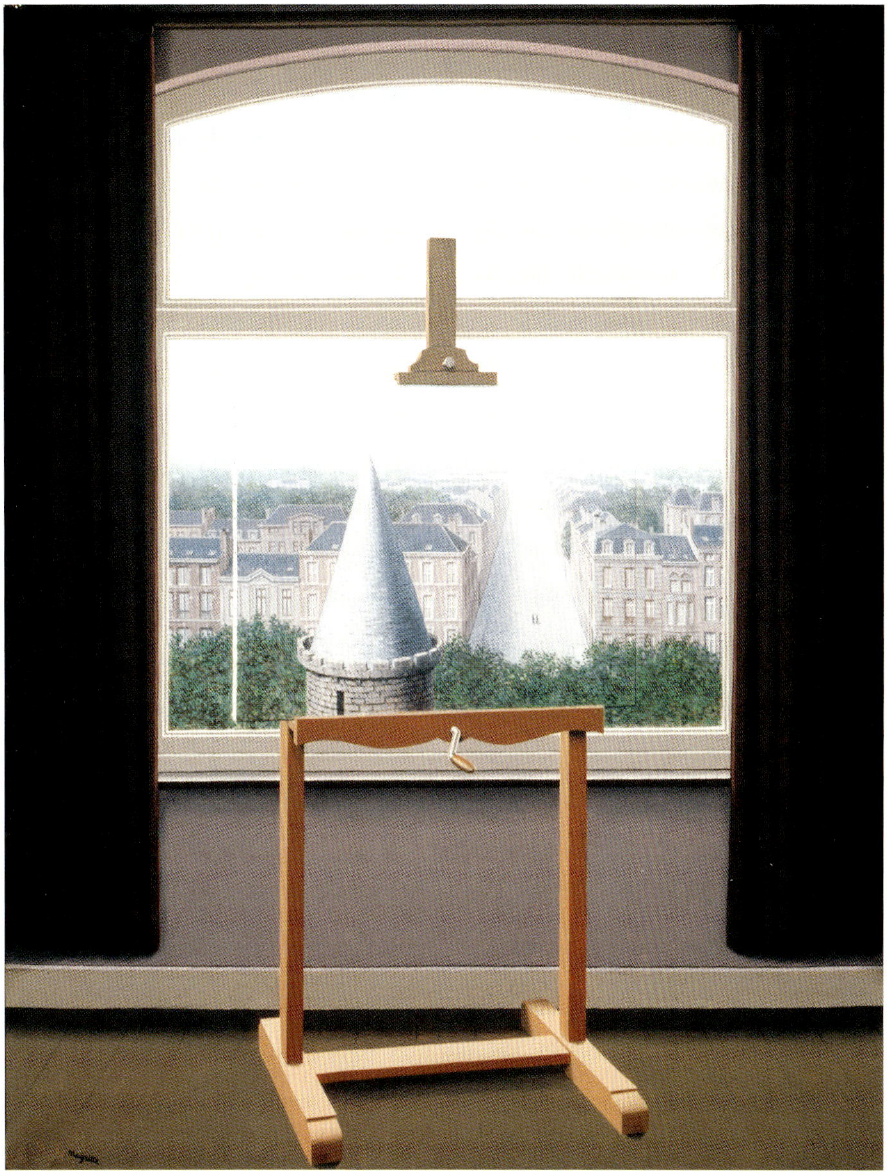

Les Promenades d'Euclide (1955)

of 'characteristics initially perceived by the senses as opposed', that the 1927 manuscript explores.[9] For example, whereas *L'Explication* (1952) is a patent demonstration of 'the possibility [...] of gradually becoming something else', as Magritte had speculated in 1927, the intellectual contrariness of *Le Bon Sens* (1945-6) is in no way anticipated in this early manuscript. Bounoure, it must be said, looks ahead to nuances of contradiction that Magritte was yet to conceive, such as that of the 'daylight and nocturnal light' of *L'Empire des lumières II* (1950).[10] Back in 1927, Magritte was still formulating the broad rudiments of a concept and was far from elaborating its specific ramifications. All he had done by

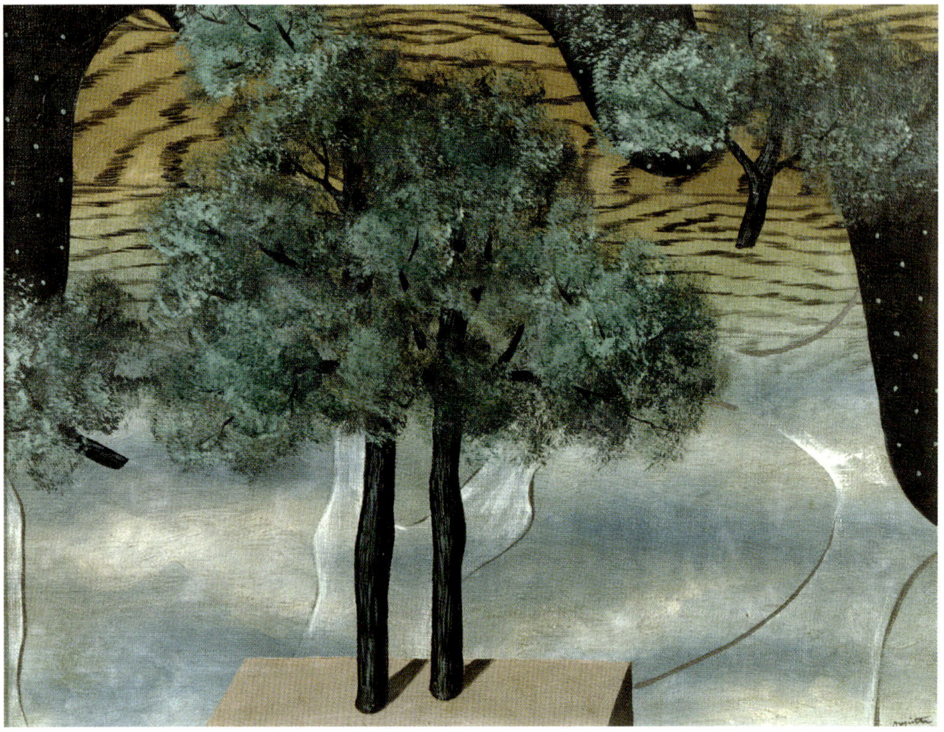

La Culture des idées (1927-8)

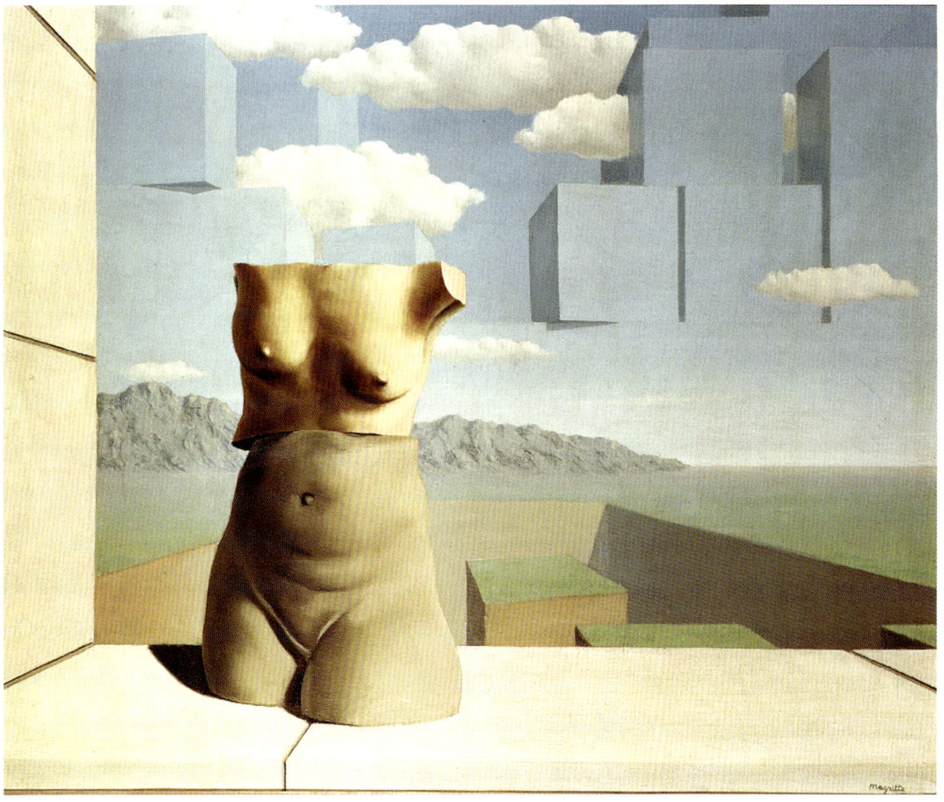

Les Marches de l'été (1938-9)

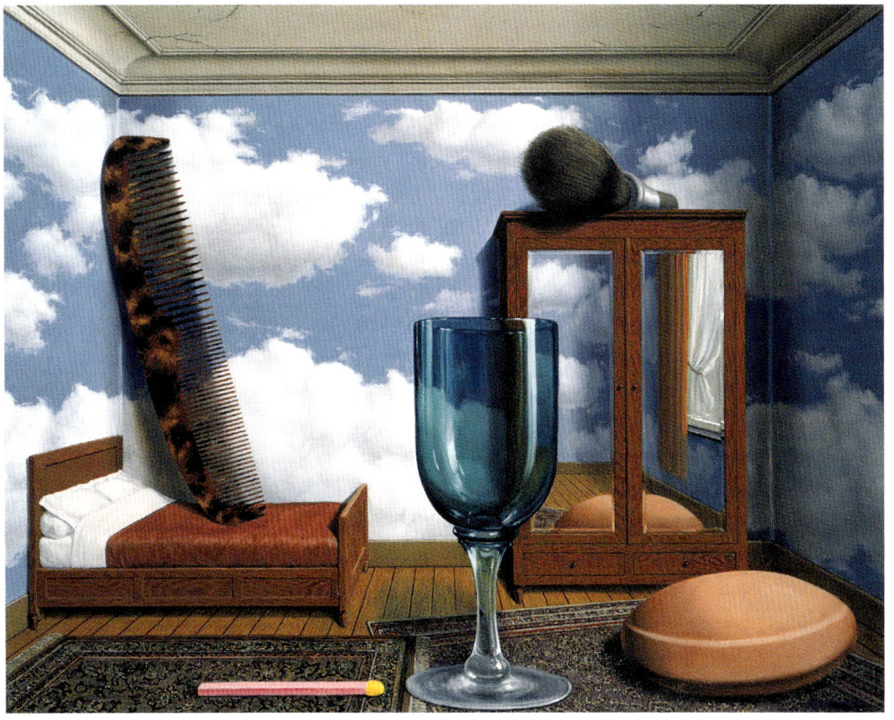

Les Valeurs personnelles (1952)

then was to argue in terms of absolutes. He had set in juxtaposition the diametric opposites of the pictorial zenith and nadir – sky and pavement.[11] By abutting these extremities of three-dimensional space, Magritte had prefigured later semantic contradictions, such as that of the vertical and the horizontal, which appears in *Les Promenades d'Euclide* (1955). In one sense, Magritte's antipodean fusion already embodied 'the antitheses of the mobile and the fixed [...] of the manipulable and the monumental, of the soft and the rigid, of the transparent and the opaque [...] the opposition between the fixed image and the fleeting image [...] the negation of the inside in favour of the outside'.[12] Magritte's sky/pavement can aptly be regarded as the 'initial opposition' to which Bounoure alludes.[13]

Where Magritte did elaborate this primal type of contradiction is in *La Doublure du sommeil* (1927-8) and *La Culture des idées* (1927-8), both of which confuse or interchange the properties of sky and pavement. For instance, in *La Doublure du sommeil* the illusion of an evening landscape is negated by a surface of planks that gradually liquefies into the sky. As there is no encasement here, but rather the suggestion of extensive space emphasized by the silhouetted hills, the *contradiction* stems from the incongruous relative scales. The relatively miniscule grain of wood is shown here as approaching the great mass of cloud formations, which transforms the planks into colossal constructions, looming beyond the horizon. The converse, however, is equally true since the sky is incised with the diminutive apertures of musical instruments and so shrinks to expanses

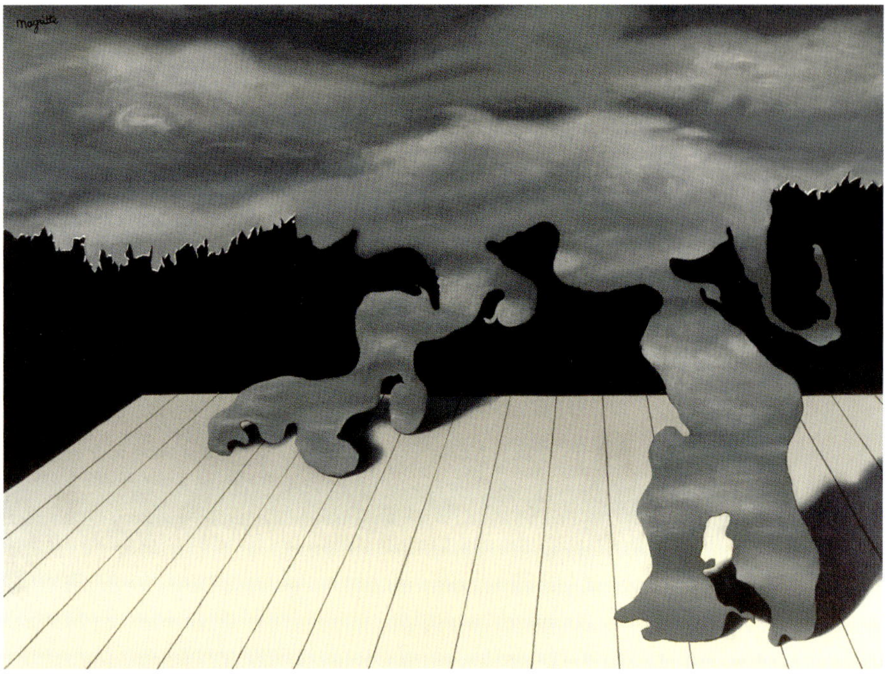

Les Muscles célestes (1927)

no larger than a few wooden planks. These conflicting readings of the sky bring about an irreconcilable tension that Magritte would go on to elaborate in *Les Marches de l'été* (1938-9), where the intrinsically impalpable sky is depicted as a stack of solid blocks, and in *Les Valeurs personnelles* (1952), in which the sky and its vaporous clouds constitute the impenetrable walls of a room.

The demarcation between the solid and the insubstantial is eliminated in yet another work of 1927, *Les Muscles célestes*. As in *La Doublure du sommeil*, there is a dark, transitional horizon, but this time it is the sky that descends onto the pavement. Magritte depicts celestial protrusions that appear to have broken away from the aerial portion of the sky in the distance, crossed a black middle distance and finally anchored themselves to the planked floor area in the foreground. What is contradicted is the depth of field that the receding orthogonals emphatically mark out. So, rather than functioning as a grid of measured surface space, the planked pavement offers only uncertainty and instability. The anatomy of its occupants is correspondingly no less equivocal: the appendages that have come down from the heavens may well have all the characteristics of solid objects – clear-cut outlines, shadows, rigidity, uprightness – but at the same time they remain the converse – nebulous, fluid, volatile. They are repositories of conflicting physical properties, where the very nature of things is nullified. Within them, substances cease to be differentiated; opposing meanings coexist and fuse. Yet, these loci of representational contradiction, at which fixed plastic interpretation ceases to be possible, are never pictorially imprecise in themselves. On the contrary, they appear as self-sufficient entities within the composition. Arguably, the celestial limbs are presented as 'escaping' the larger corpus of sky and already appear to be semi-autonomous. Untethered, as they could be imagined, they would, conceivably, turn into free units of meaninglessness that, abstrusely, would inhabit a fully articulated pictorial space. This, essentially, is Magritte's 'discovery'. His deconstruction of the pictorial plane leads to the depiction of imprecision within precision. As the 1927 manuscript reveals, works in this phase of Magritte's oeuvre can only be unravelled in terms of a dynamic, progressive procedure. At the outset there is isolation, typically via the recurrent viscous grey sludge that envelops matter and severs all its contextual ties. Then, a form of fusion occurs with dissimilar or divergent material. The ensuing irresolvable contradiction leads to a dearth of representational meaning. Finally, this zero representation, the product of self-cancelling semantic forces, assumes a life of its own. As other works would reveal, it emerges as an autonomous presence, soon to take its place in works peopled solely by entities devoid of significance, namely by the 'vague things' that had been heralded in 1927.

---

[1] The manuscript, from the collection of Mme E. DeKnop, is undated but since five of the paintings that it cites as 'these recent things' had been exhibited at Galerie L'Époque in Brussels on 7 January 1928, and since 'a nude woman with parts which also are turning into a different substance' can only be an allusion to *Découverte* (1927), a dating of 1927 is practically certain. The unspecified addressee is probably Nougé, who wrote the text for the Galerie L'Époque catalogue. Archives de l'Art Contemporain de Belgique, 9914.

[2] At this time Magritte was not consistently using words in his paintings and so the inscriptions 'planches' and 'ciel' are to be taken as a means of clarifying the drawing.

[3] René Magritte, *Écrits complets* (Paris, 1979), p. 61.

[4] Magritte, *Écrits complets*, p. 61.

[5] Magritte, *Écrits complets*, p. 61.

[6] Vincent Bounoure, 'Le Thème de la contradiction chez Magritte', *L'Œil*, 206-7 (Feb.-Mar. 1972): 4-11.

[7] Bounoure, 'Le Thème de la contradiction chez Magritte': 5.

[8] Bounoure, 'Le Thème de la contradiction chez Magritte': 2.

[9] Bounoure, 'Le Thème de la contradiction chez Magritte': 10.

[10] Bounoure, 'Le Thème de la contradiction chez Magritte': 9-10.

[11] Planks can reasonably be considered to be an allusion to Alberti's 'pavement'.

[12] Bounoure, 'Le Thème de la contradiction chez Magritte': 7-9.

[13] Bounoure, 'Le Thème de la contradiction chez Magritte': 8. This is literally an initial opposition. In his preface to Michel Foucault, *Questa non è una pipa* (Milan, 1980), Guido Almansi points out that the differentiation between 'earth/sky; land/sea' made in *Genesis* stands for the initial step in extracting a cosmic order out of 'chaos'. Only by making this and subsequent oppositions, it is argued, can separate meanings exist. On the level of pictorial construction, the sky/pavement distinction occurs as a result of one of the first construction lines, the 'centric line', according to Leon Battista Alberti, *On Painting*, trans. John R. Spencer (London, 1956), p. 58.

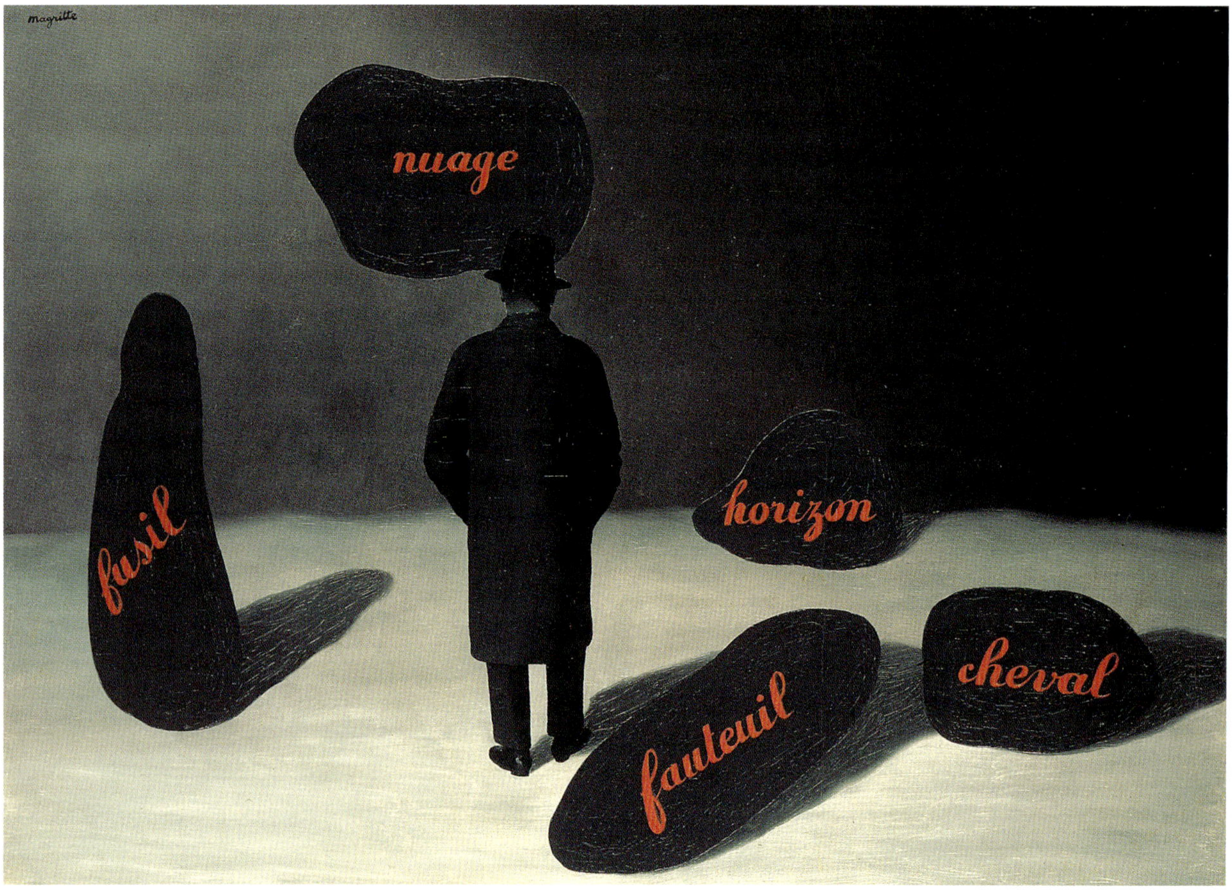

L'Apparition (1928)

Pictorial Negation

However minimally, an outline still bears hints of pictorial signification and the mere circumscription of a form is enough to establish its identity. In a further development of the dissolution, Magritte went on to deprive the pictorial element of even this evanescent fragment of meaning. Every last anatomical attribute, as Foucault observes, is compromised: 'mass is reduced, the useless name is dispensed with; Magritte elides the object'.[1] It is the most elementary of traces, those that impart the barest kind of recognisability to the object, that are now targeted. In this phase, Magritte effaces all representational precision and leaves his anatomies as equivocal traces, to which Foucault can allude only in negative terms – 'stains, shadows, silhouettes'.[2] These are little more than virtual presences, concomitants of objects, rather than objects in their own right.

A painting in which such ephemeral forms become the subject itself is *L'Apparition* (1928). In the place of recognizable objects, Magritte depicts no more than spectre-like forms. The space around them is tangible enough – a dark distant sky that meets a sandy ground at a clear horizon and a directional light source that casts heavy shadows – but apart from an anonymous, solitary figure with his back turned, pictorial content is stripped bare. The stark landscape is peopled only with indefinite entities that Robert Roseblum has aptly described as 'blobs'.[3] Anatomically, these forms are less resolved than the most minimal of linear representations, not so much incomplete, as uncertain and vacant. Magritte's 'traces', as he had termed them, do not envelop and delimit the space of an object, as would be the case for a 'circumscription', but rather stand as bereft cores. Blobs are neither shells nor skeletons. They neither conceal an essence nor are they enveloped by something more palpable. They simply point to the fact that Magritte has 'broken away from any meaning'.[4] In effect, blobs fall short of the most minimal function of the pictorial element, that of being intelligible. They amount to an elemental state. Being 'things hardly formed [...] with neither a face nor an identity', Magritte's traces can be said to precede the representational schema as a whole.[5] Anterior even to the consciously traced-out line, they hardly exceed the rudimentary notion of marking presence. Before the pictorial entity can even begin to be formed, according to Alberti, the painter conceives it in terms of a location: 'First, in seeing a thing', he wrote, 'we say it occupies a place'.[6] The 'vague things' in *L'Apparition* do no more than this.

What *can* be said of the ambiguous blob is that it constitutes the raw material of visual expression. Indeed, as Nougé pointed out, Leonardo had regarded imprecise phenomena as sources of *initial* inspiration, advising young painters

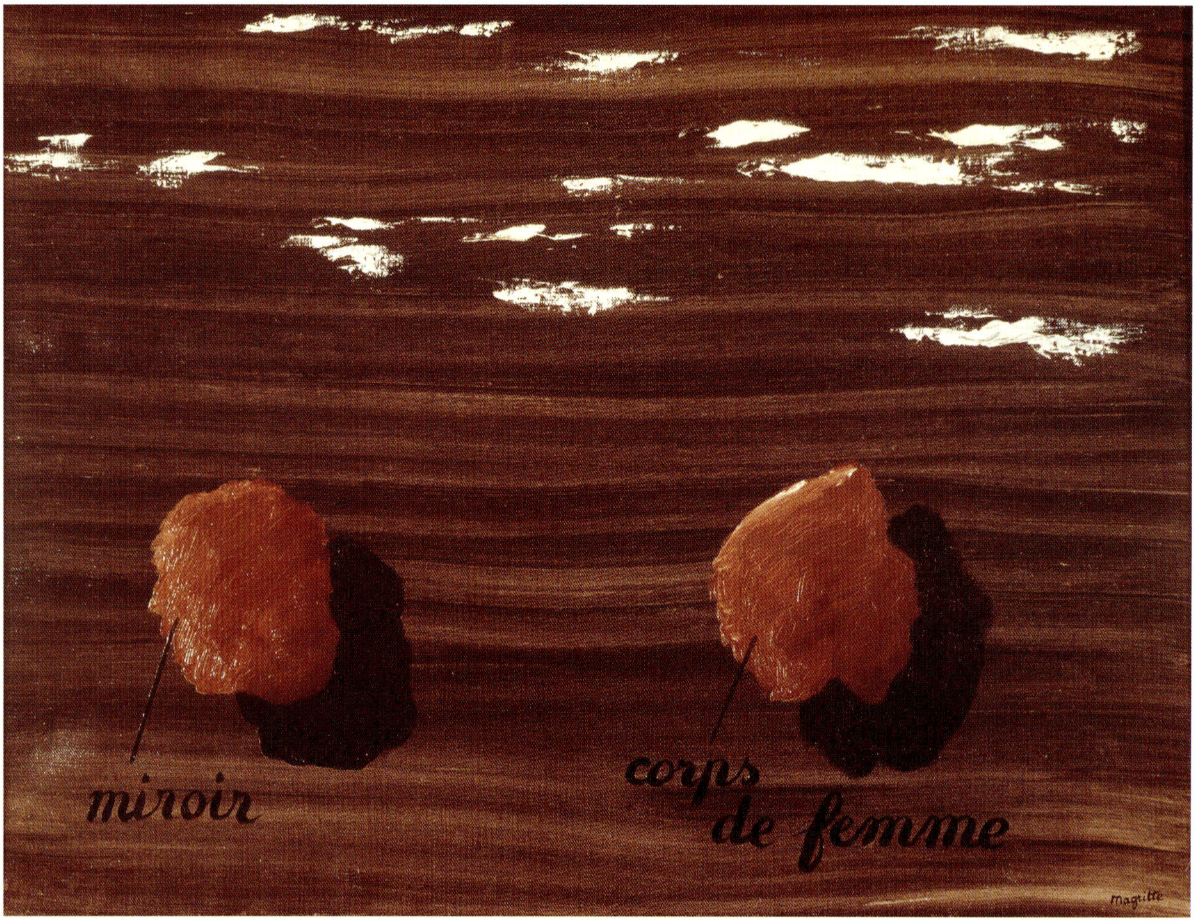

L'Usage de la parole I (1928-9)

to 'observe the cracks in old walls, the movements of clouds'.[7] For Alberti too, indefinite form had lain at the inception of anatomical representation:

> I believe that the arts of those who attempt to create images and likenesses from bodies produced by Nature, originated in the following way. They probably occasionally observed in a tree-trunk or clod of earth and other inanimate objects outlines in which, with slight alterations, something very similar to the real faces of Nature was represented.[8]

Magritte's own take on the 'clod of earth', the blobs of the late 1920s, were seen in precisely this way by Mariën; to him, they were starting points for more resolved representations, that he described as 'first signs'.[9]

In one sense, however, the blob is not quite such a return to absolute zero. Rarely is it so denuded that it is left wholly pictorially disengaged. In some way or other, it is invariably interlinked with another element, frequently the written word. In *L'Apparition* verbal elements – the words 'horse', 'armchair', 'horizon', 'shotgun' and 'cloud' – appear as though handwritten onto the blobs. Alternatively, Magritte annexes words or phrases to the blobs, as in *L'Usage de la parole I* (1928-9), in which connecting lines couple the word 'mirror' to one blob and 'woman's body' to another blob. A form of labelling takes place that appears to describe and define otherwise meaningless marks on the canvas. It would seem, therefore, that, at variance with the suggestion that blobs denote the terminal point of a dissolution of the pictorial object, these 'nondescript forms', as Magritte also termed them, are attributed at least a degree of semantic identity.[10]

In *Les Traces vivantes* (1927), however, the label 'nude woman' appears on the trunk of a tree, which indicates that words do not, after all, serve as legends for objects. Despite possible metaphorical associations, there are invariably no denotative illustrative relations between verbal elements in the paintings and the blobs with which they are coupled. This is why Foucault regards blobs as no more than 'word carriers', that is mere material supports for written inscriptions.[11] As such, blobs act like blackboards; they may be 'occupied' by words but in no way echo or confirm their referent. Indeed, as though to make this very point, Magritte not only styled his painted words in the careful, pedagogic calligraphy of a schoolmistress, but he also showed them as chalked on a classroom blackboard. As the framed blackboard on the easel of *Les Deux Mystères* (1966) demonstrates, the caption does not necessarily tie in with the image to which it refers. The lesson carefully written underneath a meticulously represented pipe is that 'this is not a pipe'. But that is not all; the label is not so much erroneous as contradictory. The verbal message counters pictorial semantic finiteness. In a drawing published in 1929 in *Variétés*, Magritte had made this point by inappropriately labelling three blobs 'character meditating on madness', 'black table' and 'open door' respectively .[12] As though emphasizing that his captions cannot possibly be taken as explanations, he gives a fourth blob two *conflicting* descriptions – 'character lying down or sitting'. Far from imparting some form of identity to the blob, words preclude it from acquiring any significance at all. In no uncertain way, for Magritte blobs remain both 'images of vague things' and 'objects that do without names'.[13] Hammacher appositely sums them up as 'nameless forms'.[14]

If blobs are meaningless pictorial units, it follows that their function must be other than *anatomical*. As the gouache of *L'Esprit comique* demonstrates, elements in a painting can be semantically depleted, whilst remaining fully operative. The 'figures' in this work are barely corporeal, stripped of content and yet they retain full animation. What the shift away from *anatomy* does not appear to do, therefore, is to lessen the alternative pictorial axis of *composition*. On the contrary, the compositional perspective appears to acquire greater prominence in such a scenario. Despite their diaphanousness, the paper cut-outs had orchestrated a whole drama, full of differentiations and nuances. The same is true of the blob. The nameless objects in *L'Apparition* may not be carriers of meaning but, as a group, they do establish a pictorial relativity. They convey information that denotes disparity; for instance, one blob is high up as opposed to another that is low down, one is upright and another lies horizontally, some are long and thin whilst others are short and portly. The blobs operate as signs of spatial differences and compositional narrative. As Goemans explained, 'Magritte separates or brings together elements without apparent plastic value and in this way *composes* a language'.[15] At this juncture of the dissolution, pictorial grammar, which had been so problematic in paintings such as *Cinéma bleu*, comes to the fore. It dominates the work and defines unambiguous and complex interrelations within it, while the anatomical object disintegrates into no more than a rudimentary mark.

✣ ✣ ✣

The definitive stage of any dissolution is when nothing remains, when the last traces of the solute are no longer present. In his nullification of the pictorial formula, Magritte too reached the point at which the subject is absented from the representational context. It is not so much a question of non-representation, as of *missing* presence. At the time Magritte was producing his denuded scenari, during the late 1920s, Willem Verougstraete had perceptively written that 'emptiness can perhaps be written about. Magritte proves it can be painted'.[16]

The mission of completely erasing the painted object, however, was one that Magritte undertook by degrees and in many works he held back from all-out representational curtailment. *Le Temps menaçant* (1929), for instance, simply *reduces* the substantiality of the object, rather than dispensing with it altogether. What are the normally solid forms of a tuba, a torso and a chair are simply denied some of their material qualities here; they are left weightless, colourless and ethereal. The three objects are shown as barely present and float in the sky as mere cloud formations that could dissipate with the slightest breeze. To all effects, they are just unstable and intangible blurs that could at any moment vanish into the thin air through which they precariously glide. Magritte prepares us for a spiriting away of the object, that he clearly had in mind and which, in *L'Inondation* (1931), begins in earnest. Again the setting is dominated by a clear blue sky, but instead of accommodating objects, even in the form of spectres, it swallows them up. The standing figure is being consumed from the top downwards and gradually fades away. It is as though the solid form were being progressively smothered and visually muffled. Magritte appears to be gradually painting out the anatomical body as though to edge it closer to total suppression.

Where pictorial vacuity becomes conclusive is in *La Voix du silence* (1928).

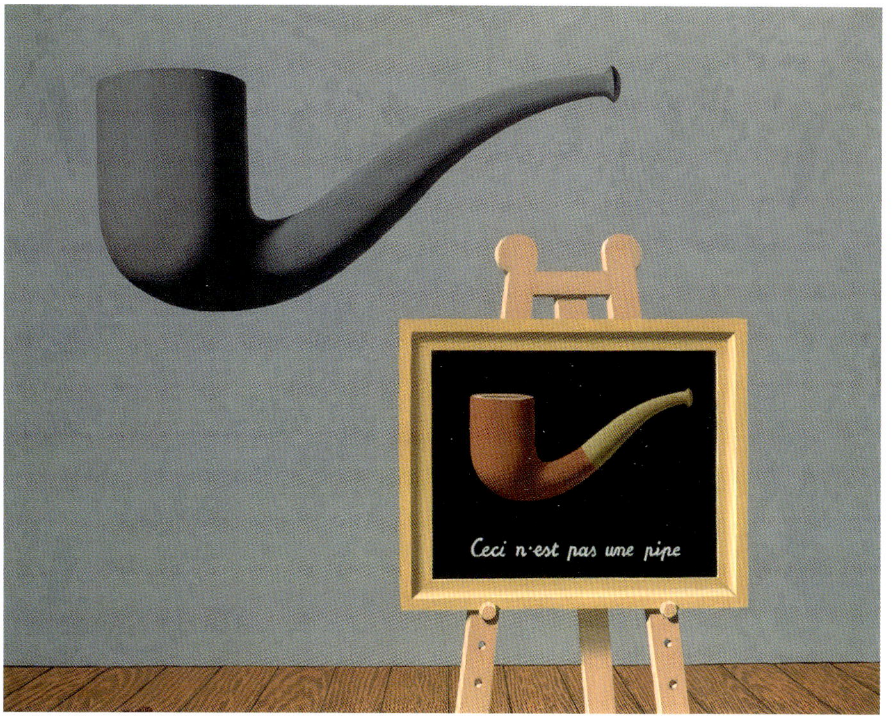

Les Deux Mystères (1966)

The title alone, 'the voice of silence', conveys the notion of definitive absence. Silence, after all, is the *elimination* of sound, not its reduction. Analogously, the work itself depicts a total suppression of the object, as opposed to its attenuation. Soundlessness precludes any sort of 'voice' and in Magritte's vacuous pictorial space represented objects are denied any form of presence. It is not that Magritte presents a visual context in which objects *cannot* exist; he does not depict a non-phenomenal world. On the contrary, he presents an unequivocal potential repository for solid form. But, he then proceeds to reveal it as bereft of anatomical content.

On the right there is an unremarkable and mundane scene – a domestic dining-room, a table, two chairs, and various ornaments, including a framed landscape painting. At face value, this is a textbook interior still-life, with a coherently composed space and solidly rendered objects; every solid form conforms to the lighting from the window on the right and, echoing the Albertian construct, the alignment of the floorboards corresponds to the orthogonals of the perspective construction. On the left of the central partition, however, where a similarly ordinary room setting could well be expected, there is nothing but darkness. *La Voix du silence* makes a sudden transition from replete banality to an inexplicable pictorial absence. Yet, the two halves of the painting are by no means contradictory. The small amount of light that permeates past the

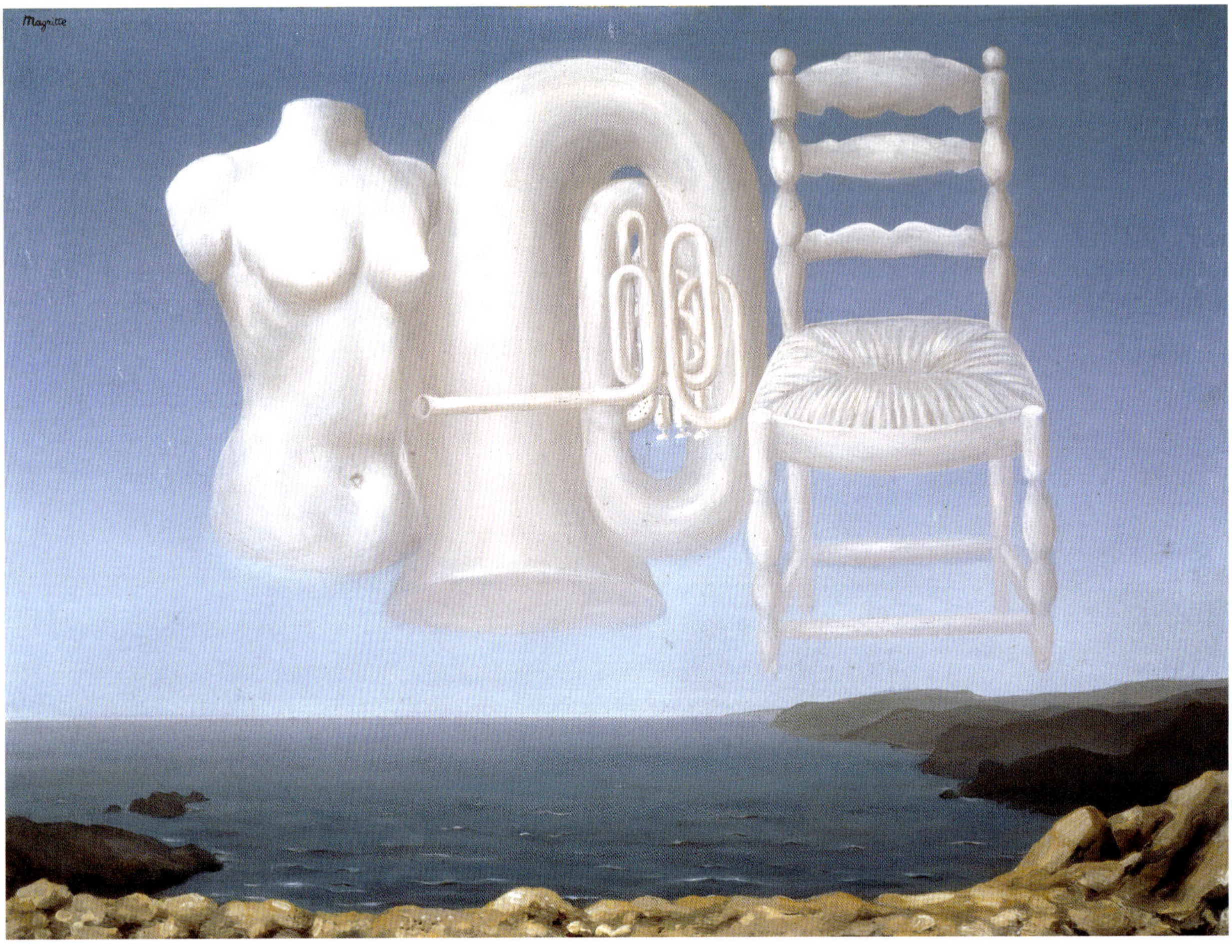

Le Temps menaçant (1929)

dividing wall shows that the pictorial space of the illuminated room, cluttered to the point of containing decorative vases and plants, is, in fact, a continuation of the darkened area. As the floorboards confirm, there is, indeed, spatial continuity between the right and the left sections of the painting. Therefore, the darkness on the left is not precluded from accommodating a further packed room. We can never know, however, whether it does or it does not. It remains a *potential* space, a potential container of objects. By contrasting the two spaces in this way, Magritte expresses what could be termed as 'pictorial dormancy'. He paints space and objects that remain unarticulated. *La Voix du silence* comprises two opposed pictorial states, one that is fully resolved and another in which space, form and light are deactivated. The darkness is charged with an uncommunicative pictorial *silence*.

What Magritte does not portray, however, is vacuity. Indeed, in concert with Nougé, Magritte was experimenting at this time with the distinctly separate notion of 'suppression of the object'.[17] In his treatise *La Subversion des images*,

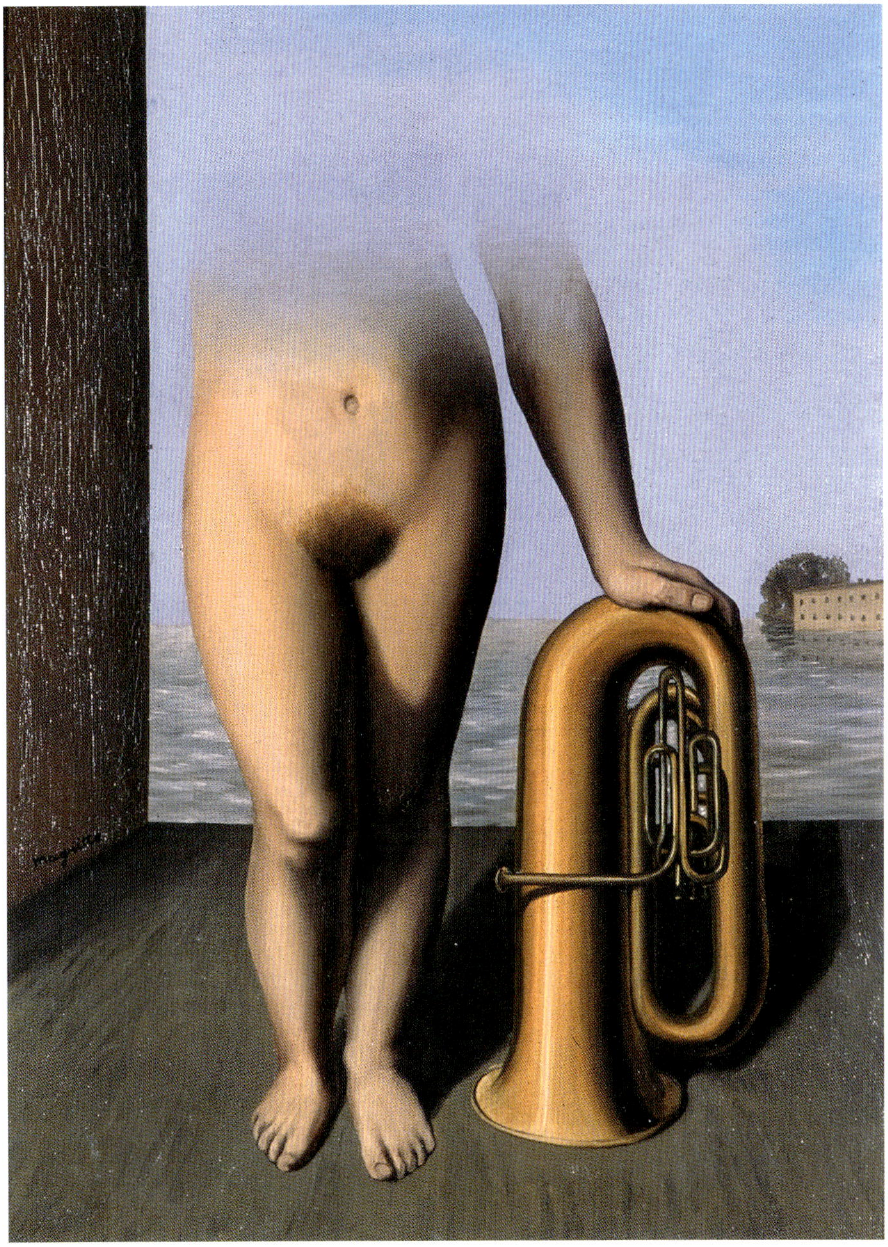

L'Inondation (1931)

Nougé had speculated on the conceptual implications of absenting elements from an otherwise undisturbed setting.[18] What he deduced was that an absence is inextricably linked to the *presence* of the complement of the missing object. In one of the examples that he cites, the removal of drinking glasses from the hands of two drinkers, he emphasizes that the situational setting should be preserved intact – 'care has been taken to remove the glasses while preserving the position of the hands'.[19] Logically, as he saw it, the absenting of the glasses

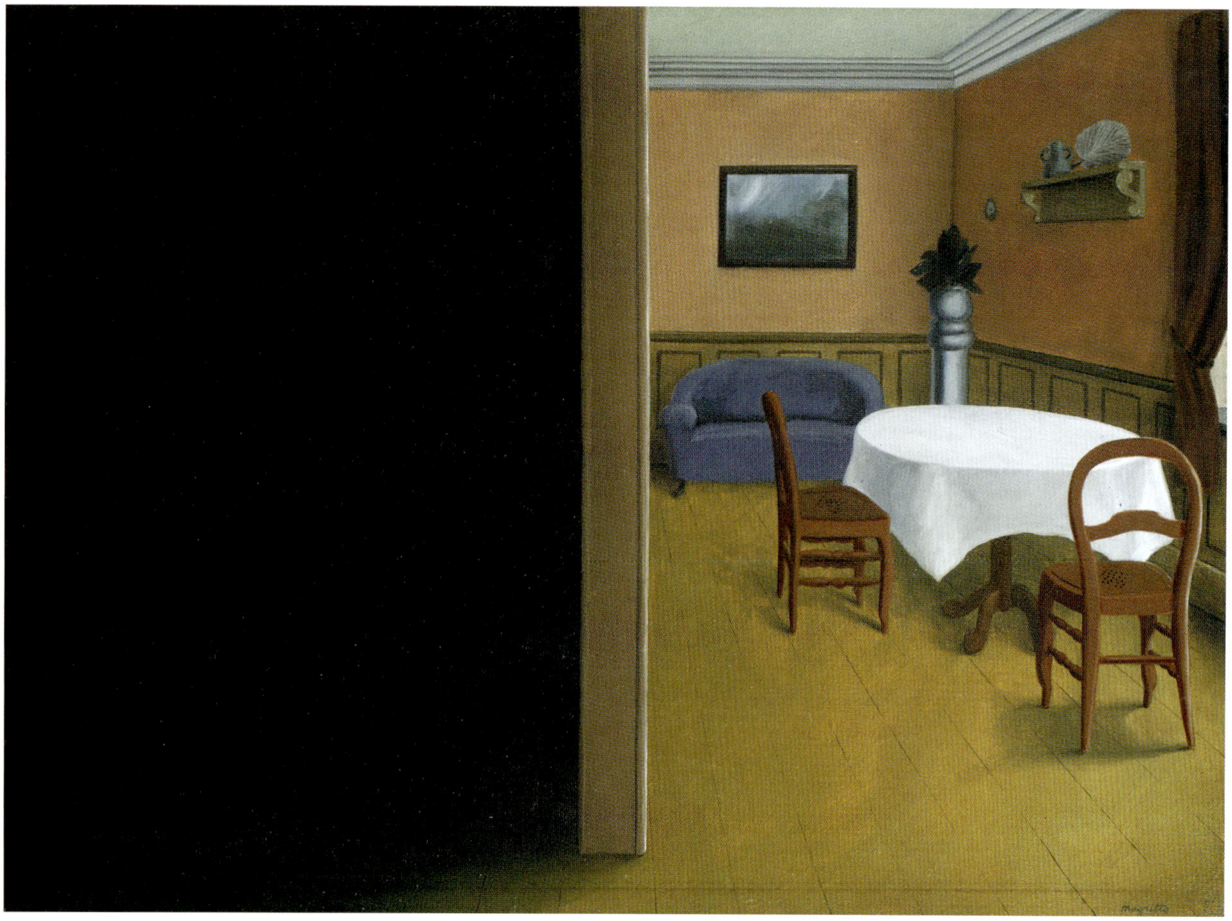

La Voix du silence (1928)

can only be expressed in terms of the presence of the clasped hands that had held them. In just the same way, the quality of vacatedness embodied by Magritte's darkened room is conveyed by the repleteness of its annexed counterpart, with which it shares a single spatial continuum. Because what emerges as visible is articulated, what is not visible remains unarticulated, rather than being non-existent; a second room is unseeable, as opposed to erased. As Douglas MacAgy put it, there is a 'felt presence' in Magritte's absences.[20] The darkness in *La Voix du silence* is just such a pregnant absence. It is a representation of a repression and functions in the same way as the obscurity of the fourth pigeon-hole in *Le Musée d'une nuit* in that it conceals a presence. As Berger argues, the process is one of inserting 'an *absence* in a statement made in a language originally and specially developed for depicting particular events in particular settings'.[21] In the words of Paul-Gustave van Hecke, it amounts to 'a negation of painting'.[22] The discourse, to return to Berger's analysis, centres on 'what is *not* shown, upon the event that is *not* taking place, upon what can *dis*appear'.[23]

What cannot be said of the darkness in *La Voix du silence* is that it imparts any kind of semantic precision. There is no sense of what it does not reveal. Imprecision and vagueness, however, are not the inevitable consequences of an absence. As *L'Homme au journal* (1927) shows, precisely the converse can equally occur. Four identical depictions of the same domestic interior are placed side by side, but only in one of these does Magritte depict the man reading a newspaper referred to in the title. In the other three the protagonist is simply not there. Nevertheless, his single appearance is enough to tell us exactly what it is that Magritte goes on to omit. One commentator aptly, although inaccurately, translated the title as 'Now, you don't'.[24] As it seems logical that the seated reader should appear with each reprise of the dining-room scenario, along with the decorative ornaments, the stove, the window and the table and chairs which are repeated, we imagine him as overlooked or 'hidden', rather than as non-extant. Indeed, Magritte was at pains to point out this very nuance:

> In the invisible it is still necessary to distinguish the invisible and what is hidden. There is a type of visible that is hidden – a letter in an envelope, for example, is an instance of hidden visible, but it is not the invisible.[25]

Like a sealed envelope, the unoccupied table is charged with potential content.

What *L'Homme au journal* does is to *point out* potential content. It impresses on the spectator that three of the repeated images are denuded. Precisely because absence is its key message, the painting does more than simply omit a pictorial element; it *shows* that there has been an omission. Lecomte goes as far as to say that absence in Magritte's work 'materializes'.[26] Indeed, even though the man reading a newspaper is not depicted in three of the four frames, he continues

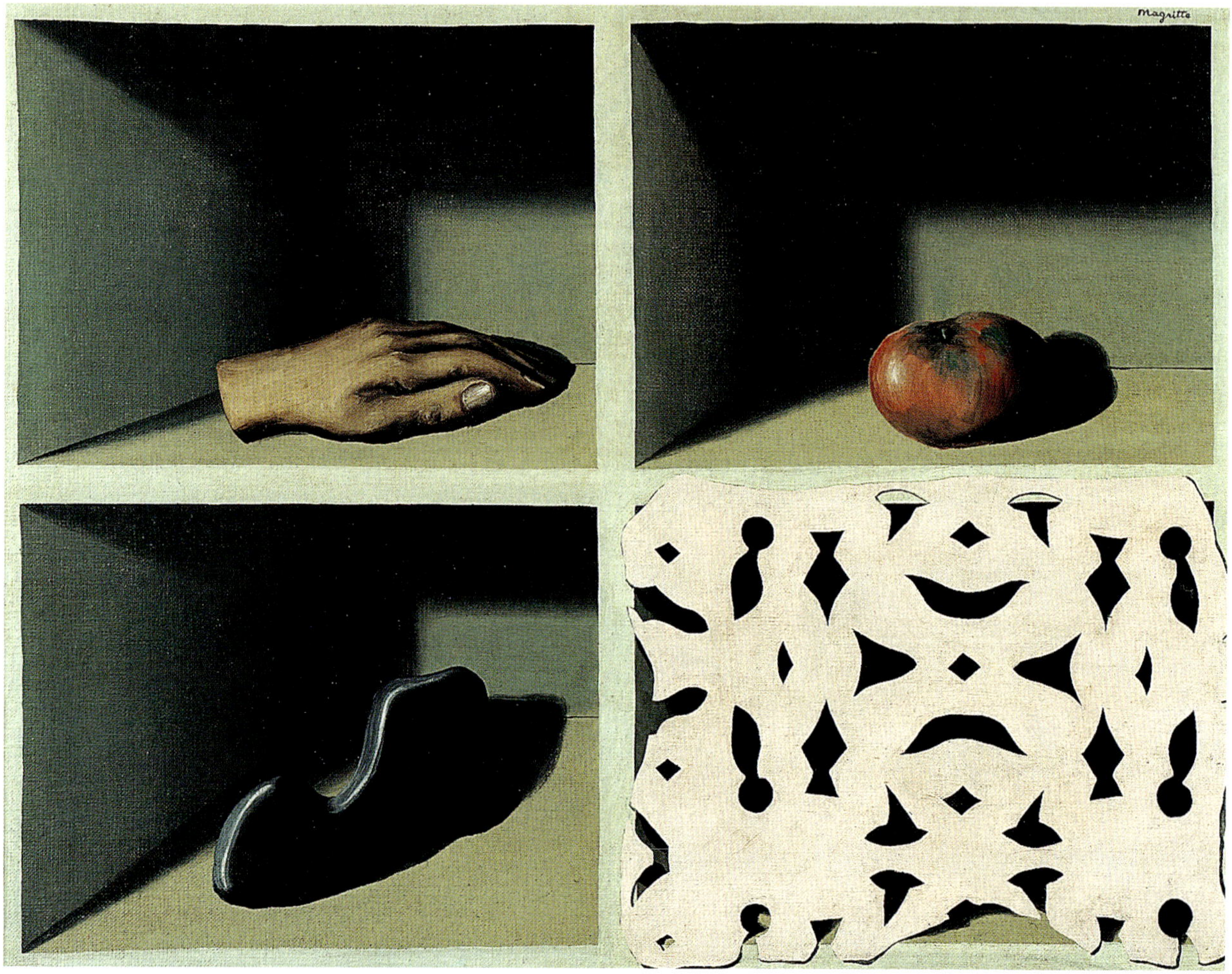

Le Musée d'une nuit (1927)

to exert a palpable non-presence in them. This same effect is conveyed in *Personnage méditant sur la folie* (1928), in which the spotlight is clearly thrown onto a point in space where nothing is present. A sombre figure is seen staring fixedly at a table-top, but, as in *L'Homme au journal*, our attention is drawn to something that is not visible. The clean white surface is patently bare. What changes here, however, is that there is no indication of what has been removed from view. In this sense, the absence is more drastic than in *La Voix du silence* or *L'Homme au journal*. It is as though, as well as giving rise to a depletion within the painting, the absence is depleted in itself. In *Personnage méditant sur la folie* the significative essence of the absence is diminished; whereas in *L'Homme au journal* Magritte had shown exactly what was missing and in *La Voix du silence* he had given a vague suggestion of what was obscured, in this case he gives no clues at all about the identity of the omission. All that can be said is that the situational context points to an omitted entity that is

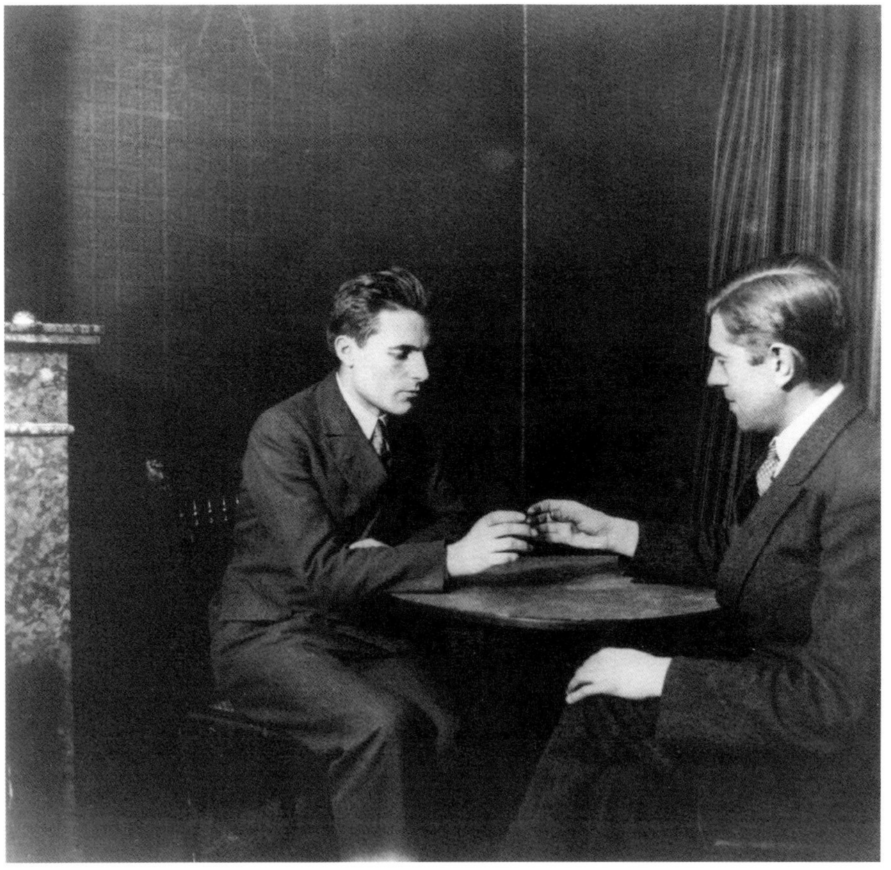

Paul Nougé, *Les Buveurs* (1929)

both finite and indeterminate. The *grammatical* scene-setting does not so much decipher a non-appearance, as it had in *L'Homme au journal*, as simply situate it. By devising forceful compositional cues, Magritte is able to negate the *semantic* object, erasing its *meaning* as well as its *presence*, whilst leaving the footprint of that negation. In this way, Magritte reaches the final stage of his dissolution, at which pictorial presence is emptied of all significance, as well as being expunged. The last three 'retakes' in *L'Homme au journal* had, at least, contained lingering denotative traces, but in *Personnage méditant sur la folie* there is total vacuity. All that the painting can do is to signal the location that accommodates this vacuity. As Enrico Crispolti suggests, the attack is on semanticity and not just pictoriality: 'his trajectory hints at the dissolution of every aspect of the visible trait, (but also) of every notion'.[27] What is sabotaged is the referent, as well as the signifier.

Yet, Magritte's semantic attenuation goes still further by eating away at the only thing that could be said to persist, the elemental notion of the *locus* of an absence. Of course, signification had been totally effaced at this juncture, but what remained was the residual, albeit paradoxical, concept of the spatial fix for the omitted entity. It is with this lingering sense of the positioning of

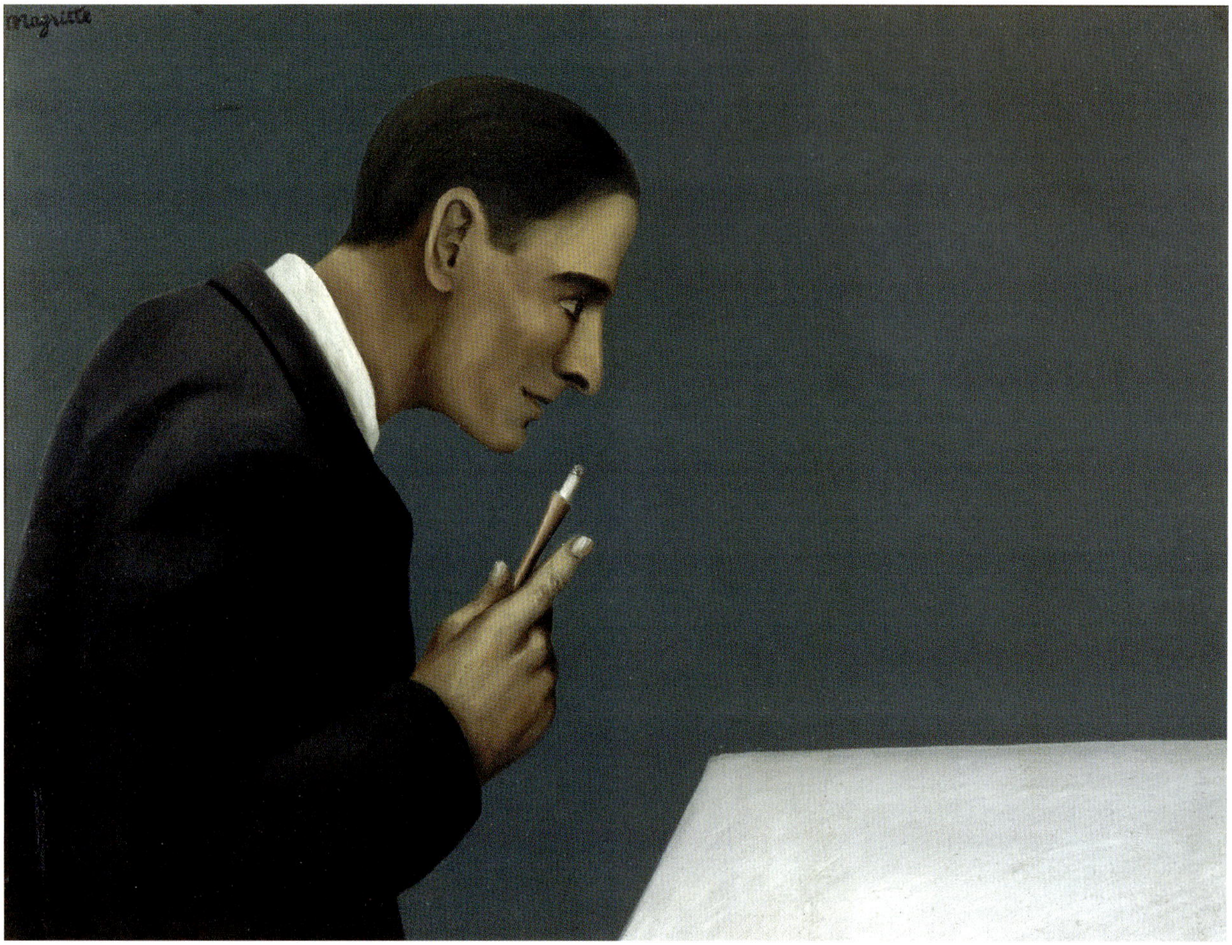

Personnage méditant sur la folie (1928)

lacunae within the painting, together with their respective implied magnitude, that Magritte's dissolution finally concerns itself. The concluding assault on unfilled space, it would seem, takes the form of a progressive contraction. The vacuity in *La Voix du silence* had occupied a whole room, whilst in *L'Homme au journal* it shrank to the size of a missing figure. Still more curtailment occurred in *Personnage méditant sur la folie*, where the unseen entity is limited to a table-top. But it is in *Le Soupçon mystérieux* (1928) that Magritte achieves his ultimate telescoping of emptiness. A motionless figure fixates on no more than a single point on the palm of his hand. The non-entity that he cannot see and merely 'suspects', as the title implies, is a pinpoint. In this climactic work, Magritte reduces an absence that is already indeterminate to miniscule proportions. The anatomical dimension regresses, therefore, to the most elementary of visual traces, the dot, and even this is expressed as a negated presence. Anatomy, in the end, ceases to have measure as well as signification. *Le Soupçon mystérieux* depicts nothingness and situates it nowhere.

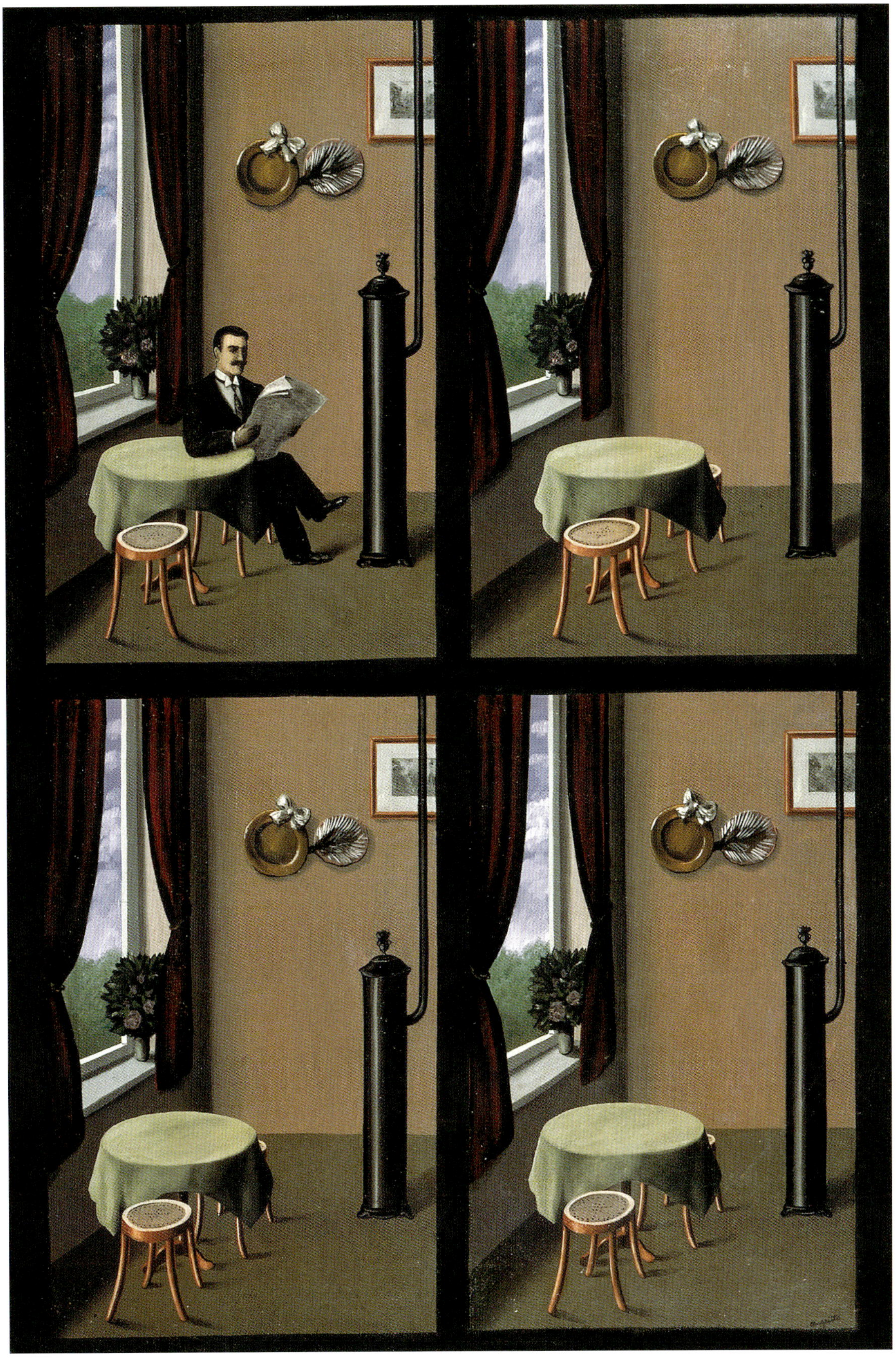

L'Homme au journal (1927)

[1] Michel Foucault, *Ceci n'est pas une pipe* (Montpellier, 1973), pp. 54-5.

[2] Foucault, *Ceci n'est pas une pipe*, p. 54.

[3] The term was coined by Robert Roseblum, in 'Magritte's Surrealist Grammar', *Art Digest* (15 Mar. 1954): 16.

[4] Robert Lebel, *Magritte, Paintings* (London, 1969): n. pag.

[5] Foucault, *Ceci n'est pas une pipe*, p. 54.

[6] Leon Battista Alberti, *On Painting*, trans. John R. Spencer (London, 1956), p. 67.

[7] Paul Nougé, *L'Histoire de ne pas rire* (Brussels, 1956), p. 236.

[8] Leon Battista Alberti, *On Painting, On Sculpture*, trans. Cecil Grayson (London, 1972), p. 121.

[9] Marcel Mariën, *René Magritte* (Brussels, 1972), p. 132.

[10] René Magritte, *Écrits complets* (Paris, 1979), p. 61.

[11] Foucault, *Ceci n'est pas une pipe*, p. 53.

[12] 9 (15 Jan. 1929): 483.

[13] Magritte, *Écrits complets*, pp. 60, 61.

[14] A. M. Hammacher, *Magritte* (London, 1974), p. 32.

[15] Camille Goemans, in Louis Scutenaire, *Avec Magritte* (Brussels, 1977), p. 23, italics my own.

[16] Willem Verougstraete, in Magritte, *Écrits complets*, p. 126, cited from *Au Large*, Brussels (2 June 1927).

[17] Paul Nougé, *La Subversion des images* (1929-30) (Brussels, 1968), p. 20.

[18] Nougé, *La Subversion des images*, p. 22.

[19] Nougé, *La Subversion des images*, p. 19.

[20] Douglas MacAgy, 'About the Art of Magritte', in exhibition catalogue *René Magritte in America*, Dallas Museum for Contemporary Arts (Texas, 1960), n. pag.

[21] John Berger, 'Arts in Society: A Way to Magritte', *New Society*, 338 (20 Mar. 1969): 450.

[22] Paul-Gustave van Hecke, 'René Magritte', *Le Centaure*, 7 (Apr. 1927): 133.

[23] Berger, 'Arts in Society: A Way to Magritte', p. 450.

[24] In David Larkin (ed.), *Magritte* (London, 1973), n. pag.

[25] Magritte, *Écrits complets*, p. 603.

[26] Marcel Lecomte, in Magritte, *Écrits complets*, p. 707.

[27] Enrico Crispolti, 'Brevi Appunti per Magritte', in exhibition catalogue *Magritte*, L'Attico (Rome, 1963), n. pag.

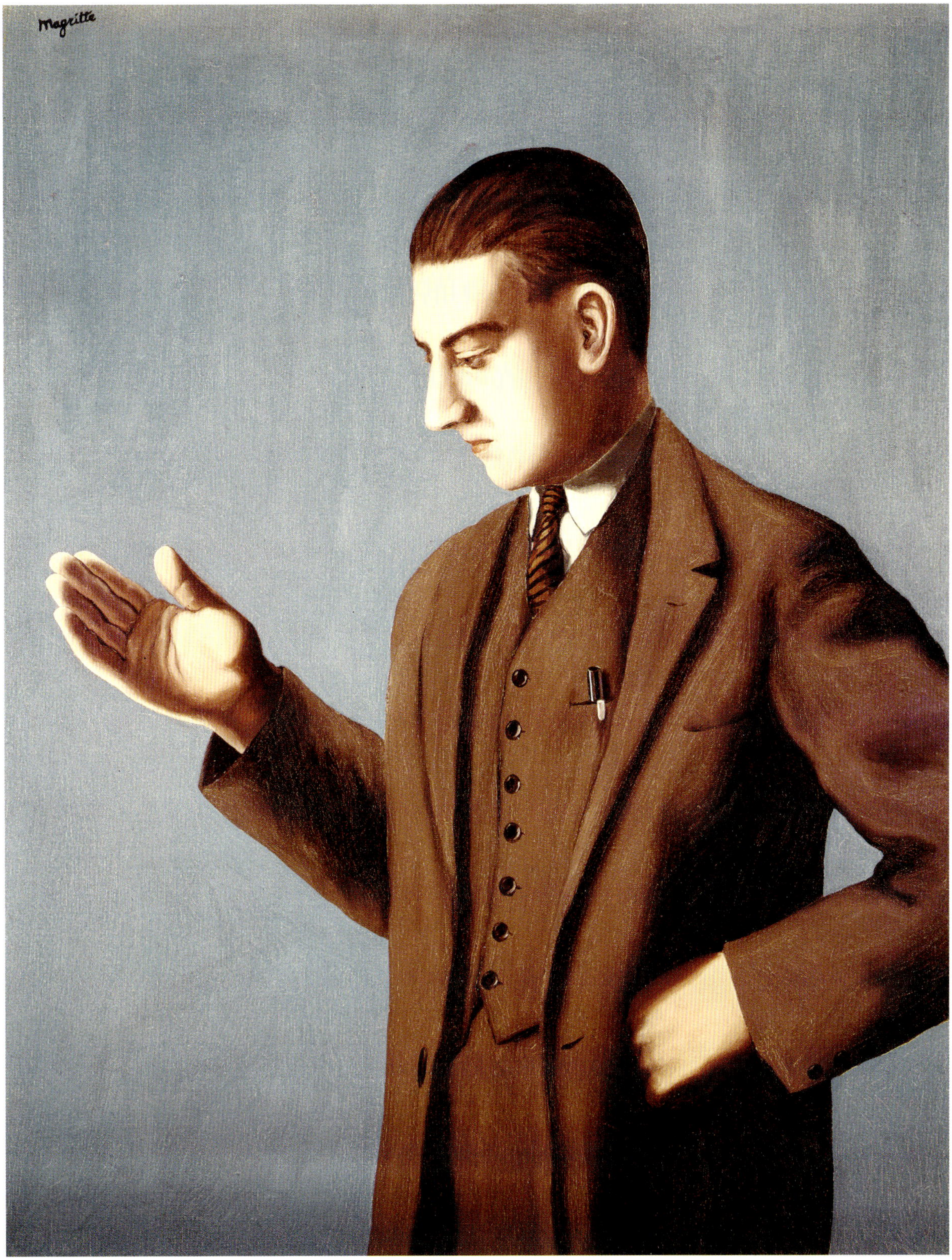

Le Soupçon mystérieux (1928)

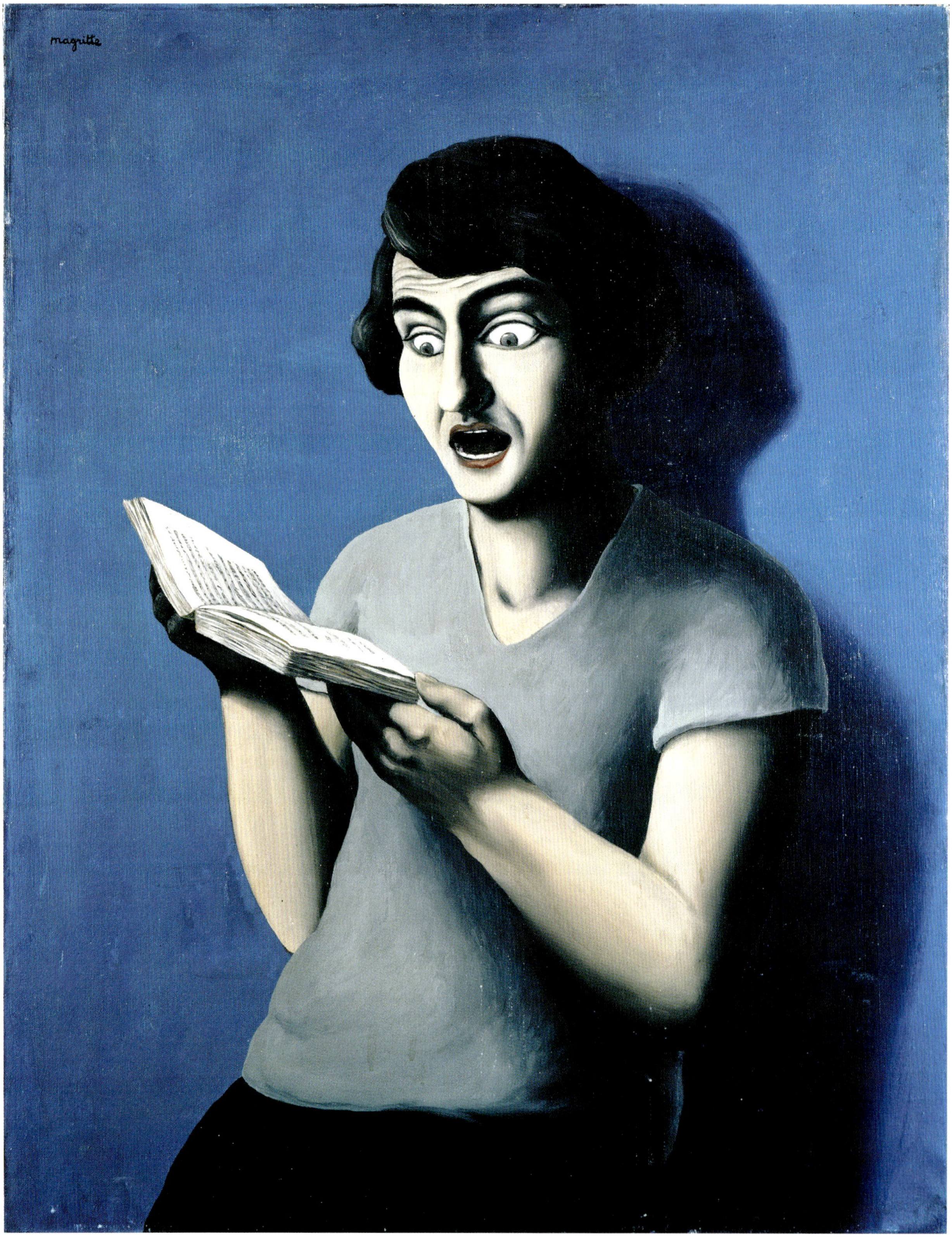

La Lectrice soumise (1928)

Beyond Representation

What Magritte demonstrated was that the representational image can be denuded of semanticity and become no more than a mark of a former presence. To all intents and purposes, he had pulled off a thorough demise of pictorial anatomy. Yet, Magritte continued to be preoccupied with the negation of the anatomical unit, which he felt could be taken beyond this seemingly decisive stage of dissolution. As he saw it, absence still retained nuances of content that could, in their turn, be eliminated as well. Accordingly, he went on to take the further step of depriving the already purged anatomical entity of the one feature that still clung to it, its erstwhile contextualization. Of course, the object had already been subjected to a definitive erasure, but what persisted nevertheless were what could be termed as its vestiges, lingering traces within the space it had occupied. It is these that Magritte proceeded to destabilize, ultimately rendering them irreconcilable with painting itself. To this end, he was to bring about a shift in the very means by which the object, albeit *in absentia*, is referred to within the painting.

The key lay in the transposition of meaningfulness, together with the way in which it is determined, from one system of signification to another. The final rigour to which Magritte subjected the semantic entity was, in fact, that of being shifted out of the confines of the schema of painting and into the antithetical domain of the verbal. But the basis of such a shift, which is denoted by the emergence of words in the early works, is to be found beyond Magritte's oeuvre, in the experiments that were being conducted contemporaneously by Nougé. In his own exploration of absence, realized through the medium of photography, Nougé had, as noted earlier, referred to 'an action carried out by means of an object, suppression of the object' and had given the example of *Les Buveurs*, in which the 'suppressed' drinking glasses of two companions had been removed.[1] A further example, *Yeux clos, bouche scellée (Les Vendanges du sommeil)*, follows the same pattern and depicts a man who is writing in full flow when, apparently, 'the pen is taken away' (21). Nougé's 'methodical exploration', which placed a conceptual distance between what we expect to see and what we are shown, continued with its second step, 'an action exercised by means of an object, modification of this object' (17, 23). Not only is the object in question now removed from the contextual setting, but it is also replaced by a totally different object: 'A woman is putting on make-up', we are told, 'the mirror is replaced by the head of a statue' (24). In other words, the *deletion* of the pictorial unit is, as in this case, superseded by its *substitution*. What results is that the original, absented object attains greater remoteness from the setting. By being replaced by an alternative, the eliminated presence is conceptually twice removed from its previous context. Engineered in this way, absence becomes more cogent than straightforward omission. More than just removing an object, Nougé denied it any direct relationship with its earlier situation. Indeed, since the scenario enters into a new relationship with a second object, the absented, first object no longer exercises a 'felt presence'.[2] In the first set of circumstances there had been a definite relationship between the context and the absence of the object, in that presence remained a potentiality; in the second situation, the primary relationship is between the replacement object and the scene. Only by inference is the original object perceived at all.

Notwithstanding, however frustrated, the relationship between the context and the original object was still one, as Nougé implied, that had originated from a *causal* association. Indeed, in both of the situations considered so far the absented object had had some *bearing* on the form of the context; as is pointed out, 'the action' had been brought about 'by means of the object'. For example, the way in which the hand is held in *Yeux clos, bouche scellée (Les Vendanges du sommeil)* could only be accounted for by the specific object 'pen'. In a further set of situations Nougé went on to suggest that the two levels of absenting objects, *suppression* and *substitution*, could equally well occur in instances where the link between the pictorial unit and its compositional context is more tenuous to begin with. Instead of being the inevitable *consequence* of the object, the action could, for instance, only be 'exercised *on* the object' (24, italics my own). The action, or pictorial context, could, therefore, just as well have been directed towards an alternative object. As the third step of his exploration, Nougé, accordingly, described a situation in which there is 'an action exercised on an object', which is then followed by a 'suppression of the object'. He gave as an example the following: 'Standing on a chair, a woman hangs her coat on thin air'.[3] As before, the object around which the pictorial context is created is omitted from the scene. This situation, however, differs from, say, *Les Buveurs* in that there is less precision about the missing item; logically, the woman could be hanging her coat on any of a number of supports. Consequently, the subject of the absence now becomes indeterminate. As there is no necessary connection between the object and the action, the removal of the object has the effect of linking a variety of alternative complements to the action. Unsurprisingly, once absented, the pictorial unit arising from this kind of context not only loses its identity, but it also leaves no clues about what could be missing. The object is not just suppressed; it is rendered indeterminable.

It therefore follows that the fourth development of Nougé's exploration can only be 'an action exercised on an object, modification of the object'. By way of example, we are told that:

> A group of people are looking at a particularly engaging and specifically located spectacle. This spectacle is substituted with a mundane wall. (24)

As in the second situation, the object is distanced from the action by being superseded by another object, in this case, a wall. Coupled to this, however, is the feature of the third situation, the lack of a unique rapport between the action and the object, which creates a scenario in which absence is both indeterminate and alienated. Formulated in this way, absence finally becomes conceptually conclusive. In earlier examples, the deduced absence had been balanced by an implicit potential presence. Here, the notion of reversing an omission or regenerating a suppression is precluded. Nougé had, as it were, operated a one-way valve: the pictorial unit is taken out of the pictorial context and is left with no way of returning. The anatomical unit, in other words, is ousted from the realm of the pictorial.

Nougé's differentiated expressions of absence, his straightforward exclusion of objects and his subsequent transmutations are, unsurprisingly, echoed in Magritte's own take on the theme. The initial phase of the first dichotomy, simple absence where there is a causal link between what is present and what is absented, is the basis of Magritte's *L'Homme au journal*, where there is precision about what is missing. The second phase of the first dichotomy, simple absence where the contextual situation is conceivably applicable to a variety of objects, occurs in *Personnage méditant sur la folie* and in *Le Soupçon mystérieux*, in both of which the absented entity is not so closely related to the situation presented. In the first case, the context compels the spectator to reconstitute the three missing newspaper readers; in the second case, the 'action' evokes a variety of possible unexpressed objects. Magritte also distinguished an intermediary stage of absence that possesses traits of both of these scenari in *La Voix du silence*, in which the spectator knows what is missing, but only in a general sense and the precise configuration of what is pictorially omitted by the shrouding darkness remains unspecified.

Magritte's rendition of the second, *compound* form of absence is signalled, as it is in Nougé's photographs, by the incongruity of the protagonists' responses to their situation. The perplexing intensity with which Nougé's gathered guests had fixated on a blank wall clearly shows that there had been a previous, more captivating focus of their attention, which has since been removed and substituted. Similarly, a woman's startled reflex in Nougé's *Femme effrayée par une ficelle* comes across as irreconcilable with an innocuous tangle of string from which she shields her eyes. In both photographs, gestural inappropriateness becomes a sign (and logically so) of 'suppression' and 'modification'. The same can be said of Magritte's *La Lectrice soumise* (1928), whose protagonist starts in horror at the sight of the pages of an open book. Seen through Nougé's schema, her disproportionate reaction betokens the erasure of a now vanished and more apposite bête noire, which would have merited the alarm we see. The absented terror has, as would appear, been replaced with a book. Magritte, however, does more than fill the void left by the suppressed object with an alternative, less appropriate pictorial element, as Nougé's formula would have prescribed. Instead, he supplants the initial cause of the protagonist's distress with a form of 'modification' that is *outside* the scope of representation, the written word. After all, the woman is now responding to what she is reading, not to what she is holding. Unlike Nougé, therefore, Magritte does not counteract the remnants of absented pictorial content with a conflicting pictorial *presence*; rather he transposes them beyond pictoriality altogether. So, whilst following the principles mapped out by Nougé, Magritte's own compounding of absence (suppression and modification) ends up as a far more radical form of decontextualization. *La Lectrice soumise* can, indeed, be seen to play out Nougé's 'modification' of a pictorial suppression, but the way in which it does so marks a change of gear in Magritte's assault on anatomy.

This is because Magritte's shift to words signals not just a *modification* of the absented pictorial unit, but also one that transcends the pictorial frame of reference. Nougé's procedure functions as a metaphorical shift; a unit in a syntagmatic sequence is first suppressed and then replaced by a substitute within the same genus. In other words, one object is replaced by another object. Modification here involves a movement within a particular paradigm, that of pictorial objects. Magritte's rationale, however, involves more than such a straightforward 'compounding' of absence. It is not so much a question of displacement along the axis of selection, as a transposition into a wholly separate syntagmatic chain. The transference is to a *parallel* system of signs. Whereas Nougé had engineered a move away from one pictorial unit and towards another, Magritte brings about a shift away from pictoriality altogether. Words, therefore, take on the role of adversaries of objects, bringing about the abandonment of the pictorial frame of reference and an engagement with an alternative system of signification, that of language, from which the visual is, logically, excluded. Words operate as negators of the pictorial, and push visual content beyond the bounds of representation.

When he labels a key, a wine glass and a guitar, 'the ocean', 'the bird' and 'the tree' respectively in a drawing of 1929, Magritte leaves us in no doubt that words in his work contest pictorial signification.[4] For him, the graphic realm is dissociated from that of images. Indeed, as he pointed out, it is necessary to 'distinguish thought constituted by words (speech) and thought constituted by [...] painting'; for him the latter is to be considered as 'another language'.[5] Michel Butor maintains that, in works of art, even when words and images are not presented as semantically conflicting, there is nevertheless a fundamental disparity between what is written and what is depicted. In his description of Juan Gris's poem-drawing *As de pique...*, in which drawings are substituted for some of the words, Butor insists that 'each of these elements has two locations

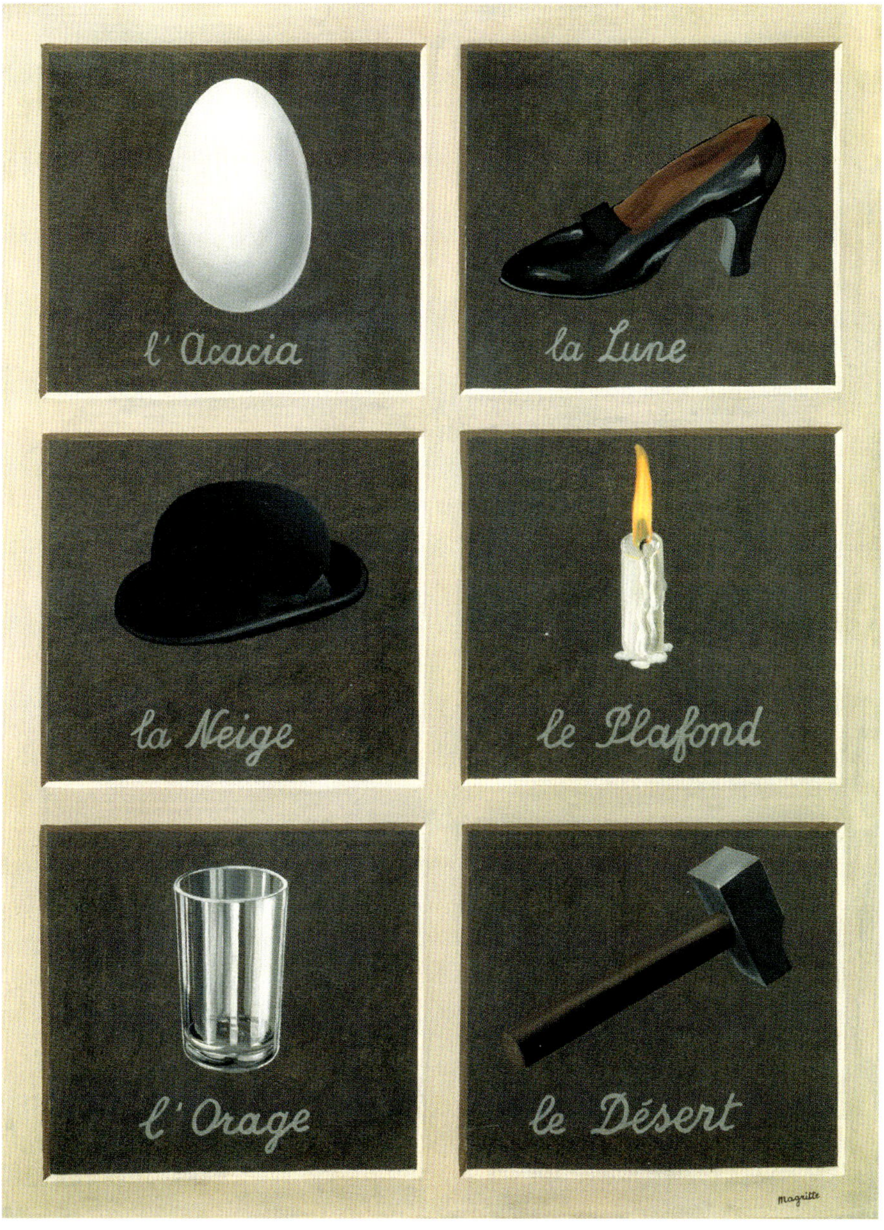

La Clef des songes (1930)

in the composition: that of its name, that of its figuration'.[6] As he explains, the 'two compositions are superimposed'.[7] Magritte made the point pictorially; in the fourth statement of his 'Les Mots et les images', a barrier in the form of a vertical line divides the verbal from the pictorial and, even though the referent of the word is the same as that of the drawing, the two alternative expressions of 'Forest' are presented as irreconcilable.[8] It is neither indicated that the word is an explanation of the image nor that the image is an illustration of the word; each simply resides in its discrete compartment, isolated from its counterpart.

Indeed, in his commentary, Magritte does not indicate that there is any essential relationship between the two 'representations' of the single meaning, but simply implies that they are annexed in a more or less incidental and even gratuitous manner: 'The image and the name of an object happen to meet'.[9] Maurice Rapin notes that Magritte established 'the difference that separates words and images [...] what is written, what is shown'.[10]

Further differentiating the verbal from the visual, Magritte was at pains to show that, in contradistinction to images, the way in which words relate to their referent is without rational foundation. As *La Clef des songes* (1930) conveys pictorially, 'the relationship between the name of an object and the object itself is only established in an arbitrary manner'.[11] Convention, as the work proposes, could just as well have associated the phrase 'The acacia' with an egg, 'The moon' with a shoe, 'Snow' with a hat, 'The ceiling' with a candle, 'The storm' with a glass and 'The desert' with a hammer. Moreover, Magritte never permitted words to enter the pictorial illusion and share the plasticity of objects. As *L'Usage de la parole I* demonstrates, the spidery inscriptions are not constituted from true substance; instead, they remain shadowless, unlike their neighbouring solidly modelled blobs. To all effects, words are present in Magritte's oeuvre in only a tenuous manner and, conceptually, linger outside pictorial space. They are in attendance and yet are never integrated in the representational narrative. According to Aragon, words in Magritte's work echo the role of collage in painting, remaining not only extraneous to the medium, but also being 'the absolute opposite of painting, beyond painting'.[12] Certainly, Magritte saw representation as a self-contained system, which, like all meaningful schemas, possesses 'frontiers', beyond which there are only 'external elements'.[13] Words, to him, were such outsiders, alien to the domain of the visible.

But words are more than just fish out of water. Their inclusion in the paintings creates a state of tension since they unremittingly gainsay the assertions of the image; even when the image affirms that we see the naked woman in *La Femme cachée* (1929), the words insist that we do not. They pressurize the visual to absent itself.[14] Through the act of bringing words into his work, therefore, Magritte edged his scenari towards the periphery of the pictorial schema. For him, words functioned as pictorial inhibitors. The progressive dissolution may have denied objects the capacity to impose their presence, but their resulting absence, logically, still resides within the pictorial. Words carry Magritte's dissolution beyond absence, to a nebulous exteriority. They fill the space left by absented objects and thwart beyond salvage the residual identity they had displaced. The verbal dimension is the ultimate barrier to pictorial meaning; its foreignness to the figurative does not just de-route the semanticity of the image, it deactivates it altogether. Acting as a pictorial doublethink, words wipe away the object and then erase the memory of its disappearance.

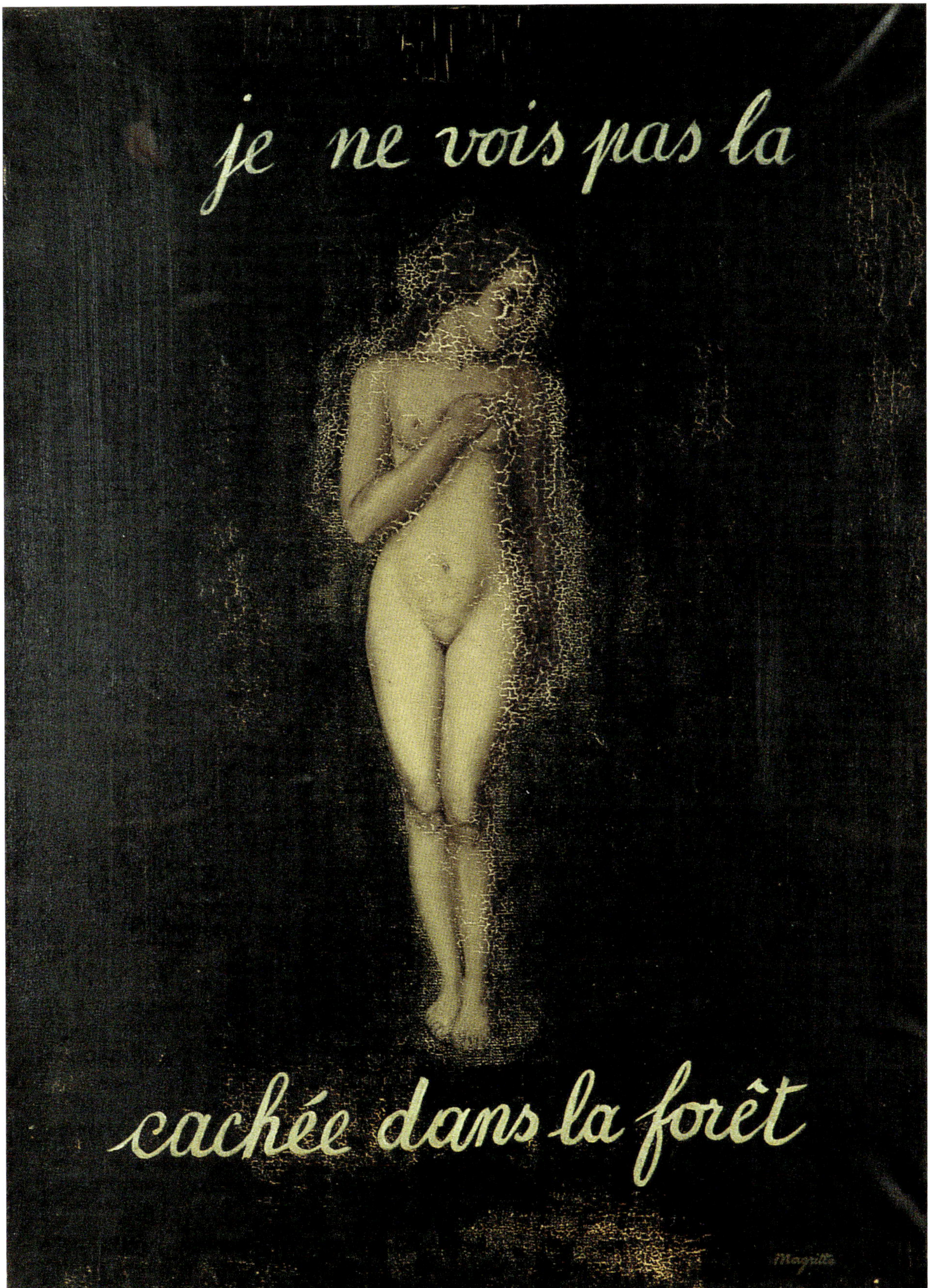
je ne vois pas la
cachée dans la forêt
Magritte

La Femme cachée (1929)

[1] Paul Nougé, *La Subversion des images*, (1929-1930) (Brussels, 1968), p. 68. Further page references are given in parentheses in the main text.

[2] Douglas MacAgy, 'About the Art of Magritte', in exhibition catalogue *René Magritte in America*, Dallas Museum for Contemporary Arts (Texas, 1960), n. pag.

[3] Nougé, *La Subversion des images*, p. 24. In order to clarify an inconsistency in Nougé's exposition, his third stage of absence is presented as the fourth and his fourth stage as the third.

[4] *Variétés*, 9 (15 Jan. 1929): 478.

[5] René Magritte & André Souris, 'Entre Musique et peinture' (1952), *Le Fait Accompli*, 67 (June 1972): n. pag.

[6] Michel Butor, 'Les Mots dans la peinture', *Répertoire IV* (Paris, 1974): 95.

[7] Butor, 'Les Mots dans la peinture': 95.

[8] René Magritte, *Écrits complets* (Paris, 1979), p. 60.

[9] Magritte, *Écrits complets*, p. 60.

[10] Maurice Rapin, *Aphorismes* (Viry-Chatillon, 1970), p. 31.

[11] Pamela Tytell, 'Lacan et l'anglais tel qu'on le parle', *Magazine littéraire*, 121 (Feb. 1977): 15.

[12] Louis Aragon, *Les Collages* (Paris, 1965), p. 54.

[13] Jean Piaget, *Le Structuralisme* (Vendôme, 1974), p. 6.

[14] *La Femme cachée* (1929) appeared in *La Révolution surréaliste*, 12 (1929): 73, as part of a montage featuring members of the surrealist grouping with their eyes shut.

Decoding

The reason why words are fundamentally extrinsic to the pictorial medium is that language and iconic representation are exclusive, distinct systems of signification. But, this does not mean that within their respective confines the two systems cannot display parallels in their internal organization. As Foucault observes, the linguistic system 'has, in its nature and in its make-up, relationships that are identical to those of representation'.[1] What follows is that there is, arguably, a correspondence between the ways in which representation can be said to 'dissolve' in Magritte's early works and the ways in which language breaks down under certain pathological conditions. The various forms of aphasic linguistic disintegration, in particular, can therefore be advanced as a model for Magritte's dissolution of the norms of representation. As with aphasia, this can be analyzed in terms of two distinct operations, compositional abatement and anatomical disarticulation. Stemming from that, Magritte's break-down of visual constructs can be apportioned, but, since aphasia is a graduated condition, it can also be calibrated. In correlation with the aphasic analogy, it can be gauged, therefore, against the rules of 'pictorial syntax' on the one hand and the principles governing the semantic make-up of the representational 'body' on the other. This binary model becomes a yardstick that measures Magritte's depleted structures in terms of the pictorial equivalents of either 'agrammatism' or 'anomia'. Moreover, in further analogy with aphasia, 'grammatical' disruption within the paintings is accompanied by a relative stability of their 'semantic' content. Conversely, and equally in keeping with aphasic distortion, the corruption of pictorial anatomy invariably occurs within cohesive compositional structures.

Agrammatism in its broadest sense is patently exemplified by the pictorial structures within *Cinéma bleu*, *La Fenêtre* and *Georgette*. Given their absence of both internal concatenation and hierarchical organization, these works can only loosely accommodate meaningful units. Pictorial content is left devoid of any rules of pictorial combination. Interrelation in such agrammatic works is either inhibited or permitted to drift outside the constraints of visual comprehensibility. The objects in *Cinéma bleu*, for instance, are 'unbridled' to such an extent that they defy the conventions of composition, in much the same way as the first stage of aphasia disrupts the contiguity of the sentence, the largest grammatical unit in language. Just as linguistic agrammatism fails to combine words by means of grammar, by virtue of the loss of connectives and conjunctions, so space, the pictorial interconnecting medium, falls short in *Cinéma bleu* of providing a unifying context for the objects contained within the painting. These objects are bereft of relational interdependence, making it impossible to quantify the relative positioning of the skittle and the curtain, for example. Not only is the degree of proximity of these objects unclear, but it also remains uncertain whether they are making contact. What is missing in *Cinéma bleu* are the 'pictorial connectives' that would resolve such ambivalence, the markers of space which, like conjunctions in language, establish the existence as well as the nature of interdependence between meaningful units. Inasmuch, *Cinema Bleu* closely corresponds to the syntactic agrammatism that marks one extremity of the aphasic spectrum. Equally paralleled in Magritte's agrammatic works is agrammatism's distinctive retention of the integrity of meaningful units. As *La Fenêtre* demonstrates, the paucity of combinational ties in no way detracts from the intelligibility of the objects themselves; despite inconsistent perspective and its resulting unviable spatial context, the hand, the bird and the curtain are far from ill-defined and appear as clearly-formed objects in credible chiaroscuro. As though making this very point, Magritte depicts two solidly modelled geometric shapes, a pyramid and a rectangular cuboid. These are the mainstays of anatomical comprehensibility *par excellence*.

In its more progressed form, however, agrammatism attacks the structure not just of sentences, but of morphemes as well. In this mode of aphasia there is a loss of inflexions and a reduction of the word to its nominal form. The meaningful unit is standardized, as it were, and its nuances, affixes, variants, tense and mood markers are lost. Correspondingly, Magritte's more compositionally disrupted works, such as *Le Dormeur téméraire* and *Le Musée d'une nuit*, are characterized by a simplification and denudation of the *pictorial* morpheme. In both paintings, Magritte depicts no more than the 'nominal' form of the object. He shows it as severed from any situational context, as no more than an inventoried or displayed item. This effectively decontextualizes the object, reducing it to the status of a prototype or specimen, wholly devoid of contextual modifications, as would be the case for words within morphological agrammatism: the sleeper's objects – mirror, bird, bowler hat, candle, ribbon and apple – all lack the pictorial inflections that would arise from insertion into a functional compositional framework. They remain as pictorial equivalents of verbal 'stems', that is to say elements of a visual lexis that are disconnected from a morphology that would allow them to operate meaningfully in the larger ensemble of a composition.

However much the links between pictorial objects may be severed or attenuated in *Le Dormeur téméraire* and *Le Musée d'une nuit*, paralleling the weakening of the grammatical ties between words in agrammatism, the correspondence between linguistic agrammatism and the dissolution of pictorial composition in Magritte's work extends further. The advanced condition of *phonological agrammatism*, in which actual word-construction is affected, is analogous to certain stages in Magritte's dissolution of anatomy, where the internal structure of the object is disrupted. Arguably though, a disruption of 'object-construction', as opposed to 'object-meaning' does occur as a final stage of the *compositional* dislocation. A closer look at *Cinéma bleu* reveals that the partially resolved objects and figures display an inadequacy of *internal* contiguity. The stage floor, for instance, cannot be said to comprise a coherent *sequence* of its parts. Through such mal-constructs, Magritte defied the norms of pictorial grammar, whilst retaining the intelligibility of individual forms. In the *internally* agrammatic works, individual pictorial meanings remain transparent, whilst the architectural relations *within* those meanings begin to crumble.

But when the wheels of Magritte's 'anomic' dissolution begin to turn it is meaning itself that comes under fire. In concert with meaning-deficient aphasia, where the resolution of words diminishes, the pictorial unit undergoes a progressive attrition in its own right. The process starts with a form of 'mollification', whereby the internal structure of anatomy is disrupted. In one sense, this deconstruction carries echoes of agrammatism in that the *contiguity* within the meaningful unit is eroded. Indeed, paintings such as *Les Idées de l'acrobate* involve a disordering of the inner 'grammar' of the body. They centre on the derangement of the *connections* between the parts of figures and could be regarded as an anomic phonological agrammatism. Both *Les Idées de l'acrobate* and *Les Impatients* do not so much fracture the 'parts' of the pictorial unit as discombobulate their configuration. Notwithstanding, this is distinct from Magritte's infractions of the rules of composition since the distortions and contortions that are imposed on the respective human figures operate on the syntax of *form*, rather than on the grammar of the pictorial *sentence*. However, as the disruption of the pictorial unit progresses from this incipient stage, the issue is less that of the object's aberrant internal arrangement and more that of its identity. In other words, the anatomical deconstruction reaches a point at which representational *meaning*, rather than representational *concatenation*, is put into question. The dissolution takes on a new direction which, as the analytical hypothesis had prefigured, pictorially equates with anomia, the aphasic demise of meaning. Indeed, it is just such an anomic bias towards the deterioration of the semantic unit that is evident in *Chasseurs au bord de la nuit* and *Le Village mental*, in both of which individual forms are stifled. Unlike the 'agrammatic' works, these paintings appear to dissolve or eat up their pictorial *subjects* much in the same way that the first stages of anomia inhibit the nominative noun-phrases of an utterance.

Just as verbal anomia results in difficulty both in identifying and generating words, so Magritte's anatomical dissolution tends towards the unintelligibility of the pictorial object. In contradistinction to the clarity and comprehensibility of a fully resolved depiction, his 'anomic' paintings conceal or mask their subjects, as in *L'Invention de la vie*, in which a shroud veils a foregrounded shape. What is shown is that the figure is *not* shown. The visual utterance becomes not just unexpressed, but also un-expressible, since finite paradigmatic selection is stymied. The pictorial presence is simply 'indicated', in a type of class of possibilities, but its precise configuration is not definitively articulated. The figure we cannot comprehend remains covered. As in the enunciations of the anomic, a prospective referent is tacitly alluded to, but remains trapped in abeyance; it makes its mark, but falls short of being actualized within the utterance.

An alternative, but equally cogent, suppression of the central subject of a painting takes the form of an attritive fragmentation of form. The dislocation of the anatomical body in, say, *Entracte* effectively deletes the semantic essence of what Magritte depicts. He, literally, excises the core, the torso in this case, and leaves only its peripherals, the anatomical members. Mirroring anomic relinquishment of verbal roots, Magritte expresses his subjects in terms of their disembodied appendages, their 'affixes', disjointed from the pictorial stems with which they normally accord. We are left with arms and legs in the place of complete bodies. But dismemberment is only part of the story and the same fundamental process also operates as an eating away of anatomical form, that neutralizes distinguishing features. *La Confidence capitale* shows disjunction, but also effacement. The degeneration involves not so much a detachment of integral parts as an erasure of nuance. What is disturbed is the basic *identity* of the object, as well as its completeness. There is a loss of definition and decipherability, as there is in anomia and, also as in anomia, semanticity or, at least, semantic precision, is diminished. By plastically compromising objects in these ways, Magritte interferes with their representational communicative value and eventually, by dint of his continual experimentation, he suppresses the very comprehensibility of the pictorial unit, leaving only blurry forms devoid of semantic content. At that point, the paintings become peopled with little more than amorphous, indistinguishable traces of meaninglessness.

Yet, however much these depleted, vague presences may be semantically ill-defined in themselves, what is far from uncertain is their status within the wider arrangement of the painting as a whole. Despite their internal paucity, the 'blobs' of the late 1920s invariably stand as clearly demarcated elements within a rigorous context of compositional interrelatedness. Just as in fluent aphasia, where semantic voids are mutually syntagmatically correlated, these nameless shapes function not as meanings, but as connected relative positions. Inasmuch, the anomic works can be said to comprise a state of virtually pure contiguity, that is to say, grammatical ties without semantic content, prepositional relationships without, or without heed to, identity. Indeed, these content-deficient paintings can be said to echo amnestic aphasic discourse, in which the similarity axis becomes virtually inoperative and the substitution set recedes to such an extent that even the verbal label cannot occur together with the visual representation. As Jakobson put it, 'a picture of an object will cause the suppression of its name: a verbal sign is supplanted by a pictorial sign'.[2] With uncanny similarity and contemporaneously with his 'disassembled' works, Magritte had commented that 'an image can take the place of a word [...] the name of an object takes the place of an image'.[3] In both proposals we are told that the symbol is divorced from its verbalized exegesis, putting meaning beyond reach. Even when Magritte does appear to be articulating meaning, and in an overt manner at that, he is, in fact, not only impeding the ascription of signification, but also de-routing the process of identification itself. Just as in amnestic aphasia, metonymical displacement confounds meaning, as opposed to failing to express it. The bird cage in *Les Affinités électives* (1933) is not so much left empty as occupied ineptly. The egg, which is paradigmatically linked to the bird, appears instead of the bird in a context that pertains to the bird, but not to the egg. A 'suppression', as Nougé would have seen it, has been 'modified', so as to result in a semantic shift. Mirroring the aphasic's 'projections from the line of habitual context into the line of substitution and selection', Magritte dislodges primary denotation with an alternative that is itself discordant with the context.[4] Just as much as the meaning-deficient aphasic, Magritte tells us only what is *not* and places the negation where it does *not* belong. Identity drifts and ends up as self-consuming.

In the final analysis, Magritte's visual dissolution can be boiled down to two distinct operations – the disruption of *encoding* on the one hand and of *decoding* on the other. The first trajectory, a form of semiological *agrammatism*, unequivocally enunciates elements drawn from the representational code but, at the same time, it confounds the structural mechanisms that tie these elements together within a cohesive *context*. The result is catalexis in pictorial encoding. The first stage of the process of encoding, morphological *selection*, remains fully resolved, whilst its second phase, syntactic *combination*, undergoes various forms of suppression. Precisely the converse is true, however, in the second type of visual derangement deployed by Magritte, pictorial *anomia*. This opposing trajectory operates by conserving contextualization, that is the mapping of relative spatial loci, whilst simultaneously eroding the ipsesity of what is contexualized. Accordingly, individual incumbents of what are invariably fully articulated compositions lose their anatomical definition and so cease to function as discrete meaningful components of the pictorial code. Magritte, however, did not stop there. He followed his course to its logical extreme and ousted these already depleted presences, by that point perceptible only as mere coordinates, from the pictorial system of signs altogether, supplanting them with words, symbols from a separate and extraneous code. These verbal usurpers finally seal the de-semanticization

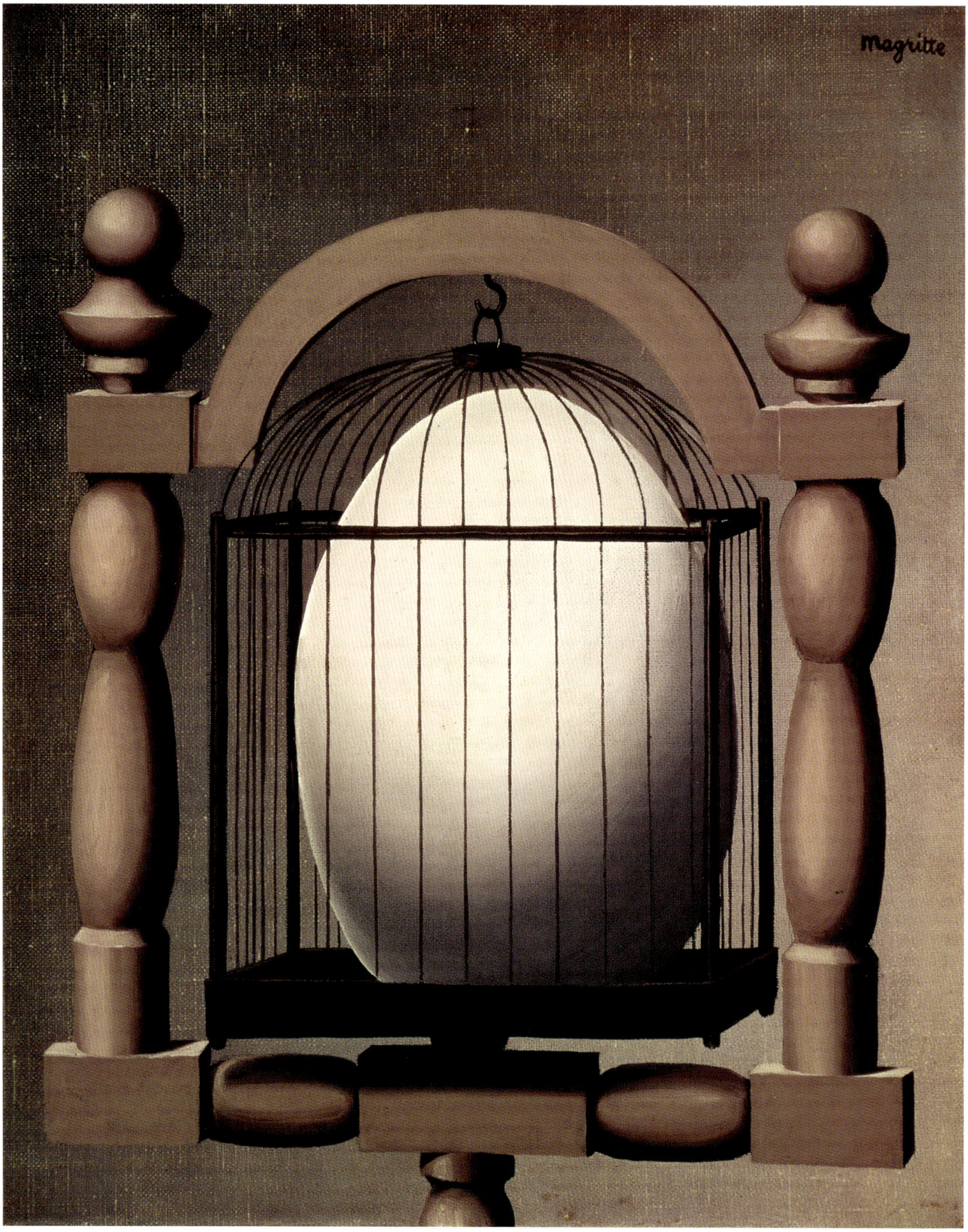

Les Affinités électives (1933)

by not only frustrating, but also overriding meaning. Quite literally, anatomy is *overwritten*. In analogy with anomia, that is decoding defective aphasia, these meaning-deficient works are characterized by an explicitly expressed matrix of *concatenation* within which, however, the second operation of decoding, the *selection* of elements from the code, is precluded. All that endures in the 'fluent' paintings is the 'support of signification'.[5] Meaning itself is eliminated.

The fact that the Albertian schema can be analyzed and, what is more, unravelled in terms that mirror the progressive degeneration of speech that occurs in aphasia, upholds the contention that visual and verbal codes share a common deep structure. What Magritte's early works reveal is that, just as much as language, the pictorial system of signs functions in terms of two structural axes, selection and combination, that are both interwoven and yet *independent* of each other. The relationship between anatomy and composition echoes the correlation between naming and grammar. But, because aphasia reveals the fundamental workings not just of language but of the intellect itself, Magritte's 'aphasic' pictorial deconstruction strips down much more than the mechanisms of picture-making. In the course of its devastation of painting, it succeeds in laying bare and crippling the elemental building blocks of visual intelligibility itself.

---

1 Michel Foucault, *Les Mots et les choses* (Paris, 1966), p. 113.

2 Roman Jakobson & Morris Halle, *Fundamentals of Language* (The Hague, 1956), p. 66.

3 René Magritte, *Écrits complets* (Paris, 1979), p. 60. The text was first published in 1929.

4 Jakobson & Halle, *Fundamentals of Language*, p. 69.

5 Roland Barthes, *Système de la mode* (Paris, 1967), p. 73.

INTERVIEWS

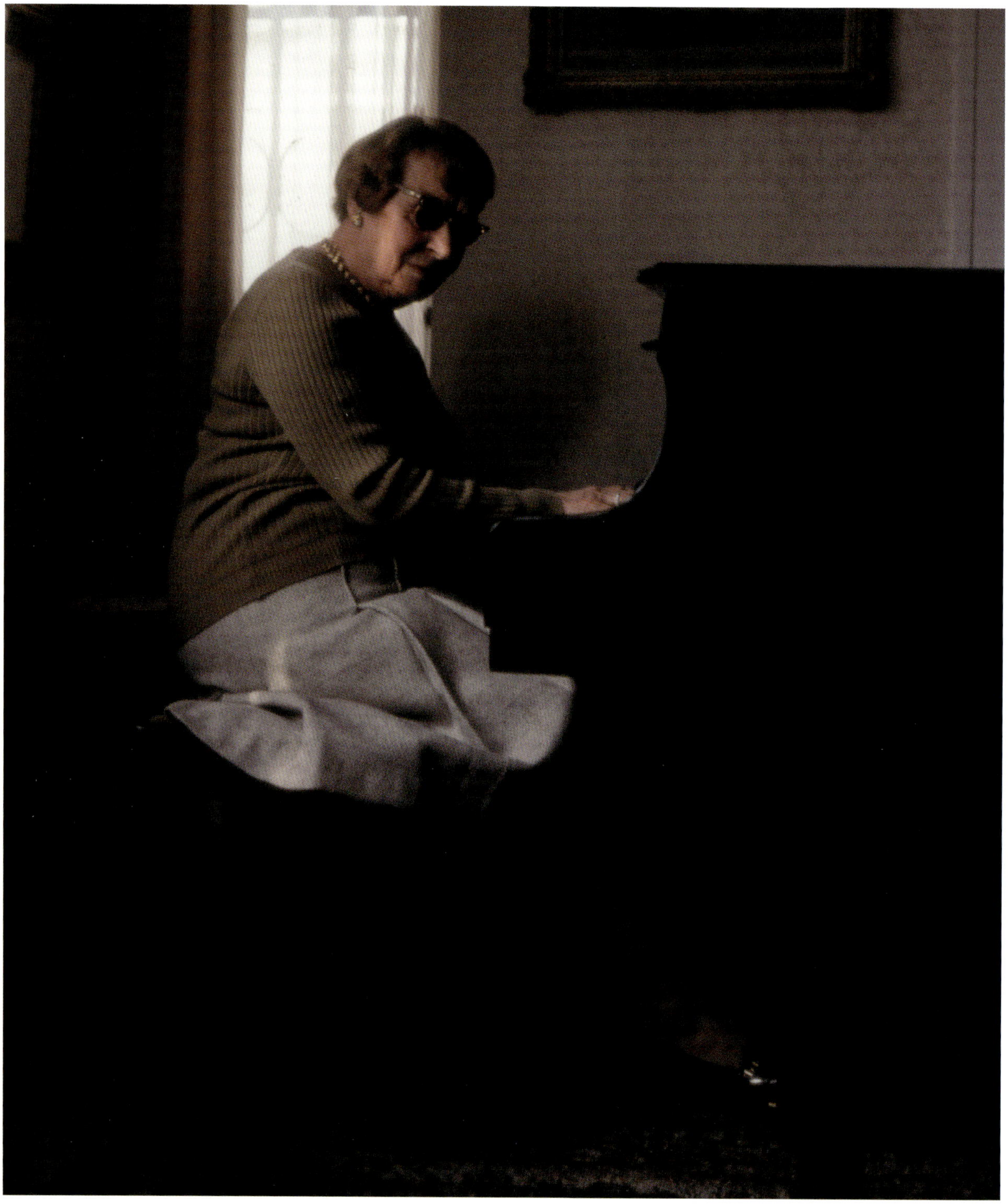

Georgette Magritte, parlour, rue des Mimosas 97, Brussels, 1981

Georgette Magritte

- Vous trouvez-vous constamment occupée par l'œuvre de votre mari ?
GM Actuellement? Je ne fais, pour ainsi dire, que ça. Il y a beaucoup de gens qui me demandent des renseignements, qui me demandent pour exposer des tableaux. Enfin, c'est toujours beaucoup de courrier, beaucoup de coups de téléphone, pour faire des cartes postales, des reproductions, des expositions, alors je suis constamment occupée de ça.

Avez-vous beaucoup d'œuvres de votre mari ?
GM Oui, assez quand même, parce que j'en ai en haut. Je vous montrerai l'atelier de mon mari si vous voulez.

*- Ce tableau (*La Pipe*, 1923) n'est-il pas de votre sœur ?*
GM Oui, j'ai maintenant des tableaux que nous avions donnés, si vous voulez, à ma sœur. Et ma sœur étant décédée les tableaux sont revenus chez moi. C'est comme ça que j'en ai assez bien. Parce qu'ici tous ces tableaux n'ont jamais changé de place, mais ceux que j'ai en haut, j'en ai un peu plus qu'autrefois. Vous savez, ce qui est resté ici, c'est le hasard. Nous n'avons pas choisi. Sauf celui-ci que mon mari a fait pour moi, expressément pour moi. (*Le Domaine d'Arnheim*, 1962). Mais les autres c'est le hasard qui a fait que [...] parce que mon mari vendait assez bien. Parfois il promettait un tableau à quelqu'un qui un an après disait 'Tiens, Monsieur Magritte, vous m'avez promis un tableau'. Alors s'il en avait fait un que j'aimais garder, il disait 'Bon, tu sais cette personne m'a demandé un tableau, en effet il y a bien un an. Je vais donner celui-là'. Et puis alors il le donnait. 'Mais je t'en ferai un autre', disait-il.

- Alors il n'avait pas l'esprit d'un commerçant ?
GM Oh non, pas du tout, ni de conservateur non plus. Ça ne l'ennuyait pas du tout que ses tableaux s'en aillent. Il pouvait les vendre, il pouvait les donner. Il en a donné beaucoup. Il voulait bien les brûler. N'importe quoi. Ça ne l'intéressait plus. Son idée était réalisée, n'est-ce pas ? Alors ce qui l'intéressait, c'était le prochain tableau auquel il pensait.

- Comment a-t-il réagi envers le succès ? Il y a une rue René Magritte, n'est-ce pas ?
GM Oui, il y a une petite rue René Magritte que moi j'ignorais quand même. C'est un ouvrier qui est venu ici qui me l'a dit. Mais il y en a aussi, à Lessines dans la ville où il est né. La maison où il est né, et on a fait une fête, on a mis une plaque – Ici est né René Magritte – et puis on a nommé une nouvelle grande

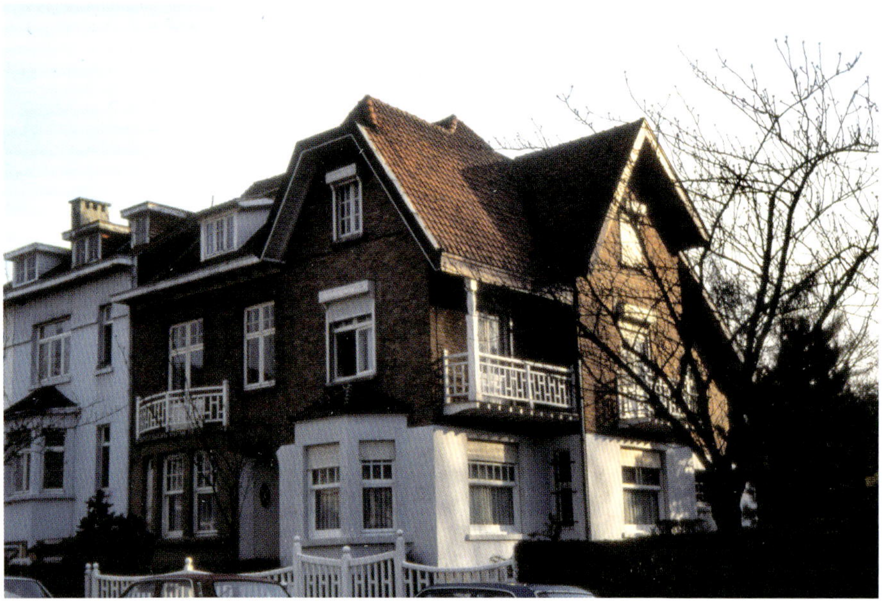

Rue des Mimosas 97, Brussels, 1981

artère. On a aussi nommé une avenue René Magritte. Je l'ai vue il y a trois ou quatre ans, au moment où ça c'est fait, mais je ne sais pas depuis si on a construit une grande nouvelle artère. On allait lui trouver un nom, peut-être 'René Magritte'. Mais je dois dire qu'on parle, je ne sais pas pourquoi, de plus en plus de mon mari. Mais lui, il n'était pas du tout sensible à ça. Je crois qu'il aurait été très ennuyé si on avait autant parlé de lui à ce moment-là que maintenant.

- Était-il accablé de beaucoup de commandes ?
GM Ah oui, des commandes. Ça il en a eu beaucoup de son commerçant qui était Iolas, qui a une galerie à New York, à Paris et une à Milan. Alors naturellement il réclamait souvent des tableaux.

- Travaillait-il lentement ?
GM Non, il travaillait assez vite. J'étais moi-même des fois étonnée parce qu'il montait dans son atelier et commençait à travailler et puis si je voulais voir il disait 'Mais non, attends un peu. Tu viendras voir quand ça sera fait'. Et je montais, peut-être, trois heures après et le tableau avait déjà l'air d'être fini. Évidemment il les travaillait, mais il peignait assez vite. Et il n'avait pas d'heures régulières. Il travaillait soit le matin, soit l'après-midi – quand il avait envie de peindre.

- Et toujours à la maison ?
GM Toujours à la maison. Il n'a jamais voulu avoir un atelier dehors. Il n'a

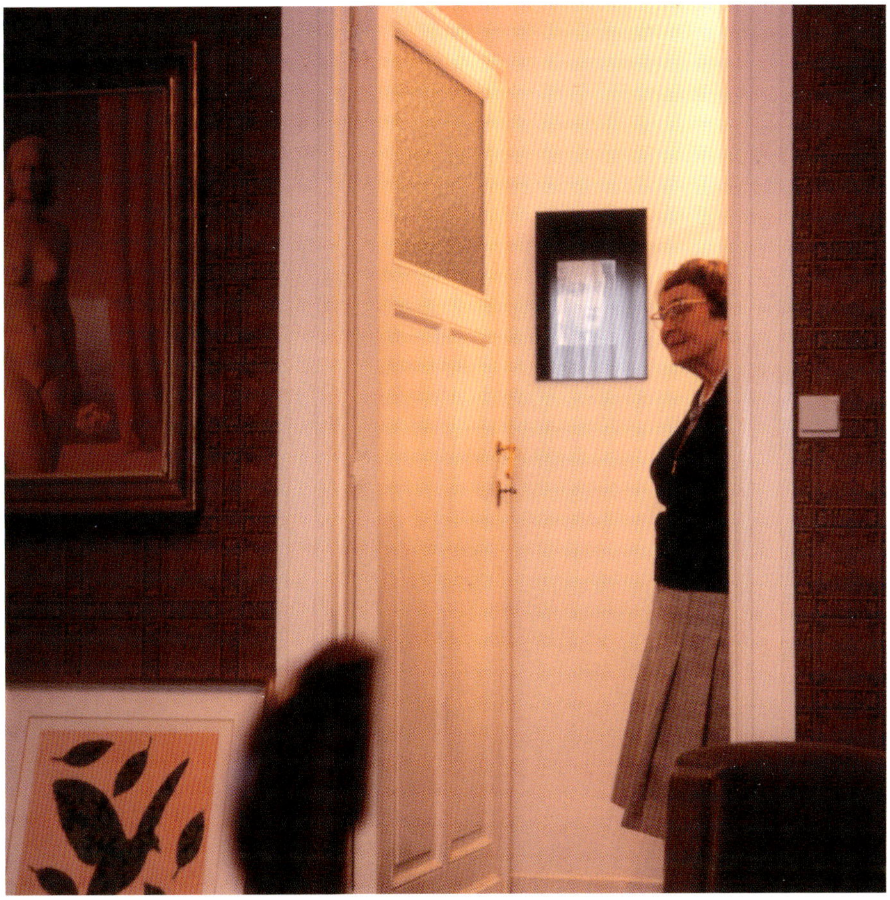

Georgette Magritte, first floor, rue des Mimosas 97, Brussels, 1981

jamais voulu avoir d'autres modèles que moi. Une fois, il en avait pris, car je lui disais 'Prends-toi un autre modèle', parce que c'est quand même un peu fatigant parfois. Alors il a pris un modèle. Il l'a renvoyé, en lui disant 'Je regrette, mais ça ne va pas'. Il m'a dit 'Tu vois, je ne sais rien faire avec un autre modèle'. Il avait ça dans l'esprit.

- *Quand vous êtes allés en Amérique, comment vous a-t-on reçus ?*
GM Ah, très bien.

- *Vous avez aimé l'Amérique ?*
GM Non. Moi vous savez, c'est beaucoup trop grand pour moi personnellement. Mon mari trouvait formidable, bien sûr. Mais, vous savez, lui ce qu'il aimait avant tout, c'était son 'chez soi'. Il disait 'Le plus beau moment d'un voyage que je fais, c'est celui où je rentre à la maison'. Et quand on allait quelque part, et qu'on lui demandait quelles étaient les choses qui l'avaient étonné, il disait 'Non, il n'y avait rien qui valait la peine des ampoules'.

- Son premier voyage à l'étranger était celui à Paris, n'est-ce pas ?
GM Oui, en vingt-sept.

- Avait-il le mal du pays à Paris ?
GM Non. Il ne se sentait pas spécialement belge. Pour lui ça n'avait pas d'importance. Il a dit 'Le fait que je suis né en Belgique ne m'intéresse pas du tout'.

- Est-ce qu'il aimait la ville de Paris ? Aimait-il se promener, ou bien travaillait-il tout le temps ?
GM Il ne travaillait pas tout le temps. Nous n'habitions pas à Paris. Nous habitions à Nogent-Le Perreux, parce que moi je n'aimais pas les villes, d'abord, et on trouvait pas d'appartement. C'était très difficile et je n'aimais pas vivre dans un petit atelier de peintre. Par exemple, nous allions chez Miró, dans l'atelier de Max Ernst, et c'étaient de grands ateliers, si vous voulez, mais je n'avais pas été habituée à vivre de cette façon. Alors nous avons cherché un appartement en dehors de la ville, mais nous passions presque cinq jours par semaine en ville, chez des amis, par exemple. On avait Goemans, qui habitait là. On allait aux Deux Magots, au Café de Flore, chez Breton, ou bien au Cyrano aux appétitifs de Breton. Pas tous les jours, parce que mon mari n'aimait pas aller dans les cafés. Il aimait recevoir lui-même plutôt qu'aller chez les autres.

- Avec lesquels des surréalistes français s'entendait-il le mieux ?
GM Parmi les Français, [...] et Éluard. Il était d'accord avec Breton, bien entendu. On allait quelquefois chez lui. Éluard venait chez nous aussi. Breton pas. Éluard venait nous voir même quand nous sommes rentrés à Bruxelles.

- Ces rencontres surréalistes, comment se passaient-elles ? Elles avaient toujours lieu dans les cafés ?
GM Pas toujours [...] c'étaient des réunions de tous les surréalistes de l'époque, dans lesquelles ils échangeaient des idées.

- Est-ce que Breton se croyait 'professeur' ?
GM Oui. D'ailleurs, vous savez, c'était le maître. Beaucoup de plus jeunes que lui étaient en admiration devant Breton. C'était un homme supérieur.

- Alors, cette question de la rupture avec Breton ?
GM Vous savez, Suzi Gablik en a parlé. Ç'a été une rupture sans l'être si vous voulez. Parce que j'avais, comme j'ai maintenant, une chaîne avec une petite Croix. Évidemment, j'étais jeune et je n'ai pas réfléchi que les surréalistes étaient contre les curés, la religion. Moi, j'avais reçu ça de ma grand-mère, étant plus jeune, et j'avais porté ça au cou, mais c'était plus petit. Alors il nous est arrivé

de prendre un taxi. Nous étions plusieurs pour rentrer chez Breton. Éluard m'a dit 'Tiens, pourquoi tu portes ça au cou ?'
'Ah!', ai-je dit, 'Quoi, ça ?'
'Bien', a-t-il dit, 'ce que vous avez à la chaîne'. Il ne voulait pas dire 'la Croix'. Il disait 'ce que vous avez à la chaîne'.
'Ah', ai-je dit, 'tiens, c'est une Croix que j'ai reçue de ma grand-mère.'
'Oh', a-t-il dit, 'Je préférerais porter un caillou.' Mais moi j'ai ri.
J'ai dit 'Un caillou, qu'est-ce qu'il est lourd à porter'. Enfin on en a fait des plaisanteries, et puis on est allés chez Breton. On était bien une dizaine, une douzaine. Il y avait Aragon, il y avait Éluard, toute la bande et assez bien qui sont morts maintenant. Il y avait beaucoup d'autres dont j'ai oublié le nom. Breton parlait et puis tout d'un coup en se promenant dans la pièce il a dit 'Oui, et parmi nous il y a quelqu'un qui porte un objet que nous détestons' [...] Enfin, il a commencé à dire [...] Mais, je ne sais pas pourquoi, je me suis sentie accusée par ce qu'il disait. Il ne m'a pas nommée. Il a dit '*quelqu'un* porte', mais, comme Éluard m'avait fait la remarque dans le taxi, brusquement je lui ai demandé si c'était pour moi. Il a dit 'Oui, et je vous demanderais de l'enlever !' Alors j'ai dit 'Non, Breton, je le ferai si je veux, mais pas sur commande. Je préfère m'en aller'. Et mon mari n'a pas eu le temps de réagir. Quand il a entendu Breton s'adresser à moi de cette façon, il a dit 'On fiche le camp'. Et on s'en va. Nous sommes partis, mais Aragon a couru derrière nous dans l'escalier. 'Allez, Magritte, revenez. Ne faites pas attention. Vous connaissez Breton.' Mais mon mari a dit 'Je préfère ne pas retourner'. Nous sommes restés donc à Paris sans voir Breton après. Alors nous sommes rentrés en Belgique. Quand nous étions encore à Paris et qu'on a rencontré Breton aux Deux Magots dans l'escalier, il s'est sauvé. Et puis, quand j'ai rencontré Breton plusieurs fois après, il était très poli, très gentil, et j'ai des lettres dans lesquelles il dit 'remets bien à ta femme'. Il avait même oublié. Quand on lui avait rappelé ce qu'il avait fait, il a dit 'Tiens, moi j'ai fait ça ?' Vous voyez, Breton était comme ça. Il fallait toujours excommunier l'un ou l'autre. C'était pareil avec Max Ernst, avec tout le monde. Alors ils se raccommodaient, si vous voulez. C'étaient des disputes sans être des disputes. Ils se séparaient. Puis ils se remettaient, parce que, quand même, ils avaient la même ligne à suivre.

- Alors c'étaient des disputes de doctrine et pas des disputes personnelles ?
GM Non, c'étaient plutôt, comme vous dites, des disputes de doctrine. Avec Max Ernst. Il s'en voulait et avec Miró aussi parce qu'ils avaient peint un décor pour les Ballets Russes et Breton était fâché pour ça.[1] Ça m'a fait rire. Pour de petites choses. Il trouvait qu'on n'aurait pas dû peindre un décor pour un ballet. Je me demande pourquoi. Et il faisait ça avec chacun.

-Votre mari a peint des décors de théâtre, n'est-ce pas ?
GM Oui, je pense. Je me rappelle notamment une pièce de théâtre de Raymond Rouleau, l'acteur de cinéma maintenant, mais qui n'avait rien de surréaliste.[2] Mon mari était jeune à ce moment-là, et il faisait ce qui lui plaisait.

- Avez-vous été choquée par ses toiles ?
GM Choquée ? Non. J'ai eu un choc quand même, mais il y a très longtemps, ça. J'étais seule et mon mari avait peint dans mon absence une fenêtre de l'intérieur par laquelle on voit un oiseau. Et il y a une main qui veut attraper cet oiseau. [*La Fenêtre*, 1925]. Il a fait un tableau *Une Jeune Fille mangeant un oiseau* (1927), mais cela ne m'a pas choquée.

- On dit qu'il était un homme calme, mais on voit beaucoup de violence dans ses toiles – Une Jeune Fille mangeant un oiseau, Le Ciel meurtrier.
GM Je sais que mon mari ne se fâchait jamais. Je n'ai jamais vu mon mari vraiment en colère. Il ne se disputait pas. Il disait ce qu'il avait à dire et c'était tout.

- J'ai lu qu'une fois il a donne un coup de pied à un invité.
GM Oui, mais ce n'était pas par méchanceté. J'avais une amie qui avait comme ami un monsieur. Vous savez c'était un monsieur qui s'habillait encore un peu comme autrefois, avec de longs cheveux et c'était un monsieur de quarante-cinq ans. Mon mari était beaucoup plus jeune. On dit aussi qu'il a frappé une femme, mais ce n'est pas vrai. On invente toujours. Lui, il était très sage. Il ne cherchait pas à se débattre.

- Quels autres artistes aimait-il ?
GM Les cubistes. D'ailleurs, il a fait quelques essais cubistes en 1924 [...] Mais, vous savez, Mesens, qui était plus jeune, allait beaucoup à Paris. Il allait chez Erik Satie à Paris et revenait avec ses musiques [...]

- On voit beaucoup de partitions dans ces tableaux.
GM Ah oui.

- Et les partitions, d'où les a-t-il prises ?
GM Pour ses collages ? Ça c'est un mystère.

- Il a fait beaucoup de dessins publicitaires et beaucoup d'entre eux étaient pour des maisons de couture.
GM Oui, mais mon mari n'était jamais en rapport direct avec la maison.

- Est-ce qu'il s'intéressait aux étalages, aux vitrines, aux questions de mode ?
GM Je ne sais pas, mais il trouvait que la mode c'était bête. Il a même dit que si ces imbéciles se mettaient dans la tête de mettre des bosses aux femmes, alors tout le monde se mettrait une bosse dans le dos. Il trouvait ça inutile. Il trouvait inutile même de faire de nouveaux meubles.

- Est-il allé à l'exposition de l'Art Déco en 1925 ?
GM Non, il n'aimait pas ça. Il n'aimait pas le symbolisme non plus. Beaucoup de gens disaient que dans sa peinture il y a un symbole, et c'était surtout ça qu'il ne voulait pas. Il disait qu'il n'y avait aucun symbole. Le symbole est une représentation d'une idée ou d'un sentiment.

- C'étaient des solutions de problèmes ?
GM C'étaient des solutions de problèmes.

- Étiez-vous là quand il a vu l'œuf dans la cage ?
GM Oui, forcément. Il avait cru voir un œuf. Nous avions un canari et quand ils dorment ils se roulent en boule. Et alors il avait vu ce canari et il avait cru voir un œuf. Alors il l'a peint. Et, en effet, il y a un rapport direct entre l'oiseau et l'œuf.

- C'était en 1933 ou en 1936 ?
GM J'en sais rien.

- Il y a deux 'Ligne de vie', une qui donne la date 1933 et l'autre 1936.
GM C'est vrai ? Ça, je ne savais pas. Vous voyez, il y a eu la guerre. Avant la guerre c'était une période, et après la guerre, c'était encore une autre période. Mais finalement on ne se rappelle plus ce qui était avant la guerre ou après la guerre [...] quant à l'époque Vache, c'est une chose qui lui est venue comme ça. Il n'a rien vendu [...] (*La Pipe*, 1923) c'est le seul tableau qui est comme ça (en relief). Probablement, je ne m'en souviens plus, je suppose qu'avant de peindre ça il avait fait un autre tableau parce que vous voyez il y a des rides. Comme il n'avait pas beaucoup d'argent il a repeint une toile. C'est peut-être qu'elle ne lui convenait pas. C'est dommage qu'elle est un peu abîmée comme ça, mais lui il n'y attachait pas d'importance.

- La maison a été toujours comme ça, bien arrangée, impeccable ?
GM Oui. Mon mari n'aimait pas le désordre, je dois le dire. Vous savez, ces bibelots, ce n'est pas mon mari. Quand il voyait un bibelot dans un magasin, il disait, par exemple, 'Quelle belle petite pendule', et il l'achetait pour moi. Mais lui personnellement ne les choisissait pas. Ça ne l'intéressait pas.

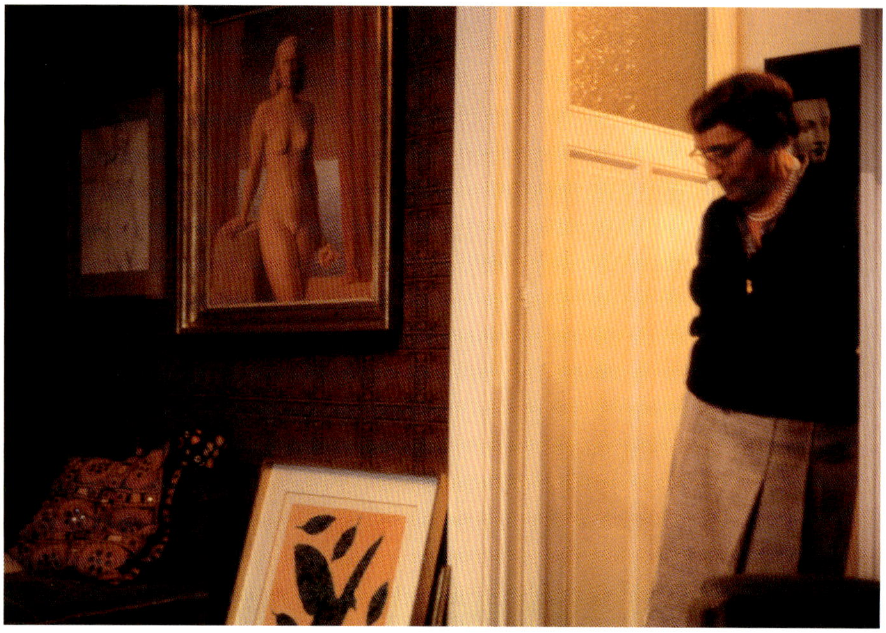

Georgette Magritte, first floor, rue des Mimosas 97, Brussels, 1981

Évidemment il aimait mieux un bel objet que n'importe quoi. Par exemple, il aimait un piano à queue. En fait il aimait un grand piano. Autrefois, chez mes parents, j'avais un piano droit quand j'étais jeune. Après, lui il a trouvé que c'était plus beau, un piano comme ça. C'est pour ça qu'il l'a choisi [...] Ça vous connaissez [*La Dame*] ? Il avait fait ça pour s'amuser, comme il avait fait le petit œil qui est là-bas, mais pour nous [...] Tout le monde est touché par ce tableau [*L'Empire des lumières*]. Combien de personnes m'ont dit 'Nous sommes allés à la campagne ou à la mer et il y avait un ciel Magritte'. Avant, ils n'auraient pas remarqué ce ciel. Mais maintenant mon mari le leur a fait voir. Et ce n'est pas mon mari qui a fait un ciel, mais c'est le ciel qui est devenu un ciel Magritte [...] J'ai connu mon mari quand j'étais très jeune. J'avais douze ans, à la foire de Charleroi. Évidemment j'étais jeune. Lui il allait à l'athénée. Moi j'allais en classe, et on se rencontrait toujours à la sortie des écoles. Un jour il a dit qu'il se souvenait de moi à cette époque, et il a fait d'après son souvenir une fille, un visage de fille très jeune. Ça c'est des années trente.

11 March 1981, rue des Mimosas 97, Brussels

---

[1] Sergey Diaghilev's *Romeo et Juliette* of 1926. Max Ernst created the decor for the second act and Miró was responsible for the first act.

[2] Raymond Rouleau directed and appeared in the stage production *Amitié de Michel Mourguet* at Théâtre du Marais, Brussels, which opened on 1 January 1931.

- Are you constantly dealing with your husband's work?

GM At the moment? I do nothing but, so to speak. There are lots of people who want information, who ask if they can exhibit paintings. So, there are always lots of people writing and telephoning about producing post cards and reproductions and mounting exhibitions. I am constantly kept busy with these things.

- Do you have many of your husband's works?

GM Yes, a reasonable amount, because some are upstairs. I could show you my husband's studio, if you like.

- Doesn't this painting [La Pipe, 1923] *belong to your sister?*

GM Yes, I now have paintings that we had given, as it were, to my sister. And, since she has now died, the paintings have come back to me. That's how I come to have a fair amount. You see, all these paintings have always been here, but, as for those upstairs, I have a few more than previously. You know, it's by chance that certain paintings have remained here. It's not that we chose them. Except for this one, that my husband painted especially for me [*Le Domaine d'Arnheim*, 1962]. But, as for the others, it's by chance that [...] because my husband's work sold fairly well. Sometimes he would promise someone a painting and a year later that same person would say 'Oh, Mr Magritte, you promised me a painting'. So then, if there was one that I had liked and had kept for myself, he'd say 'You know, someone asked me to do a painting well over a year ago. I'll give him this one'. And then he'd give it to him. 'But I'll paint you another one', he'd say.

- So he didn't think like a businessman?

GM Oh no, not at all. Nor did he think like a museum curator. He wouldn't mind at all when his paintings would leave. He might sell them or give them away. He gave a lot away. Sometimes he wanted to burn them. Anything was possible. He'd stop being interested in a work once it was finished. His idea had been realized, hadn't it? All he'd be interested in then was the painting that was coming next.

- How did he react to success? There's a rue René Magritte, isn't there?

GM Yes, there is a small street named René Magritte about which I didn't know. A workman who came here told me about it. But there is another in Lessines, the town where he was born. They had a ceremony at the house where he was born and erected a plaque – 'René Magritte was born here' – and then they named a major road after him. There is also an avenue René Magritte. I saw it three or four years ago when it was named, but I don't know whether they have since built a major trunk road. A name had to be found and it was perhaps 'René Magritte'. But I must say that people are talking more and more about my husband and I don't know why. But that sort of thing made no impact on him. I think he would have found it tedious if people had talked as much then about him as they do now.

- *Was he overwhelmed with many commissions?*
GM Certainly commissions. He had many from his dealer, who was Iolas. He has galleries in New York, Paris and Milan. So, obviously, he often requested paintings.

- *Did he work slowly?*
GM No, he worked fairly quickly. I used to be surprised sometimes because he would go up to his studio and start working and then, if I wanted to have a look, he would say 'No, wait a bit. You can come up when it's finished'. I would go up perhaps three hours later and the painting looked as good as finished. Obviously, he would rework them, but he painted rather quickly. Nor did he follow a routine. He would work either in the morning or in the afternoon – whenever he felt like painting.

- *And always at home?*
GM Always at home. He never wanted to have a dedicated studio. He never wanted models other than me. He did take one once, since I kept saying 'Take another model'. It is, after all, tiring sometimes. So he took a model. He sent her away, saying 'I'm sorry, but it's not working'. He said 'You see, I can't manage anything with another model'. It was a fixation with him.

- *What reception did you get when you went to the States?*
GM Oh, a very good one.

- *Did you like the States?*
GM No, you know, personally I found it far too big. My husband found it amazing, without a doubt. But, you know, what he liked best were his home comforts. He used to say 'The best part of a trip for me is the moment I get home'. And when he'd go on a trip somewhere and was asked what he had found surprising, he'd say 'No, there was nothing worth getting blisters for'.

- *His first trip abroad was the one to Paris, wasn't it?*
GM Yes, in 1927.

- *Was he homesick in Paris?*
GM No. He didn't feel particularly Belgian. For him that wasn't important. He

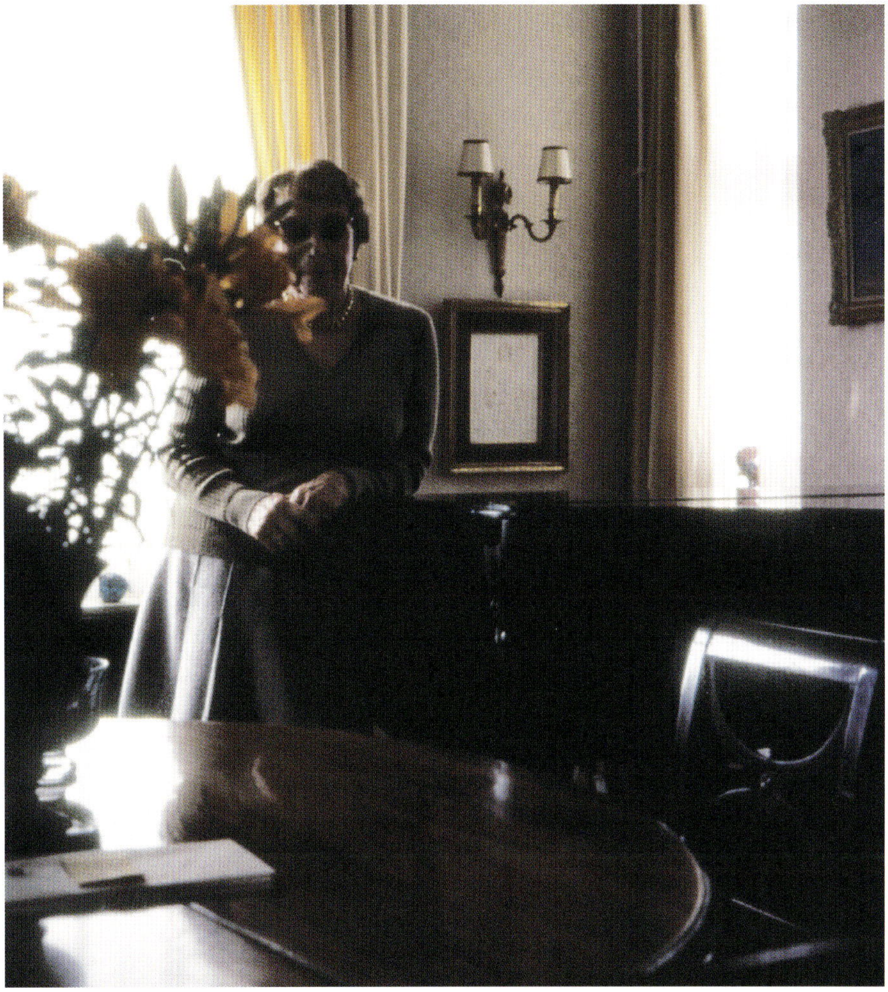

Georgette Magritte, parlour, rue des Mimosas 97, Brussels, 1981

said 'I'm not at all interested in the fact that I was born Belgian'.

- Did he like Paris as a city? Did he like taking strolls, or did he work all the time?

GM He didn't work all the time. We didn't live in Paris. We lived in Nogent-Le Perreux, firstly because I didn't like cities and, secondly, we couldn't find an apartment. It was very difficult and I wouldn't have liked to live in a small painter's studio. For example, we used to go and see Miró or Max Ernst in their studios, and these were large studios, so to speak, but I hadn't been used to living like that. So we looked for an apartment outside the city, but we spent nearly five days a week in the city, seeing friends, for example. We knew Goemans, who lived there. We used to go to the Deux Magots or Café de Flore. We used to visit Breton or go to Le Cyrano for Breton's drinks get-togethers. Not every day, because my husband didn't like going to cafés. He preferred to invite people home, rather than going to see them.

- *With which of the French surrealists did he get on with best?*
GM With the French, [...] and Éluard. He got on with Breton, of course. We'd go to his apartment sometimes. Éluard used to visit us too. Breton never did. Éluard used to come to see us even when we moved back to Brussels.

- *What happened during these surrealist gatherings? Did they always take place in cafés?*
GM Not always [...] they were meetings of all the surrealists of the time, in which they exchanged ideas.

- *Did Breton see himself as the 'teacher'?*
GM Yes. Besides, you know, he was the master. Many of the younger ones admired Breton. He was a cut above the rest.

- *So, what of this issue of the split with Breton?*
GM You know, Suzi Gablik has spoken of it. It was, so to speak, a split without being a split. Because I had then, as I do now, a chain with a small Cross. Obviously, I was young and I hadn't thought about the fact that the surrealists were anti-clerical, anti-religion. It had been given to me by my grandmother much earlier when I was young and I had worn it around my neck, but that one was smaller. So, one day, several of us had taken a taxi to go to Breton's apartment. Éluard said 'Now then! Why are you wearing that thing around your neck?'
'Oh?', I said, 'What "thing" do you mean?'
'I mean', he said, 'the thing you are wearing on the chain'. He didn't want to say 'the Cross'. He said 'the thing you are wearing on the chain'.
'Oh', I said, 'well, it's a Cross my grandmother gave me as a gift.'
'Oh', he said, 'I'd rather wear a stone.' I just laughed. I said 'A stone would really weigh me down'. So, we made a joke of it, and then we got to Breton's apartment. There were ten or twelve of us. There was Aragon, there was Éluard, a sizeable group and quite a few who are now dead. There were many others whose names I've forgotten. Breton was speaking and then, as he was walking up and down in the room, he suddenly said 'Yes, and among us there is someone wearing an object we detest' [...] he ended up by saying [...] I don't know why, but I felt I was being accused by what he was saying. He didn't mention me by name. He said '*someone* is wearing', but, as Éluard had mentioned it to me in the taxi, I suddenly asked him if he was referring to me. He said 'Yes, and I would ask you to remove it!' I then said 'No, Breton, I'll do it if I want, but I won't be told. I prefer to leave'. And my husband didn't

have the time to react. When he heard Breton talking to me like that, he said 'Let's get the hell out of here'. And we left. We left, but Aragon ran after us down the stairs. 'Come on, Magritte, come back. Don't take any notice. You know what Breton's like.' But my husband said 'I prefer not to go back'. We therefore stayed on in Paris without seeing Breton again. Then we moved back to Belgium. When we were still in Paris and happened to meet Breton on the stairs of the Deux Magots he ran away. I later met Breton on several occasions and he was very polite, very kind, and I have letters in which he writes 'regards to your wife'. He had even forgotten. When we reminded him about what he had done, he said 'Really? Did I do that?' You see, Breton was like that. He always had to excommunicate someone or other. It was the same with Max Ernst, with everyone. Then they would patch things up, so to speak. These were arguments without being arguments. They split up. Then they got back together, because, after all, they were all singing from the same hymn sheet.

- So these were doctrinal arguments and not personal arguments?
GM No, they were mostly, as you say, doctrinal arguments. With Max Ernst. He had it in for Miró too because they had painted the set for the Ballets Russes and, as a result, Breton was angry.[1] It made me laugh. For such little things. He felt it was wrong to paint a ballet stage set. I can't imagine why. And he was like this with all of them.

-Your husband painted theatre sets, didn't he?
GM Yes, I believe so. I particularly remember a play by Raymond Rouleau, who is now a screen actor, which had, however, nothing surrealist about it.[2] My husband was young at that time and he did what he liked.

- Have you been shocked by his paintings?
GM Shocked? No. I did, however, have one shock, but that was a long time ago. I was alone and, when I had been out, my husband had painted a window seen from the inside through which a bird was visible. And there's a hand trying to catch this bird [*La Fenêtre*, 1925]. He painted *Une Jeune Fille mangeant un oiseau* (1927) [Young Girl Eating a Bird], but that hadn't shocked me.

- He's often described as a calm man, but there is a lot of violence in his paintings. – Une Jeune Fille mangeant un oiseau, Le Ciel meurtrier.
GM I can tell you that my husband never got cross. I have never seen my husband truly angry. He never argued. He said what he had to say and that was it.

- I once read that he kicked a guest.
GM Yes, but it wasn't malicious. I had a friend who was acquainted with a

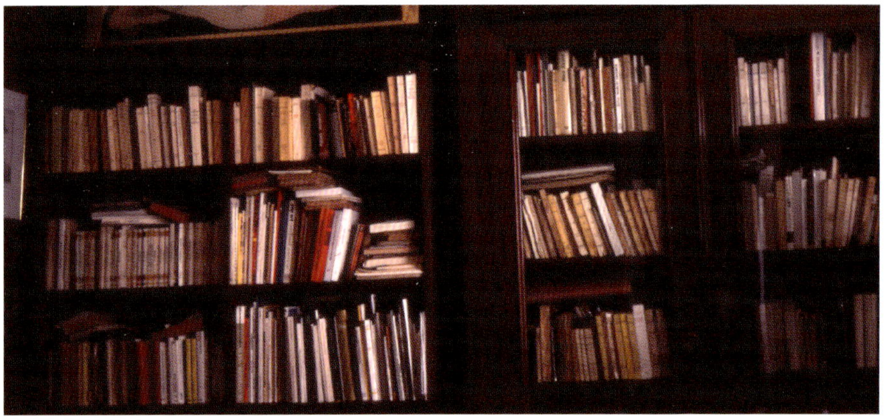

Bookcase, first floor study, rue des Mimosas 97, Brussels, 1981

certain gentleman. He was a forty-five-year-old gentleman who still dressed, you know, in a slightly old-fashioned way and had long hair. My husband was a lot younger. Rumour has it that he also hit a woman, but that's not true. People always make things up. He was very well-behaved. He didn't go round looking for arguments.

- *Which artists did he like?*
GM The Cubists. Besides, he experimented a bit with Cubism in 1924 [...] But, you know, Mesens, who was younger, often went to Paris. He used to go to see Erik Satie in Paris and came back with his scores [...]

- *There's a lot of sheet music in his paintings.*
GM Oh yes.

- *Where did the sheet music come from?*
GM The ones he used in his collages? That's a mystery.

- *He did a lot of drawings for advertisements and many of these were for fashion houses.*
GM Yes, but my husband was never directly employed by the fashion houses.

- *Was he interested in shop window displays, shop windows, questions of fashion?*
GM I don't know, but he thought that fashion was daft. He even said that if these idiots got it into their heads to put humps on women, everyone would go round like hunchbacks. He didn't see the point. He didn't even see the point of making new, modern furniture.

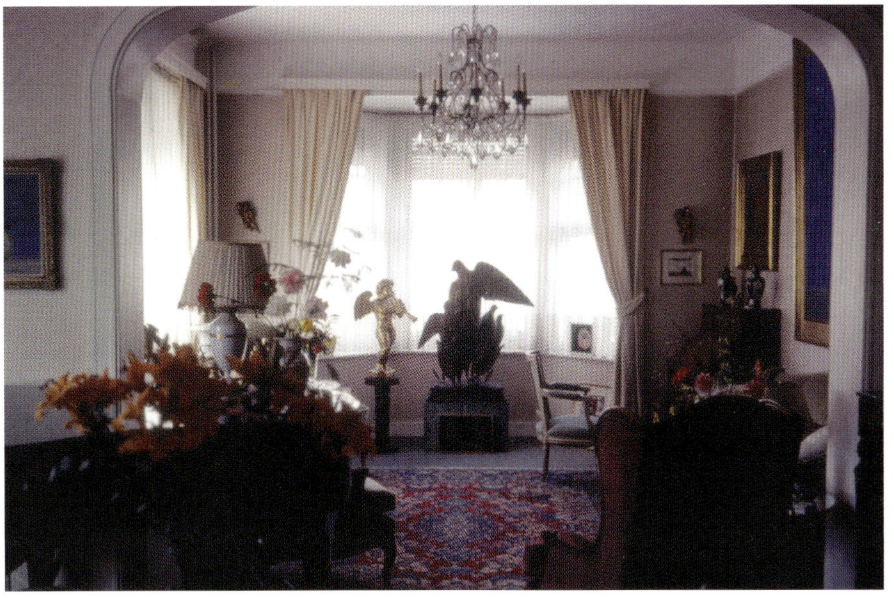

Parlour, rue des Mimosas 97, Brussels, 1981

- *Did he go to the Art Déco exhibition in 1925?*
GM No, he didn't like that. He didn't like symbolism either. Many people used to say that there were symbols in his paintings, and that's precisely what he objected to. He used to say that there weren't any symbols. A symbol is a representation of an idea or an emotion.

- *Were they solutions to problems?*
GM They were solutions to problems.

- *Were you there when he saw the egg in the cage?*
GM Yes, naturally. He thought he saw an egg. We had a canary and when they sleep they roll themselves up in a ball. And so he saw this canary and thought he had seen an egg. So he painted it. And, indeed, there is a direct link between a bird and an egg.

- *Was it in 1933 or 1936?*
GM I've no idea.

- *He wrote two 'Ligne de vie'* [*Lifeline*], *one in which he gives the date 1933 and another in which he cites 1936.*
GM Really? I didn't know. You see, there was the war. Before the war was one period, and after the war, it was another. In the end you can't remember what came before or after the war [...] as for the Vache period, it was a flash in the

pan. He didn't sell anything [...] This [*La Pipe*, 1923] is the only painting that's like this [in relief]. I can't remember now, but I suppose he had probably painted something different before painting this, because you can see some raised lines. Since he didn't have much money he repainted a canvas. Perhaps he didn't like it. It's a pity that it's a bit damaged, but he didn't care about things like that.

- Has the house always been as tidy and immaculate as this?
GM Yes. My husband didn't like untidiness, I must say. You know, these ornaments are nothing to do with my husband. When he would see an ornament in a shop, he'd say, for example, 'What a lovely little clock', and he'd buy it for me. But he wouldn't buy them for himself. He wasn't interested in them. Obviously, he preferred a beautiful object to something run-of-the-mill. For example, he liked grand pianos. In fact, he loved concert-grands. Years ago, at my parents', I used to have an upright piano when I was young. Later my husband felt a piano like this one was more attractive. That's why he chose [...] Do you know this [*La Dame*]? He painted this to amuse me, since he had painted the small eye there, but just for us [...] This painting has an effect on everyone [*L'Empire des lumières*]. The number of people who have said to me 'We went to the countryside or to the beach and there was a Magritte sky'. They wouldn't have noticed the sky previously. But now my husband has made them see it. Not that my husband had painted that sky; it's more that the sky had become a Magritte sky [...] I met my husband when I was very young, at the Charleroi fair when I was twelve. Needless to say I was young. He was at secondary school. I was in the lower school, and we always used to meet after school. One day he said he was thinking of me in those days and he painted a girl from memory, the face of a very young girl. This is from the thirties.

---

1 Sergey Diaghilev's *Romeo et Juliette* of 1926. Max Ernst created the decor for the second act and Miró was responsible for the first act.

2 Raymond Rouleau directed and appeared in the stage production *Amitié de Michel Mourguet* at Théâtre du Marais, Brussels, which opened on 1 January 1931.

Louis Scutenaire & Irène Hamoir

- En 1945 Mesens a dit 'Magritte fut «surréaliste» autant en 1925 que, par exemple, en 1936'. Voyez-vous quand même un écart entre les années vingt et les années trente ?
LS Je crois qu'en 1936 il soignait plus la peinture qu'il ne la soignait en 1925. Dans les débuts Magritte voulait s'occuper de l'anti-peinture, c'est-à-dire peindre violemment, peindre mal, ne pas rechercher l'effet esthétique, tandis que plus tard il a recherché un peu cet effet.

- Quand il est revenu de Paris pensez-vous que sa peinture a changé ?
LS Il ne me semble pas. Je crois qu'il a continué à peindre comme il avait commencé à peindre à Paris. Je ne vois pas la différence.

IH Il y a une différence dans la présentation, dans la technique.

LS Entre ce qu'il faisait à Perreux et ce qu'il faisait à Bruxelles ?

IH Entre ce qu'il faisait dans les années vingt et ce qu'il faisait après.

LS Oui, vingt, bien sûr. Mais à Paris il a déjà commencé à peindre 'mieux', d'une façon plus délicate, plus fine, moins violente, brutale.

- Vous avez dit, vous-même, en 1942, que 'Magritte n'a pas eu le désir de servir la peinture'. Comment s'en est-il servi alors ?
LS Il s'est servi de la peinture pour faire de l'anti-esthétisme et de l'anti-peinture. C'est la révolution par des moyens picturaux.

- Y a-t-il de magrittisme, c'est-à-dire est-ce que la peinture de Magritte est tout à fait arbitraire ou est-ce qu'il y a, au niveau le plus fondamental, un système qui rend l'œuvre cohérente ?
LS Je pense qu'il y a une œuvre très cohérente et pas arbitraire du tout. C'est le contraire même de l'arbitraire. La peinture de Magritte a toujours été pensée. Elle a suivi une filière très cohérente.

- Alors il n'y a pas d'automatisme dans sa peinture.
LS Non, pas du tout.

- Je pense à l'affaire des faux Magritte. Est-ce que cela démontre qu'il y a, en

fait, quelque chose qui lie les peintures, une formule ?
LS Cette exposition de gouaches [New Smith Gallery, Bruxelles, 18 novembre–18 décembre 1970] c'était la fausseté même. C'était d'une grossièreté de facture extraordinaire. Magritte avait une facture violente mais pas grossière, pas laide, pas maladroite.

- *On a pu comprendre que ce n'était pas Magritte.*
LS Oui, bien sûr. Cela sautait aux yeux. C'était évident, l'évidence même. Je pense, par exemple, qu'un peintre pourrait copier une toile de Magritte de façon que cela paraisse un vrai, mais je ne vois pas quelqu'un inventant une toile de Magritte et que cela apparaisse comme vrai.

- *Il y a un système fondamental.*
LS Il y a quelque chose. Je ne sais pas très bien exprimer quoi, mais il y a quelque chose qui montre que c'est un Magritte ou que ce n'est pas un Magritte. On peut copier si on est un habile copiste, cela bien sur, ou même faire plus que l'imiter. Par exemple on pourrait copier *Découverte* et ajouter un petit objet ou l'autre, ou un décor derrière, mais [...] je vous quitte pour cinq minutes pour voir une course de cyclisme à la télévision. (D'après M. DeKnop, Louis Scutenaire était un grand amateur des courses de cyclisme.)

- *Vous a-t-il parlé de l'Académie ?*
LS Non. Je sais qu'il était à l'Académie quelques années et il paraît qu'il était un élève peu assidu, mais lui il n'en parlait pas. Il ne parlait pas volontiers de ce qui s'était passé avant le moment où il parlait. Il n'aimait pas son passé et alors il n'en parlait pas.

- *Que devrait-on entendre par la phrase de Magritte 'La pensée inspirée ressemble au monde' ? Pour moi, c'est assez obscur.*
LS Pour moi aussi. Ça peut vouloir dire cent mille choses. Je n'ai jamais parlé philosophie avec Magritte.

- *Magritte aimait la musique, il écoutait souvent des disques. Est-ce que* L'Assassin menacé *est un autoportrait ?*
LS Je ne crois pas. Je pense que c'était plutôt inspiré par la lecture des romans policiers de *Fantômas*.

IH Le phonographe fait étrange comme le fameux parapluie sur la table. C'est un objet insolite, le gramophone, et il était là probablement parce qu'il est insolite. Il adorait jouer avec les objets insolites.

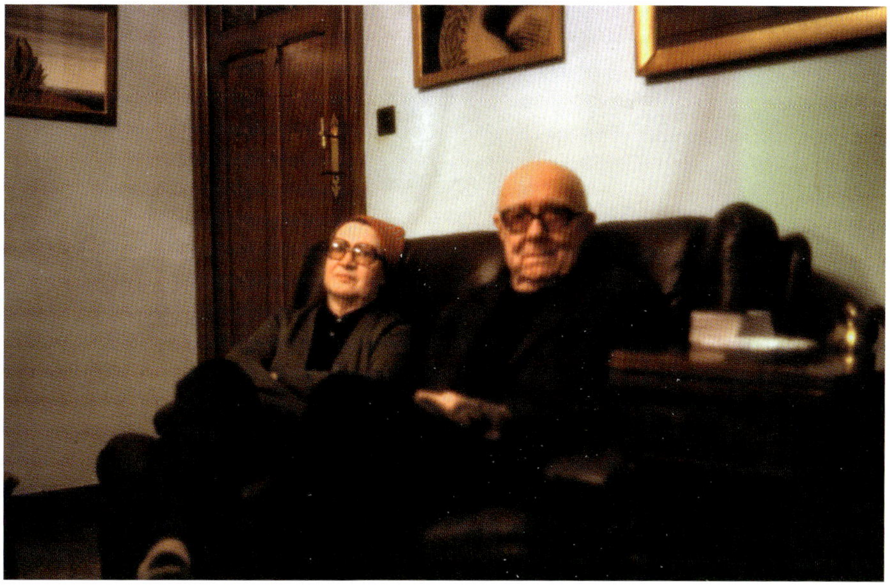

Irène Hamoir and Louis Scutenaire, rue de la Luserne 20, Brussels, 1981

LS C'est-à-dire qu'il adorait placer les objets d'une façon insolite dans un décor qui ne l'était pas, ou le contraire.

- C'était un homme calme qui détestait la violence. Ne pensez-vous pas qu'il y a quand même une violence latente dans son œuvre qui se démontre des fois ?
LS Mais si. Elle est toute violente, son œuvre. Même dans la toile la plus calme, il y a de la violence chez Magritte, toujours. De ses gouaches qui ont l'air gentil saute une violence extraordinaire. C'est ce qui me plaît dans la peinture de Magritte, sa violence.

- Comment les problèmes se posaient-ils ? Est-ce qu'on lui en a proposé ?
LS J'imagine qu'il y a des gens qui lui ont proposé des problèmes. Je crois qu'en général il les repoussait. Il ne s'intéressait qu'aux problèmes qui lui venaient à l'esprit, sans l'intervention d'autrui. Les gens qui disent qu'ils ont inspiré Magritte mentent ou se trompent. Il est possible que des gens lui ont proposé des idées et que Magritte ait fait tout autre chose. Je ne lui en ai jamais parlé, mais je l'ai tellement fréquenté que je ne le vois acceptant la proposition d'une autre personne pour une toile.

IH Mariën est dit lui avoir donné des sujets de peintures, mais un ou deux. C'est pour ça que la question a peu d'intérêt. S'il a accepté les idées d'autrui c'est vraiment fort peu. Mariën lui à proposé une ou deux idées. Maurice Rapin est dit aussi lui avoir fait des propositions. Claude Spaak est dit avoir proposé un sujet, mais c'est si peu de chose. En général il n'acceptait pas les idées des gens. Ça c'est sûr.

Souvent des gens lui en proposaient à des réunions auxquelles nous allions et ...

LS Il arrivait à Magritte de réclamer des idées à des gens et ces gens se fatiguaient à en trouver et lui n'en faisait rien, bien sûr. C'était une sorte de jeu. Il avait un grand ami qui s'appelait Colinet. Lui a donné parfois des idées, mais Magritte en avait assez. C'était pourtant de très belles idées en général. Magritte n'aimait pas ce qui venait d'autrui.

- Peut-on dissocier la période Vache du reste de son œuvre ?
LS Je pense que oui, tant par l'aspect que par la volonté beaucoup plus révolutionnaire et plus violente qu'il y avait dans son œuvre précédente, et dans son œuvre postérieure. Ça c'était Magritte tel qu'il me semble le connaître. C'est Magritte tout nu. Je crois que c'est la seule période de sa vie où il a été vraiment heureux avec sa peinture et en conformité avec lui-même. C'était une réaction contre la vie telle quelle est, la vie sociale que nous vivons et qui ne lui plaisait tellement pas.

- C'était sa première exposition à Paris.
LS C'était sa première exposition personnelle. Il avait peut-être participé dans des expositions collectives mais de cela je n'en sais rien.

- Alors il n'avait pas tellement envie de plaire aux Français ?
LS Certainement pas du tout. Il n'a pas gardé un bon souvenir de la France ni des Français. Il a voulu d'ailleurs les heurter. Il y a un certain monsieur du Centre Pompidou qui nous a dit que Magritte avait fait à Paris une expédition punitive. Je trouve la formule magnifique.

- Est-ce que Magritte a dépassé les cubistes avec son usage des mots dans ses tableaux ?
LS Oui, c'était une autre volonté, une autre démarche. Je pense que les cubistes utilisaient les mots comme moyens décoratifs, comme moyens picturaux, tandis que Magritte les employait comme moyen philosophique, une sorte de pensée plutôt que visualisation. Je crois que l'intention était toute autre.

- Pensez-vous qu'il avait l'esprit analytique ?
LS Je pense que oui, mais il n'avait pas les fondements qu'ont les linguistes. Je pense qu'il avait cet esprit analytique sans avoir la technique scolaire de l'analyse.

- Dans ses textes sur la 'ressemblance' il se sert des expressions 'en fait' et 'en droit', qui proviennent de la terminologie légale. Vous avez été avocat et je me demande si c'est vous qui les lui a proposées.

LS Non.

IH Magritte s'est servi de beaucoup d'expressions. Il avait le goût de la philosophie sans en avoir les moyens. En ce qui concerne la peinture il en avait les moyens. En ce qui concerne la poésie il en avait les moyens. Il n'avait pas les moyens de faire de la philosophie, mais il adorait en faire.

13 March 1981, rue de la Luserne 20, Brussels

- *In 1945 Mesens said 'Magritte had been as much a "surrealist" in 1925 as, for example, he had been in 1936'. Do you, nevertheless, see a demarcation between the twenties and the thirties?*
LS I think that in 1936 he painted more meticulously than in 1925. At the start, Magritte wanted to focus on anti-painting, that is to say painting violently, painting badly and disregarding aesthetic niceties, whereas he later paid a little attention to the aesthetic aspects of his work.

- *Do you think his painting changed when he came back from Paris?*
LS I don't think so. I think he continued to paint in the way in which he had started to paint in Paris. I don't see that there is a difference.

IH There is a difference in the overall appearance and in the technique.

LS Between what he was doing in Perreux and what he was doing in Brussels?

IH Between what he was doing in the 1920s and what he did later.

LS Yes, of course. But in Paris he had already started to paint 'better', in a manner that was more delicate, more attentive to detail, less violent and brutal.

- *You yourself said in 1942 that 'Magritte did not want to serve painting'. How did he use painting therefore?*
LS He used painting to make anti-aesthetic, anti-painting statements. It's revolt by pictorial means.

- *Is there a Magrittism, by which I mean is Magritte's painting inherently without logic or is there, at the most fundamental level, a system that makes his oeuvre coherent?*
LS I think that his is an extremely coherent oeuvre, which is in no way arbitrary. I'd go as far as to say that it's the opposite of arbitrary. Magritte's painting has always been well thought out. It has followed a very coherent course.

- *So there is no automatism in his painting.*
LS No, not at all.

- *I'd like to turn to the affair of the fake Magrittes. Does it show that there is, in fact, something that interlinks the paintings, a formula?*
LS This exhibition of gouaches (New Smith Gallery, Brussels, 18 November – 18 December 1970) was the epitome of fakery. The execution of the works

showed an extraordinary crudeness. Magritte's technique was violent, but not shoddy, ugly, inept.

- It was evident that these were not by Magritte.
LS Yes, of course. It was blindingly obvious. It was as clear as it could be. I think, for instance, that a painter could copy a Magritte in such a way that it would look genuine, but I don't see that someone could invent a new Magritte and pass it off as an authentic work.

- There is an underlying system.
LS There is something. I don't know how to express what that is, but there is something that shows that it is a Magritte or that it is not a Magritte. Granted, a skilful copyist can easily copy, or even go further than imitating. For example, it would be possible to copy *Découverte* and add some or other little object or a background scene, but [...] excuse me for five minutes. I have to watch a cycling race on television. [According to M. DeKnop, Louis Scutenaire was passionate about cycle racing.]

- Did he talk to you about the Académie?
LS No. I know that he had been at the Académie for a few years and it seems he wasn't a conscientious student, but he didn't talk about it. He was never happy to talk about what had happened prior to the moment in which he was speaking. He did not like his past and so he didn't talk about it.

- What is to be understood by Magritte's phrase 'Inspired thought resembles the world'? To me, it's quite obscure.
LS To me too. It could mean a thousand things. I've never discussed philosophy with Magritte.

- Magritte loved music, he often listened to records. Is L'Assassin menacé *a self-portrait?*
LS I don't think so. I think it was more inspired by his reading of the *Fantômas* detective novels.

IH The gramophone creates strangeness like the famous umbrella on the table. It's a bizarre object, the gramophone, and it was probably there because it is not what you would normally expect. He loved playing with surprising objects.

LS That is to say he loved staging objects in an unusual way in a setting which was not unusual, or vice versa.

- He was a calm man who detested violence. Do you not think that there is, nevertheless, a hidden violence in his works, which sometimes emerges?
LS Precisely so. His work is all violent. Even in Magritte's most serene painting there is violence and that's always the case. An extraordinary violence leaps out of gouaches that appear harmless enough on the surface. That's what I like in Magritte's painting, its violence.

- How did the 'problems' arise? Had some been suggested to him by others?
LS I imagine that there are people who had come up with suggestions for 'problems'. I think, generally, he took no notice. He was only interested in problems that occurred to him without external intervention. Those who say that they have inspired Magritte are either lying or mistaken. It is not beyond possibility that ideas could have been suggested to Magritte and that he went on to do something completely different. I've never spoken to him about this, but I was so close to him that I cannot see that he would ever have accepted another person's suggestion for a painting.

IH Mariën is supposed to have given him subjects for paintings, although no more than one or two. This is scarcely an issue. Even if he had accepted the ideas that came from others, it was only on extremely rare occasions. Mariën suggested one or two ideas. Maurice Rapin is also said to have made suggestions. Claude Spaak is said to have suggested a subject, but it was something minor. In general, he did not accept ideas from other people. That is certain. People often tried to make suggestions at the gatherings which we attended and ...

LS Sometimes Magritte would ask people for ideas and then they would go to a lot of trouble to come up with something. Magritte, of course, would totally disregard the ideas. It was a sort of game. He had a close friend called Colinet. He had sometimes given Magritte ideas, but Magritte had enough of his own. To be fair, these had been very good ideas on the whole. Magritte disliked what came from others.

- Would it be reasonable to separate the Vache period from the remainder of his oeuvre?
LS I think so, as much on the level of appearance as on the level of their intent, which was far more revolutionary and violent than anything that had come before or would come after. It revealed Magritte as I knew him to be. It was Magritte stripped bare. I think it was the only period in his life when he was truly happy with his painting and at one with himself. It was a reaction against life as it really is, against the societal context within which we live and which he found objectionable.

- It was his first Parisian exhibition.
LS It was his first solo exhibition. He may have taken part in group exhibitions, but I couldn't tell you.

- So he wasn't very interested in pleasing the French.
LS Absolutely not. He didn't come back with good memories of either France or the French. Besides he wanted to offend them. A certain gentleman at the Centre Pompidou told us that Magritte had gone to Paris to make a punitive foray. He couldn't have expressed it better.

- Did Magritte's use of words in his paintings go beyond what the Cubists had done?
LS Yes, he had a different aim and approach. I think the Cubists used words in a decorative way, as pictorial elements, whereas Magritte used them as a philosophical apparatus, as a means through which to express thoughts, rather than as a visual device. I think his intention was wholly different.

- Do you think he thought in an analytical way?
LS I think so, but he didn't have the theoretical grounding of the linguisticians. I think he had that sort of analytical mind without having the technique of scholarly analysis.

- In his texts on 'ressemblance' he uses expressions such as 'de facto' and 'de jure', which come from legal terminology. You have been a lawyer and I wonder whether you had suggested these terms to him.
LS No.

IH Magritte used a lot of terminology. He had a taste for philosophy, but lacked the means to elaborate it. As far as painting went he possessed the means. As far as poetry went he had the means. He didn't have the means to elaborate philosophical thought, although he loved doing so.

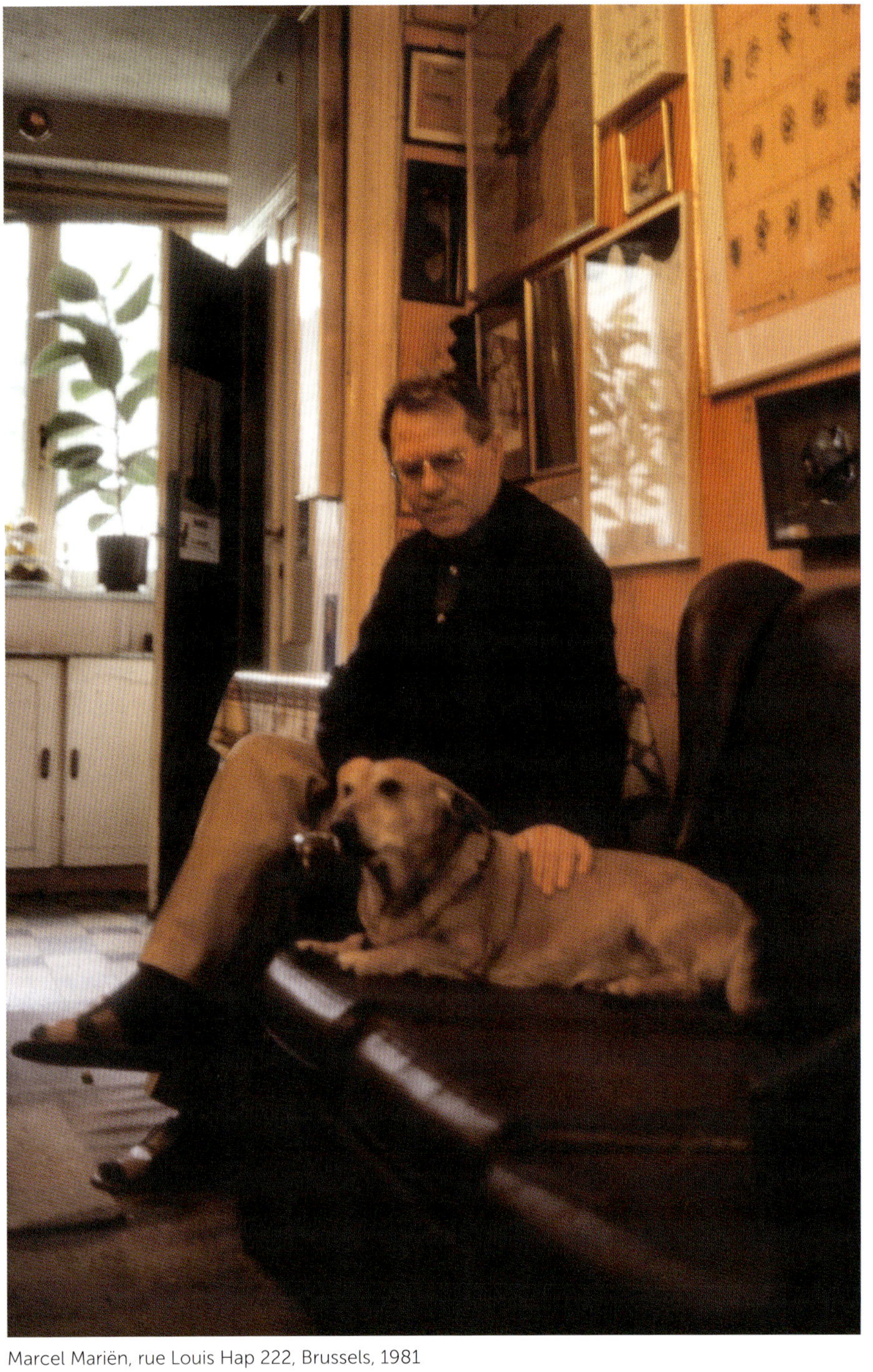

Marcel Mariën, rue Louis Hap 222, Brussels, 1981

MARCEL MARIËN
FIRST INTERVIEW

- Avez-vous été influencé par Magritte ?
MM Oui, si on veut. La pipe, ça s'appelle 'La Fausse Compagnie'. Il y a un miroir. C'est une demi-pipe, la demi-*Trahison des images*.

- On a dit souvent que Le Jockey perdu *est le premier tableau achevé de Magritte.*
MM Non, c'est le tableau que lui préférait. C'est un tableau que lui-même préférait à beaucoup d'autres, mais avant ça il y a un autre tableau, qui d'ailleurs vient d'être vendu, je crois, à Londres, que moi j'ai publié, qui n'a jamais été reproduit ailleurs, je crois. Il s'appelle 'Nocturne'. C'était un tableau dans un tableau, mais qui est en oblique, et à l'intérieur du tableau il y a une maison qui brûle, et il y a un oiseau qui sort du tableau et qui va dans l'autre espace du tableau, et ça c'est antérieur encore au *Jockey perdu*. C'est peut-être une toile qui est la plus surréaliste des premières. C'est un tableau de 1925. Donc *Le Jockey perdu* est un tableau pour lequel Magritte avait une préférence personnelle et c'est pour ça qu'il le citait plus volontiers, mais c'est évidemment un tableau parmi les premiers, mais il y avait tous les tableaux de l'exposition du Centaure (1927). C'étaient tous à peu près du même moment.

- Je pense plutôt au Cinéma bleu.
MM Là je crois avoir découvert que c'était sous l'influence du film *L'Inhumaine* (1924) de Marcel L'Herbier.[1] C'est un classique du cinéma de l'époque et qui a fait beaucoup de bruit parce qu'il y avait un climat moderne. Si on voit ce film, je l'ai vu il y a deux ou trois ans à la télévision, on est très frappé par la ressemblance qu'il a avec les tableaux de Magritte de cette époque – l'homme blanc, le personnage de femme. Ce n'est pas seulement parce que c'était la mode à l'époque, mais aussi une certaine composition et présentation. C'est très frappant. Je crois qu'il y a eu une sorte d'influence.

- Pensez-vous que Magritte a été influencé par les étalages, la mode ?
MM Non, je ne crois pas. Mais il y a une autre influence, si on veut parler d'influences, que moi j'ai relevée, qui est le sol avec des croix, des lignes.

- Le sol polygonal ?[2]
MM Oui, ça se trouve dans le film *Docteur Caligari*, où il marche sur un sol qui est plissé comme ça, je pense.[3] J'étais frappé par ça, surtout que c'est un film qui a eu beaucoup d'influence à l'époque. Quand j'ai revu ça, j'étais frappé par ce fait que le sol – il n'y a pas seulement l'architecture, ça c'est propre au

film – mais le sol curieusement entreligné qu'on voit dans plusieurs tableaux de Magritte, *Après le Bal* et dans les collages de 1926. Oui, c'est ça. C'est peut-être un accident mais ça m'a frappé.

- Vous croyez que c'est une déformation du 'plancher' de la perspective ?
MM Oui, mais c'est aussi dans le film. Je n'en tire pas de conclusions. Il y a plus d'influence pour moi de l'esprit des Mack Sennett, chez Magritte, si on peut parler d'influences.

- Et l'Académie, il vous en a parlé ?
MM Non, je ne crois pas que cela ait eu d'influence. La seule fois qu'on en a parlé c'était pour dire que c'était un peu inutile parce qu'on apprenait le dessin comme un écrivain doit apprendre la grammaire.

- Il ne tenait pas aux règles académiques et classiques ?
MM Non, il se servait de la peinture et d'autre part il y avait très peu de peintres qu'il aimait. Un jour je lui ai posé la question de ce qu'il aimait en peinture. Il y en avait très peu. Il a cité *Le Cimetière juif* de Ruysdael. C'est un tableau assez tourmenté. Et alors les tableaux de Lionello Balestieri. C'était moi qui ai trouvé ces choses parce que c'était très, très rare, ces choses. Je possédais des cartes postales. Il avait aussi de l'intérêt pour des choses comme Botticelli, mais il ne se souciait pas beaucoup de ce que les autres faisaient. Alors il n'aimait même pas le genre de Klee, Miró. Il détestait ça.

- Je me demande quel genre d'homme il était, son caractère, parce que van Hecke a dit en 1927 que son monde était silencieux, calme et froid.
MM C'était dans son monde pictural.

- Oui, mais je vois beaucoup de violence, de sang, et de couleurs dans son œuvre.
MM Violence, non, parce qu'il détestait la violence. Évidemment il aimait les romans policiers, mais en général il détestait la violence.

- Et la violence dans L'Assassin menacé*, son traitement du corps de la femme, par exemple ? Il le découpait.*
MM Ça dépend de quoi, parce que *L'Évidence éternelle*, ce n'est pas dans le sens du découpage. C'est dans un autre sens. Il y a *L'Assassin menacé* où il y a une femme assassinée. Là, c'est le personnage qui est distrait, qui écoute un disque pour ne pas s'occuper de la femme assassinée, pendant que tout autour on attend pour le guetter. Sinon, je ne vois pas de même qu'on a une tendance à le mettre toujours parmi les peintres érotiques. Il n'y a rien d'érotique chez lui.

- *Et* Les Idées de l'acrobate ?
MM Ce n'est pas dirigé contre la femme. C'est un tour d'image. Cela n'a pas une incidence psychologique ni sociale.

- *Alors il était comme l'on dit ?*
MM Très calme, très rangé. Il se couchait très tôt, ne buvant pas d'alcool, supportant très mal l'alcool. Quand il en buvait, il était malade.

- *Fumait-il une pipe ?*
MM Non, jamais, mais il a fumé la cigarette et je crois qu'il l'a abandonnée.

- *Dans* Clarté *en 1945, on a écrit, 'Communiste, Magritte l'est depuis longtemps. Et il ne s'est pas contenté d'être communiste au fond de son cœur : il l'a manifesté souvent, parfois avec scandale, par ses tableaux, par ses articles, par ses déclarations'.*
MM Ça c'est l'époque où il a été officiellement admis dans le parti communiste après la guerre. Évidemment il a été toujours du côté communiste à l'époque. Il a fait des déclarations, mais il n'a rien fait de très, très spectaculaire. Le texte, qui s'appelle 'L'Art bourgeois', a été écrit pour le journal du parti communiste et ça a été refusé. Je me souviens à cette époque-là il a proposé des affiches. C'était le moment où on allait destituer le roi. Il y avait une campagne contre le roi Léopold en Belgique. Il a fait un projet d'affiche et il a été refusé. Il n'avait jamais de contacts. D'abord parce qu'on se trompait sur la véritable nature des communistes, qui étaient complètement dirigés par Staline. On croyait qu'il y avait une sorte d'autonomie locale, mais il n'y avait rien à faire. Alors il y a eu de petites relations comme ça. J'ai moi-même raconté qu'il y avait un tableau qui a été discuté dans la préface que j'ai écrite pour *Les Manifestes*. Alors là je raconte qu'il y a eu une exposition sur l'art social. Il y avait un tableau de Magritte représentant un fusil dans une chambre et du sang qui coule le long du fusil. C'est le seul tableau dont tout le monde a parlé en le critiquant, en l'attaquant. C'était toujours comme ça avec les communistes. A l'époque il fallait peindre des ouvriers malheureux avec de grands drapeaux rouges, de sorte qu'il n'y a jamais eu de grande activité. Il y avait une sorte de rapport très lointain, sans beaucoup d'importance.

- *La Société de Mystère, est-ce qu'elle existait ?*
MM Ça c'était une invention de Waldberg. On peut dire que c'était un rapport entre des gens, un rapport très étroit, des gens qui étaient comme une société, mais qui n'avaient même pas de nom.

- *Ce n'était pas qu'ils travaillaient ensemble ?*
MM Non, au contraire, c'étaient des relations régulières, comme des amis qui se

rencontrent, mais qui, au contraire, s'étaient très souvent perturbées parce qu'il y avait des troubles, des disputes, qui duraient parfois plusieurs années. Avec Nougé il y avait des genres d'éruptions. Quand je l'ai rencontré en 1937, déjà Nougé et Magritte ne se voyaient pas. Puis ils se sont revus un jour en 1938 et puis ils se sont de nouveau brouillés. Puis ils se sont revus après la guerre. Ils se sont de nouveau brouillés. Quand ils se sont brouillés la dernière fois j'ai publié la lettre de rupture. C'était en '52, 3, 4, et alors ils ne se sont plus revus jusqu' à la mort de Magritte. Donc c'était loin d'être une 'société'. Mais il y a eu une sorte de centralisation que Nougé avait apportée, surtout avant Magritte. Avant le groupe surréaliste, comme l'on dit, il y a eu déjà deux groupes – Mesens, Magritte d'un côté, Nougé, Goemans, Lecomte de l'autre. Et alors quand ils se sont rencontrés à la fin de 1926 il y a eu un groupe uni, qui a fait des choses. Alors Magritte a été toujours entouré par Nougé et les autres. Chaque fois qu'il faisait une exposition il était un peu le centre à cause de ses activités. Les autres activités étaient beaucoup plus invisibles parce qu'il y avait peu de publications. Il y a eu des relations plus importantes avec le groupe français à partir du moment où Magritte est venu à Paris.

- *Il est allé voir Dalí ?*
MM Oui. Il était venu parce que Goemans était marchand à Paris. Il avait une galerie. Il a été le premier à exposer Dalí et alors Dalí a invité Goemans et Goemans est venu avec Magritte, sa femme, et Éluard et Gala, qui était encore avec Éluard.

- *Est-ce que Magritte a parlé de Dalí ?*
MM Il m'a un jour dit que si Dalí n'avait pas rencontré Gala, il serait un homme qui ne ferait rien et qui resterait assis sans rien faire. C'était elle qui le poussait à travailler. Cela n'empêche qu'il avait quand même déjà au départ une activité très bruyante, même avant d'être véritablement lancé.

- *On dit que c'était à cause de Georgette que Magritte n'a plus peint de tableaux Vache.*
MM Ah non. Il n'en a plus peint parce que c'était pour une seule exposition. Il avait fait ça comme une manifestation et alors il n'avait absolument rien vendu. C'était sa première exposition à Paris à cinquante ans et il ne vendait rien du tout, ce qu'il savait d'avance, mais il n'allait pas continuer. S'il a dit ça sur le moment cela ne veut pas dire qu'il en avait l'intention. En réalité, il a recommencé à faire des tableaux après comme il faisait avant, également abandonnant l'époque 'Solaire'. Cette époque 'Solaire' avait tout de même traîné jusqu' à là. C'était en fait la fin de l'époque 'Solaire', la peinture à la Renoir. C'est venu comme un défi, parce qu'il était connu sans être connu. Il n'avait jamais fait d'exposition

personnelle à Paris. Il n'avait jamais rien eu. Peut-être il y a eu de petites choses à l'époque où il était à Paris avec Goemans, mais on n'est pas très sûr. Donc à l'âge de cinquante ans il y a un bonhomme à Paris qui est dans une galerie tout à fait en dehors du circuit habituel des galeries intéressantes qui propose de faire une exposition. Alors il invente, rien que pour cette exposition, toute la période Vache. C'était déjà au moment où il faisait des tableaux dans l'esprit de la peinture dite 'Renoir', mais c'était déjà la fin et alors après la période Vache il a repris une peinture mieux achevée. Il a abandonné la technique impressionniste. En fait il avait cru en la période 'Solaire', mais personne ne le suivait. Même ses amis trouvaient ça moins bon. Alors il a laissé tomber.

- C'était une façon de se moquer des acheteurs ?
MM Oui.

- A ce temps-là vivait-il de sa peinture ?
MM Mal, parce que ce n'est qu'en 1948 qu'il a eu son premier contrat avec l'Amérique. Il y avait une exposition à la Hugo Gallery. Ça a commencé seulement à ce moment-là. Mais c'était encore au point où il fait des choses commerciales et Georgette a toujours travaillé chez sa sœur régulièrement. Donc je dirais que le véritable succès de vente a commencé en 1960, même plus tard, en 1962 avec l'exposition rétrospective à Knokke. C'est très court. Il est mort en 1967. Il n'y a eu que cinq ans. Et alors c'est allé très, très fort. Je crois qu'on a vendu un tableau de lui à un million de francs belges en 1966. C'était la limite. Il n'a pas été dans la misère, mais il n'était pas dans une situation très brillante.

- Qu'est-ce qu'elle faisait Georgette ?
MM Sa sœur avait un commerce de fourniture artistique et elle aidait sa sœur. Elle allait travailler l'après-midi. Il avait probablement des toiles gratuites et des pinceaux. La sœur avait aussi beaucoup de toiles qu'elle avait reçues. Elle est morte il n'y a pas longtemps et le mari, donc le beau-frère, a tout redonné à sa belle sœur. Il y avait beaucoup de tableaux anciens. Avant, elle [Georgette] n'avait que des tableaux récents parce que tout était vendu au fur et à mesure. Mais depuis qu'elle a reçu des choses de sa sœur, elle a *L'Esprit comique*. Il y a un tableau très mystérieux qui représente une pipe, de 1924, qu'on ne comprend pas très bien – une simple pipe peinte en 1923 ou en 1924. C'est un tableau assez bizarre.[4]

- Dans les textes de Magritte le lecteur pourrait croire mieux comprendre les tableaux, mais est-ce que c'est une façon de se moquer du lecteur qui tache de comprendre son œuvre ? Par exemple, 'La Ressemblance' ?

MM Ah oui, la fin. Je crois justement qu'il ne se moquait pas. Il voulait qu'on prenne ça très sérieusement. Mais là je me perds un peu parce que c'est très obscur. Ça c'est une période où il s'aventure dans une espèce de philosophie. D'ailleurs, on s'est un petit peu séparé sur ces choses-là. Mais dans d'autres textes avant, par exemple, dans sa conférence, je trouve que c'est plus clair. Après, quand il s'est mis à définir la ressemblance et les images, la poésie et le mystère, c'était incompréhensible.

- C'était, en fait, un peintre, pas un philosophe ?
MM Oui. Enfin on peut peut-être dire qu'il faisait de la philosophie avec la peinture. En tout cas si on le considère sur le plan de ce qu'il écrit alors c'est très obscur. Il essayait de dire quelque chose, mais je ne pense pas qu'il arrivait à le dire. Il n'est pas le seul. Il y a tant de philosophes qui essayent de dire quelque chose sans rien dire.

- Pensez vous qu'il a été influencé par Nougé ?
MM Oui. Il a eu une sorte d'influence morale qui a surtout duré pendant toute l'époque dont on parle (1920-1930), depuis le début. Mais on ne peut pas dire qu'il a eu une influence directe sur ses œuvres parce que c'était une invention. Nougé l'a conseillé, si on veut. Il lui donnait des appréciations. On ne peut pas dire que vraiment il l'a influencé au sens où il a dit qu'il faut peindre ça ou ça. Par exemple, il est arrivé qu'il lui dise 'Il faudrait que tu songes à faire' – parce qu'on parlait toujours du *problème* – 'le problème du piano', et alors Magritte a fait *La Main heureuse*. Mais ce n'est pas une influence de Nougé. C'est Nougé qui a dit c'est intéressant de voir ce qu'il faudrait faire avec un piano. Donc on ne peut vraiment parler d'influence.

- Il ne lui a pas proposé une méthode scientifique ?
MM Non. C'est-à-dire qu'il a créé une sorte d'appareil doctrinal, si on veut, à partir de la peinture. Où Nougé a joué un grand rôle c'est dans l'idée des titres, le titre étant donné comme une protection contre le fait que les gens pourraient concevoir ça comme plaisanterie. Le titre donnait toujours un appui poétique à l'image. C'est une tendance que Magritte a toujours conservée, qui venait de Nougé, l'importance du titre. Avant ça ses titres étaient comme tous les titres qu'on donne. En général, le titre c'est une chose rapide sans beaucoup d'importance, tandis qu'avec Nougé il y avait vraiment soutien. Il précisait dans *Les Images défendues* que les tableaux n'ont pas vraiment besoin d'un titre mais que c'est un moyen d'empêcher que le spectateur les néglige, soit indifférent. En tout cas il l'empêche de considérer ça comme une chose secondaire ou sans importance. Sur ce point-là je dirais que ça c'est une influence. Un grand nombre des titres sont de Nougé, mais Magritte a donné

des titres. Le cas que je connais c'est la carotte avec la bouteille. Magritte tenait beaucoup à ce que ça s'appelle 'L'Explication' parce que des gens demandaient toujours 'Qu'est-ce que cela veut dire ?' Il a montré une carotte et une bouteille et à côté une bouteille qui devenait une carotte. Alors à cette époque-là Magritte ne voyait pas Nougé. Ils s'étaient brouillés. Moi je racontais à Nougé les tableaux de Magritte. Je faisais un petit croquis et lui donnait les titres, et moi je transmettais les titres. Pour celui-là Nougé avait tout de suite trouvé 'Discours de la méthode'. Mais Magritte tenait à son 'Explication' parce que c'était plus direct, plus terre à terre et c'est comme ça que j'ai transmis d'autres titres, entre autres 'La Folie Almayer'. C'était un titre que Nougé a donné, un titre de Conrad. Il y avait aussi un autre tableau qui est la Terre et une pomme, *L'Autre Son de cloche*, titre de Nougé. Moi je transmettais les titres et tout de suite Magritte acceptait. Il y a eu d'autres cas comme ça.

- Il y a, en fait, un autre tableau qui s'appelle 'Discours de la méthode'. Pour revenir à la période Vache, pensez-vous que c'était une façon de se libérer du système, de 'l'appareil doctrinal' qu'il s'est imposé lui-même ?
MM Non. Ça lui est venu comme ça. Il avait comme ça des élans, des fantaisies. C'est venu du fait que c'était un homme de cinquante ans qui n'avait même pas eu une seule exposition à Paris.

- Il y a beaucoup de violence quand même dans la période Vache.
MM Oui, et alors c'est prophétique. A cette époque-là c'était quelque chose d'absolument fou. C'était délirant. C'était vraiment inadmissible. Après, avec le Pop Art, cette sorte de chose est devenue tout à fait acceptable, parce qu'on peut tout faire maintenant. A ce moment-là c'était impensable. Même la peinture 'traditionnelle', si on peut dire, de Magritte n'était absolument pas admise. Il n'y avait à ce moment-là que des peintres abstraits dans toutes les galeries et tout ce qui était surréaliste était considéré comme une chose totalement dépassée, méprisée, rejetée. Alors, en plus de ça, il faisait encore de la peinture Vache. Dans le livre d'or il y avait 'Ridicule' et alors en dessous Éluard avait écrit 'Rira bien qui rira le dernier'.

9 March 1981, rue Louis Hap 222, Brussels

---

[1] *L'Inhumaine*, Dir. Marcel L'Herbier, Cinégraphic & Georgette Leblanc, 1924.

[2] José Vovelle, *Le Surréalisme en Belgique* (Brussels, 1972), p. 77.

[3] *Das Cabinet des Dr. Caligari*, *The Cabinet of Dr Caligari*, Dir. Robert Wiene, Decla-Bioscop (Germany), Goldwyn Distributing Company (US), 1920.

[4] André Blavier gives the date 1923, *Ceci n'est pas une pipe* (Verviers, 1973), p. 23.

- *Have you been influenced by Magritte?*
MM Yes, you could say that. The pipe is called 'False Company'. There is a mirror. It's a half pipe, a half *La Trahison des images.*

- *It's often said that* Le Jockey perdu *is Magritte's first accomplished painting.*
MM No, it was his personal favourite. He liked it over and above many others, but there was another work before it, which, as it happens, has just been sold, in London, I think, which I had published and which, I think, had never previously been reproduced. It's called 'Nocturne'. It was a painting within a painting, but which is at an angle, and within the painting there is a house on fire, as well as a bird coming out of the painting and entering the other space of the painting, and that was before even *Le Jockey perdu.* It's perhaps the most surrealist of his early works. It was painted in 1925. Therefore *Le Jockey perdu* was a work Magritte himself liked particularly and that's why he would often refer to it whenever the opportunity arose, but it's obviously only one of the early works, whereas there were all the works shown at Le Centaure exhibition (1927). They were all done more or less at the same time.

- *I'm thinking more of* Cinéma bleu.
MM As far as that work goes I believe I've discovered it was heavily influenced by the film *L'Inhumaine* (1924) by Marcel L'Herbier.[1] It was a cinema classic of the time, which got a lot of media attention because it had a modern feel. If you watch the film, which I did two or three years ago on television, you are struck by its similarity to the paintings Magritte was producing at the time – the white man, the way of depicting women. It's not just that it was fashionable then, but there was also something about the composition and the settings. It's striking. I believe there was a sort of influence.

- *Do you think Magritte was influenced by shop window display, by fashion?*
MM No, I don't think so. But there is another influence, if we must talk of influences, which I discovered, concerning crosses or lines on the ground.

- *The ground as polygons?*[2]
MM Yes, you see that in the film *Dr Caligari* in which he walks on ground which has these types of folds, I think.[3] I was struck by this, particularly since it was a very influential film at the time. When I watched it again I was struck by the ground – there is more than the buildings, which are unique to the film – the ground with strange criss-cross lines on it, which appears in several of Magritte's paintings, *Après le Bal* and in the collages of 1926. Yes, that's it. It may be an accident, but it struck me.

- Do you think it's a distortion of the 'pavement' of the perspective construction?
MM Yes, but it's also in the film. I'm not drawing any conclusions from it. In Magritte's work there is more influence, for me, from the spirit of Mack Sennett films, if we must talk of influences.

- And the Académie, did he talk to you about it?
MM No, I don't think that had had an influence. The only time he talked about it was to say that it was a bit useless because they had to learn to draw in the way someone who writes has to learn grammar.

- He didn't think much of academic, classical rules?
MM No, he made use of painting and, besides, there were very few painters whom he liked. One day I asked him what paintings he liked. There were very few. He cited *The Jewish Cemetery* by Ruysdael. It's a fairly tortured work. And, as well, works by Lionello Balestieri. I was the one to glean these things, which were very, very obscure. I had some postcards. He was also interested in such things as the work of Botticelli, but he didn't worry much about what his contemporaries were doing. In fact, he didn't even like artists such as Klee, Miró. He hated that sort of thing.

- I keep wondering what type of man he was, his personality, because in 1927 van Hecke said that his world was silent, tranquil and cold.
MM That was a description of his pictorial world.

- Yes, but I can see lots of violence, blood and colours in his work.
MM Violence, no, because he hated violence. Obviously he liked crime novels, but, in other circumstances, he hated violence.

- And the violence in L'Assassin menacé, *his treatment of the female body, for example? He routinely sliced it up.*
MM It depends what we are referring to, because *L'Évidence éternelle* is not meant to be a slicing up of the body. It's something else. Take *L'Assassin menacé*, in which there's a murdered woman. Here, it's the protagonist who is preoccupied, who listens to a record to avoid dealing with the murdered woman, while, all around, others are waiting to pounce on him. Apart from that, I frankly can't see why there's a constant tendency to regard him as an erotic painter. There is nothing erotic about his work.

- And *Les Idées de l'acrobate*?
MM It's not directed against women. It's a visual pun. It has no psychological or social connotation.

- So he was just as he is described?
MM Very calm, very tidy. He went to bed very early, didn't drink, couldn't hold his drink. When he did drink he was ill.

- Did he smoke a pipe?
MM No, never, but he smoked cigarettes and I think he gave up.

- In Clarté *in 1945 we find the following: 'A Communist is what Magritte has been for a long time. What is more, it's not enough for him simply to be a true Communist: he has often demonstrated his commitment, sometimes by creating a stir, in his paintings, in his articles, in his public statements'.*
MM That was at the time he had been officially admitted to the Communist Party after the war. Obviously he had always had Communist leanings at that time. He made statements, but didn't actually do anything very, very spectacular. The text, which is entitled 'L'Art bourgeois', had been written for the Communist Party newspaper and was not accepted for publication. I remember that at that time he had put forward ideas for posters. It was the time that the king was going to be deposed. There was a campaign in Belgium against King Léopold. He had drawn up a design for a poster and was turned down. He never had the right contacts. To begin with, people were mistaken about the true nature of the Communists, who were wholly under Stalin's control. People thought there was a sort of local autonomy, but there was nothing of the sort. So, there were minor interactions like these. In the preface I wrote for *Les Manifestes* I commented on a particular painting. On that point, I explained that an exhibition on social art had been held. It included a work by Magritte, depicting a gun in a room and blood running down the length of the gun. It was the only work everyone talked about, criticising and attacking it. It was always like that among the Communists. At that time you had to paint wretched peasants with large red flags, with the result that there was never any significant activity. There was a sort of very distant rapport, which never amounted to much.

- Did The Society of Mystery exist?
MM That had been invented by Waldberg. It would be fair to say that this refers to the relationship of a group of people, a very close relationship, a group of people who were like a society, but who didn't even have a name for themselves.

- Wasn't it that they were working together?
MM No, on the contrary, they frequently met up, just like friends would, but they would also very often clash because they'd be at odds with one another, they would have arguments which, sometimes, lasted several years. In the case of Nougé there were what could be termed 'eruptions'. When I met Magritte, in

1937, he and Nougé were no longer on speaking terms. Then one day in 1938 they met up again and it wasn't long before they quarrelled again. Then they met up again after the war. They quarrelled once again. When they quarrelled for the last time I published the letter that consolidated the split. It was in '52, 3, 4, and from that point they didn't see each other, even once, right up to Magritte's death. So, you see, it was far from being a 'society'. But there was a sort of centralization that Nougé had brought, particularly before Magritte. Before the surrealist group, as it is termed, there already existed two groups – Mesens, Magritte on the one hand and Nougé, Goemans, Lecomte on the other. And so when they all met up at the end of 1926 a united group resulted, which achieved a great deal. From then on Magritte had always been surrounded by Nougé and the others. Every time he had an exhibition he became the focal point, because of what he did. Other activities were far more unseen, since there were very few publications. There were more significant relations with the French group once Magritte had gone to Paris.

- *Had he gone to see Dalí?*
MM Yes. It happened because Goemans was a dealer in Paris. He had a gallery. He had been the first to give Dalí an exhibition and so Dalí invited Goemans to his home and Goemans went with Magritte, his wife, and Éluard and Gala, who was then still with Éluard.

- *Did Magritte talk about Dalí?*
MM He once said that if Dalí hadn't met Gala he would have been a man who achieved nothing and sat around all day without doing anything. She was the one who pushed him to work. That still doesn't mean that, at the start, he wasn't already attracting a lot of attention, even before he had properly risen to fame.

- *According to some, it was because of Georgette that Magritte didn't paint any more Vache works.*
MM Not at all. He didn't paint any more of them because these were done for a single exhibition. He did these as a protest and, as a result, he sold absolutely nothing. It was his first exhibition in Paris, at the age of 50, and he didn't have a single sale, as he well knew in advance, but he had had no intention of continuing. If, on the spur of the moment, he had said that he would continue, it doesn't mean he meant it. As it turned out, he subsequently resumed painting in his usual style, which also meant that he abandoned his 'Sunshine' phase. This 'Sunshine' phase had, indeed, gone on up to that point. It was, in fact, the end of the 'Sunshine' phase, his Renoiresque style. It amounted to a defiant gesture, because he was known without being known. He had never had a solo exhibition in Paris, not once. He may have shown works in a minor way with

Goemans when he was in Paris, but that's just guesswork. So, when he gets to 50, along comes some Parisian chap from a gallery which is in no way part of the influential galleries circuit and offers him an exhibition. So, with nothing but this exhibition in mind he dreams up the whole of the Vache period. This came when he had been doing his Renoiresque works, but the phase was coming to an end, so, after the Vache period, he resumed a more accomplished style. He abandoned his Impressionist technique. He had, in fact, genuinely believed in the 'Sunshine' period, but no one else had. Even his friends didn't think much of it. So he gave up.

- *Was it a way of cocking a snook at art buyers?*
MM Yes.

- *Was he making a living from his painting at that time?*
MM Barely, because it was not until 1948 that he had his first commission from the States. He had an exhibition at the Hugo Gallery. Things really got going from then on. But up to then he was doing commercial work and Georgette was still working regularly for her sister, who had a business. So I'd say that he started selling successfully from 1960, even later, in 1962 with the retrospective exhibition at Knokke. It was a short period of time. He died in 1967. There were only five years. That's when things went sky-high. I think one of his works sold for one million Belgian Francs in 1966. That's as far as it went. He wasn't a pauper, but he wasn't excessively wealthy either.

- *What did Georgette do?*
MM Her sister had an artists' materials shop and she helped her sister. She worked in the afternoons. He probably got free canvases and paint brushes. The sister had been given lots of paintings. She died recently and her husband, that is Georgette's brother-in-law, gave them all back to his sister-in-law. There were lots of early works. Previously, Georgette only had recent works, since everything had been sold in dribs and drabs. But when she was given the works that had belonged to her sister she had *L'Esprit comique*. There's a very mysterious painting of 1924 depicting a pipe, which people don't understand very well – a simple pipe painted in 1923 or 1924. It's quite an odd work.[4]

- *You would think that reading what Magritte wrote might be a way understanding his paintings better, but are these texts his way of scoffing at those who try to delve into the meaning of his oeuvre? Take the text 'La Ressemblance', for instance.*
MM Oh yes, ultimately. Ironically, I think he was not poking fun. He wanted his writings to be taken very seriously. But I have trouble following them because of their extreme impenetrability. This is a phase during which he ventures into

a kind of philosophy. What's more, we didn't totally see eye-to-eye on such things. But in other, earlier, texts, such as his lecture, for example, I find it easier to understand what he meant. Later on, when he set about defining resemblance and images, poetry and mystery, he became incomprehensible.

- *He was, in fact, a painter, not a philosopher?*
MM Yes. Essentially, one could perhaps say he was expressing philosophical ideas through painting. Whichever way you look at it, if he is approached via what he wrote, then he becomes very difficult to fathom. He kept trying to say something, but I don't think he managed to. He is not alone. There have been numerous philosophers who have tried to say something and ended up saying nothing.

- *Do you think he was influenced by Nougé?*
MM Yes. He had a sort of moral influence, primarily during the whole of the period we're concerned with (1920-1930), right from the start. But it would not be true to say that he had had a direct influence on his works because these came from Magritte's own imagination. Nougé gave advice, so to speak. He would give him critiques. It cannot be said that he truly influenced him in the sense that he dictated what should or should not be painted. For example, he once said to him 'You should think about solving' – because they would always be talking about a *problem* – 'the problem of the piano', and so Magritte painted *La Main heureuse*. But this wasn't his being influenced by Nougé. All Nougé had done was to say it would be interesting to see what should be done with a piano. Therefore, we can't really talk of an 'influence'.

- *Didn't he put forward a scientific methodology?*
MM No. That is to say, he created a sort of doctrinal apparatus, so to speak, based on painting. Where Nougé played a major role was in the idea behind the titles, which were given to protect the works from being taken as jokes. The title always gave the image a poetic slant. The idea that the title was important, which had come from Nougé, was one that Magritte always hung on to. Up to that time his titles were like all other titles. Generally, titles are given in a cursory manner and don't matter much, whereas with Nougé they really involved a lot of thought. In *Les Images défendues* he wrote that paintings don't really need titles, but they act as a way of focusing the attention of the spectator and creating an impact. In any case, the spectator is prevented from considering the title as something secondary or unimportant. On this particular point I would say that there *is* an influence. A great many titles are Nougé's, but Magritte did find some titles. One case I know about is that of the carrot and the bottle. Magritte was keen for it to be called 'The Explanation' because people always asked what it

meant. He painted a carrot and a bottle and beside them put a bottle turning into a carrot. At that time Magritte was no longer seeing Nougé. They had quarrelled. I would go to Nougé and describe Magritte's paintings. I'd do a little sketch and he'd give the titles, which I would then pass on to Magritte. For this painting Nougé had immediately come up with 'Discours de la méthode' [Discourse on the Method].[5] But Magritte was keen on his own 'Explanation' because it was more direct, more down-to-earth. That's how I transmitted other titles, such as 'La Folie Almayer', among others. That was a title that Nougé had given, one of Conrad's texts. There was also another painting titled by Nougé, which was of the Earth and an apple, *L'Autre Son de cloche*. I would transmit the titles and Magritte accepted them without hesitation. There were other instances like that.

- There is, in fact, another painting called 'Discours de la méthode'. To return to the Vache period, do you think that it was a way of freeing himself of his self-imposed 'doctrinal apparatus'?
MM No. It was just one of those things that came to him. Things would come to him out of the blue, fantasies. It happened because he was a man of fifty who hadn't even had a single exhibition in Paris.

- There is, even so, a lot of violence in the Vache period.
MM Yes, and it turned out to be prophetic. At that time it was regarded as something totally mad. It was over the top. It was really inadmissible. Later, with Pop Art, that sort of thing became completely acceptable, because anything can be done now. At that time it was unthinkable. Even Magritte's traditional painting, if we can call it that, was absolutely not admissible. At that time all the galleries were only showing the abstract painters and everything which was surrealist was regarded as totally old hat, it was despised, rejected. So, in addition to all that, he had the gall to produce his Vache paintings. Someone wrote 'Ridiculous' in the visitors' book and so underneath Éluard added 'He who laughs last, laughs the loudest'.

---

1 *L'Inhumaine*, Dir. Marcel L'Herbier, Cinégraphic & Georgette Leblanc, 1924.

2 José Vovelle, *Le Surréalisme en Belgique* (Brussels, 1972), p. 77.

3 *Das Cabinet des Dr. Caligari*, *The Cabinet of Dr Caligari*, Dir. Robert Wiene, Decla-Bioscop (Germany), Goldwyn Distributing Company (US), 1920.

4 André Blavier gave the date 1923, *Ceci n'est pas une pipe* (Verviers, 1973), p. 23.

5 The inevitable clumsiness of any translation from the French is due to the fact that Descartes' treatise is invariably referred to by an abbreviated title. The complete title is *Discours de la méthode pour bien conduire sa raison, et chercher la vérité dans les sciences* (Discourse on the method of correctly conducting one's reason and of seeking truth in the sciences).

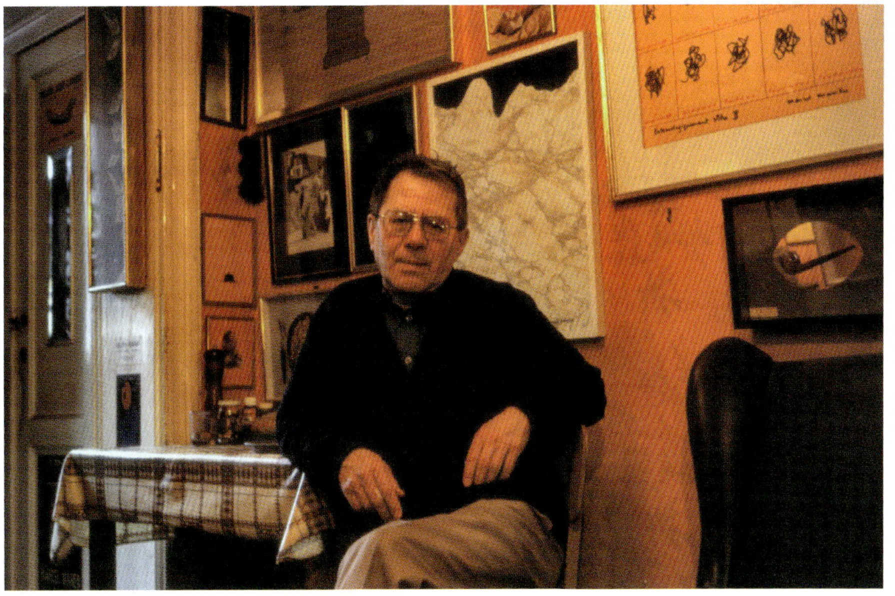

Marcel Mariën, rue Louis Hap 222, Brussels, 1981

Marcel Mariën

SECOND INTERVIEW

- Votre vie a été très active.

MM Oui, mais j'étais beaucoup sans rien faire. J'ai passé une grande partie de ma vie sans rien faire. J'ai eu des périodes où je n'ai pas pu écrire. Je faisais autre chose. C'était un long combat : je ne pouvais pas renoncer à écrire et en même temps je ne pouvais pas faire ce que je voulais. J'ai commencé à écrire vers maintenant. Je n'ai jamais écrit avant. J'écrivais un peu par accident. Le cas de Nougé est assez différent, mais quand même similaire. Par exemple, la plupart des choses qu'il a écrites sur Magritte, c'étaient toujours à l'occasion d'une exposition. C'est Magritte qui le poussait à écrire s'il ne voulait pas écrire. Quand les choses ont pris un tour plus important il a fait *Les Images défendues*, qui étaient destinées à un livre mais toujours à l'instigation de Magritte. Plusieurs textes qu'il a écrits sont aussi des textes qui sont nés des circonstances. Il aimait bien dire qu'il était un écrivain de circonstance. Moi, dans un sens aussi, j'ai eu des périodes de facilité puis des autres périodes de silence, de difficulté.

-Vous avez été marin ?

MM Oui, j'ai été mess-boy.

- Magritte, ou plutôt sa vision poétique, fait partie de notre culture. La publicité s'en sert et il y a une rue René Magritte. Est-ce que son surréalisme a été remplacé par une autre contestation, plus violente, peut-être ?

MM Actuellement, si c'est sur le plan des mœurs alors il faut dire que tout est fait, tout est permis. Il n'y a plus d'ambition. Quand on n'a pas d'ambition c'est presque une forme naturelle de vie parce qu'on va d'une chose à l'autre. Alors, évidemment, j'ai sauté sur les occasions. J'ai eu l'occasion de partir en Amérique, même si c'est pour d'autres raisons. Puis, un jour, j'avais l'occasion d'aller en Chine. Chaque fois, j'ai attrapé l'occasion. Je n'ai pas réfléchi. Je n'ai pas hésité.

- Vous vous êtes décrit comme un 'croyant'.

MM Ça c'est une liste qui commence 'J'ai été. Je pourrais être...' Évidemment, j'étais croyant en marxisme. C'est dans un sens général.

- Mais vous ne croyez pas à l'Homme ?

MM C'est à dire je ne crois pas qu'il y ait une explication du monde. De toute façon c'est absurde puisque le monde n'est pas terminé alors ce serait absurde de dire qu'il y a une explication.

- Si 'il y a des salauds sur la terre', comme l'a dit le vieillard dans L'Imitation du cinéma, *ce sont qui ?*

MM Ah, ça c'est tout le monde. Oui. C'est qui qui dit 'Vae victis', malheur aux vaincus ? C'est la même chose.[1]

- Est-ce qu'on peut faire un rétrécissement d'objets ?[2]

MM Oui, mais je n'ai pas pensé à en faire. Mais il faut avoir des instruments spéciaux, des matières très faciles à travailler.

- Je ne parle pas du côté technique.

MM Ah oui, évidemment.

- Alors vous n'avez pas une conception du rétrécissement qui s'applique uniquement à l'image ?

MM Non, mais c'est simplement une expérience qui est limitée et que je ne considère pas comme une chose qu'il faudrait continuer.

- Dans votre 'Jeu de la vie' où est le surréalisme ?

MM C'est très difficile. Je vais peut-être répondre à ça parce que je suis en train d'écrire sur cette question.

- Magritte, comment a-t-il joué le 'Jeu de la vie' ?

MM Sur le plan de ce qu'on appelle 'la vie', d'une façon assez résignée. C'est un jeu qui s'est passé dans sa peinture. Moi j'ai certainement fait beaucoup plus d'action que lui parce que j'ai bougé. Je n'ai pas vécu d'une manière continue comme ce qu'on appelle la vie bourgeoise. Ça ne diffère pas tellement parce qu'on peut considérer qu'un industriel qui se lance, mettons Henry Ford, qui commence ouvrier et qui fait l'empire des Ford, est un aventurier. C'est exactement la vie d'aventurier, avec tous les dangers, que ça comporte, les risques, des tas de choses. Et un peintre qui fait tout comme Magritte a fait également une chose qui est une aventure. En dehors de quoi il y a la vie quotidienne. Je ne pense pas que l'aspect quotidien de la vie dans le cas de Magritte puisse être considéré comme important, ou de la critiquer, comme l'on a fait d'habitude, comme une chose bourgeoise. Ce n'était pas tout à fait ça. Il n'avait pas besoin nécessairement, pour faire sa peinture, de s'habiller comme un pauvre et de traîner dans des cafés à Paris jusqu' à minuit, comme font certains artistes. De sorte que c'est plutôt un aspect presque pervers d'avoir une vie très régulière. C'est comme Kant qui avait une vie régulière. C'est un peu comme ça qu'il faut voir la vie de Magritte.

- *Avec vous c'est l'envers.*
MM Oui, dans un sens, mais j'ai aussi quand même une conception assez, même très, disciplinée. Je me lève à une heure précise, je ne traîne pas, etc. C'est peut-être plus pittoresque. La vie elle-même tend à être régulière.

- *Et votre biographie ?*
MM Oui, d'abord ça tient à toutes sortes d'accidents, mais ça tient en partie parce qu'à un certain moment j'ai vécu avec une femme et que j'ai dû m'en séparer. Je n'avais pas de métier. Je n'avais pas un métier fixe et je n'avais pas de problèmes de ce côté-là. Si c'est sur le plan de l'invention poétique, là évidemment il n'y a pas grand-chose, sauf peut-être dans le domaine du cinéma. En peinture je ne vois pas ce qui dépasse Magritte actuellement ou ce qui continue l'élan de Magritte. En poésie c'est assez trouble aussi. Je crois qu'il a eu un accident qui s'est produit à un certain moment. C'est que la tendance poétique a été rejetée par la tendance politique. Il y a toute une chose qui s'est passée en partie à cause de la guerre et déjà un peu avant la guerre et qui fait que toute la jeunesse intellectuelle s'est mise à s'intéresser beaucoup plus à la question politique. Alors il y a eu le phénomène existentialiste et, après, cela a continué et toujours la politique a pris une grande importance dans ces histoires. Disons qu'à l'origine les surréalistes étaient peut-être parmi les premiers à s'intéresser aussi à la politique, mais tout de même en la considérant comme une chose secondaire, tandis qu'après, c'est devenu presque primordial. Enfin on a tout ramené à la politique. Je ne sais pas si on dévie un peu de la question, mais je veux dire c'est ça je crois la grande différence et c'est peut-être pourquoi le surréalisme

est un peu resté sur le côté, comme une chose passée, parce que cette politique est devenue tellement importante, même dans les mouvements. Je ne sais pas si vous connaissez ça, la revue *Tel Quel* à Paris – des gens autour de Roland Barthes et Philippe Sollers. Bien qu'ils soient en marge de la politique, ils ont quand même fait quelque chose qui est tout à fait différent et qui pour moi n'est pas intéressant, mais qu'eux considèrent comme l'avant-garde actuellement.

24 March 1981, Antwerp

---

1 In 387 BC an army of Gauls led by Brennus attacked and captured all but one of the Roman hills, which was besieged. When the Romans complained about the way in which their gold was being measured out to meet the ransom, Brennus angrily retorted 'Woe to the vanquished', making it clear that the conquered have no rights.

2 The technique of 'rétrécissement' was devised by Marcel Mariën and involved 'shrinking' photographs of figures by cutting away parts of the image. The procedure is referred to above in the chapter 'Elastic Form', endnote 3.

- You've had an eventful life.

MM Yes, but I also spent a lot of time doing nothing. I spent a great deal of my life doing nothing. There were periods when I couldn't write. I did other things. It was a long battle: I couldn't give up writing and at the same time I couldn't do what I wanted. I recently started to write poetry. I was previously never a writer. I used to write a little by accident. In Nougé's case it was quite different, but still similar. For example, most of his texts on Magritte were invariably prompted by an exhibition. It was Magritte who kept pushing him to write whenever he didn't want to. When Magritte started getting well-known, Nougé wrote *Les Images défendues*, which was intended to be a book, but only at Magritte's instigation. Several of the texts he wrote also arose out of specific circumstances. He liked saying he was a writer of circumstance. I too, in a sense, had periods when I could write easily and others when I was silent, when I found writing difficult.

-You were a sailor?

MM Yes, I was a mess-boy.

- Magritte, or rather his poetic vision, is now part of our popular culture. Advertising makes use of it and there is a street named after him (rue René Magritte). Has surrealism been replaced by another form of contestation, a more violent one perhaps?

MM Nowadays, if we're talking about our way of life then it has to be said that we can do anything, nothing is off limits. There's nothing left to achieve. When there's nothing to strive for, life can be lived in a way that is more or less natural, just going from one thing to another. So, obviously, I grabbed opportunities that came my way. I had the opportunity of going to the States, even if it was for other reasons. Then, one day, I had the opportunity of going to China. Every time, I seized opportunities. I didn't think twice. I didn't hesitate.

- You described yourself as a 'believer'.

MM This is a list which begins 'I have been, I could be ...' Obviously, I had been a believer in Marxism. The word is used in its general sense.

- But don't you believe in Man?

MM That's to say, I don't believe there's an explanation for the world. In any case it's an absurd thought since the world hasn't come to an end and so it would be absurd to say that it has an explanation.

- If 'there are bastards on this Earth', as the old man in L'Imitation du cinéma *said, who are they?*

MM Ah, that's everybody. Yes. Who was it who said 'Vae victis', woe betide the vanquished. It's the same thing.[1]

- *Can the rétrécissement be made with an object?*[2]
MM Yes, but I haven't thought of doing it. But you need special tools, materials that can be easily worked with.

- *I'm not speaking about practical technique.*
MM Yes, that's clear.

- *So your conception of the rétrécissement is not restricted to the image?*
MM No, but it's just a limited experiment, which I don't think should be carried on.

- *In your 'Jeu de la vie' [Game of Life] where is the surrealist quality?*
MM That's difficult to say. Perhaps I'll be giving the answer, since I'm currently writing about just that.

- *How did Magritte play the 'Jeu de la vie'?*
MM On the level of what we call 'life', in a fairly resigned manner. It's a game that was played in his paintings. I myself have certainly been more active than he had been because I've moved around. I haven't lived in a steady way, in a way we call a bourgeois lifestyle. The two are not that different since an industrial tycoon starting out, take Henry Ford for instance, who began as a factory worker and ended up creating the Ford empire, is an adventurer. This is precisely the life of an adventurer, with all the dangers that that entails, the risks, a mass of things. And a painter who has followed a course like Magritte's has equally pulled off an adventure. Beyond this there is everyday life. I don't think that what Magritte did in his day-to-day life can be considered as important. Nor should it be criticised, as it so often is, as being bourgeois. It wasn't totally like that. In order to paint as he did he didn't need to dress like a tramp and hang around in Parisian cafés until midnight, as certain artists do. People expect that so much that it becomes quite perverse to have a very routine lifestyle. Kant had a similarly routine lifestyle. It's a bit like that that Magritte's life should be viewed.

- *In your case the opposite is true.*
MM In one sense, yes. But I do, nevertheless, have an approach to life that is fairly disciplined, even very disciplined. I get up at the same time every day. I don't dawdle around, etc. My life is perhaps more colourful, but, essentially, it tends to be a routine existence.

- And your biography?

MM Yes, to begin with, it results from all sorts of accidents, but part of the story is that at one point I lived with a woman and we had to go our separate ways. I had no profession. I had no steady job and that didn't cause a problem. If we're talking on the level of poetic invention, clearly nothing much has been achieved, except perhaps in the realm of film-making. As far as painting in general goes, I can't see that there's anything at the moment that improves on Magritte or that carries on from where he left off. In poetry, things are rather problematic too. I think that by accident events took a certain course at a particular point in time, with the result that the poetic trend was ousted by the political current. A great shift had occurred, partially because of the war, but also because of what was already happening just before the war, which meant that all young intellectuals increasingly turned their attention to political issues. The Existentialist phenomenon came about and then it took hold. From then on politics took centre-stage in intellectual circles. Let's not forget that, at the start, the surrealists had perhaps been among the first also to take an interest in politics, albeit by giving it a secondary importance. Afterwards, however, it assumed an almost primordial significance. In the end, everything came to be viewed in terms of politics. I'm not sure if we are straying a bit from the question, but I'd like to say that this, I think, is the big difference and is perhaps why surrealism has been somewhat sidelined as something outmoded. This was because political thinking had become crucially important, even in artistic movements. I don't know if you are familiar with this, the *Tel Quel* journal in Paris – the circle of Roland Barthes and Philippe Sollers. Although they are on the margins of politics, they have, nevertheless, done something totally different. To me it doesn't amount to much, whilst they consider it as the current avant-garde.

---

1 In 387 BC an army of Gauls led by Brennus attacked and captured all but one of the Roman hills, which was besieged. When the Romans complained about the way in which their gold was being measured out to meet the ransom, Brennus angrily retorted 'Woe to the vanquished', making it clear that the conquered have no rights.

2 The technique of 'rétrécissement' was devised by Marcel Mariën and involved 'shrinking' photographs of figures by cutting away parts of the image. The procedure is referred to above in the chapter 'Elastic Form', endnote 3.

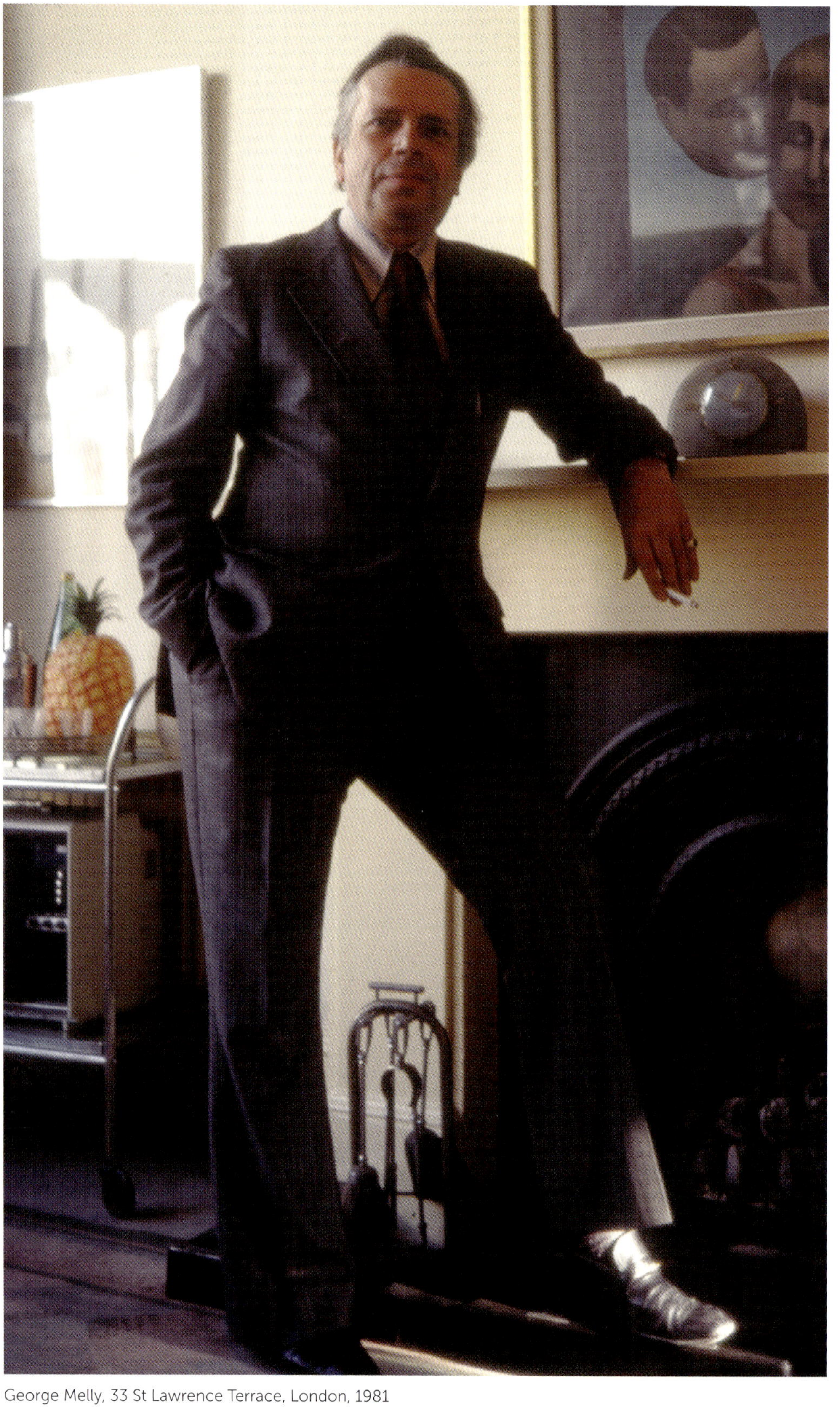

George Melly, 33 St Lawrence Terrace, London, 1981

George Melly

- How did you become associated with Mesens?

GM I became interested in surrealism when I was still at school, aged about fifteen or sixteen. I came upon Herbert Read's book and when I joined the Navy I linked up again, funnily enough, with a school friend who was also in the Navy. As an Able Seaman, he had discovered there was a surrealist group in London, which I did not know at that time. We sent off for their various publications, notably *Message from Nowhere* which was a little pamphlet produced during the war, and it had the address of the surrealist group. I was starting to write surrealist poems and he was making collages so we sent them off from the naval camp to the surrealists and got a reply from the secretary, who was called Simon Watson Taylor, saying if I was ever in London to go and see him, which I did when I was stationed at Chatham. He invited me to a surrealist séance, as they called them. It sounds more mysterious than it is. It means meeting in French. So I went to the Barcelona Restaurant in Beak Street, which is where the surrealists were meeting once a week, on Mondays I think, and I met Mesens for the first time. He was rather taken with me because I was in naval uniform and very enthusiastic, and we became great friends. In consequence, he suggested when I was demobbed from the Navy that I went to work for him at the London Gallery, which he was starting up again. He had run it before the war. It had closed down during the war and he was opening it again. So I did. When I had left the Navy I had six months in Liverpool, pretending to learn shorthand and typing, and then came to London and worked for him.

- Mesens seems to have been an ambassador between Brussels and London.

GM That was one of his roles all his life. He was an ambassador between Brussels and Paris, and then between London, Brussels and Paris. He was very much a travelling salesman, as it were, of surrealism. In his secondary role as art dealer, he was able to promote and push the artists in whom he believed. He also had to sell artists he did not believe in particularly in order to keep body and soul together. He was always a tremendous enthusiast for Magritte at a time when everybody disliked him intensely, and he persisted in that. And by the end of his life, of course, he had seen the tide turn. Then everybody was mad about Magritte.

- Mesens wasn't just benevolent towards Magritte, though.

GM He hoped to sell and get his percentage, but nevertheless he hoped to sell those artists in whom he believed. Frequently, and indeed at the end of the war particularly (before the war was another matter: surrealism was considered a smart novelty and so people tended to buy them if they had a lot of money), when nothing could have been less fashionable, less in the swim, less right than the surrealists, he persisted obstinately in pushing them, because he believed in them. He remained a surrealist after all, and so one could scarcely claim that he was opportunistic at that time in showing Magritte. He would have done better to show John Minton or John Craxton, the latter of which he did show in order to pay for the shows where he showed Magritte and Ernst and others. The fact that history in its arbitrary way swung back the spotlight onto the surrealists towards the middle of the sixties, not much before, (probably the whole psychedelic, swinging London thing reanimated people's ideas in art of the imagination as opposed to a sort of stylized factual art) meant that, in the end, Mesens was a very rich man. But after the war the London Gallery was doing so badly that he frequently had to take his salary in a picture from stock. So it was an heroic struggle, really.

- It strikes me that Mesens and Magritte seem to be temperamentally incompatible. Magritte was a non-drinker, and his lifestyle was conventional even to the point of going to bed early, whereas Mesens is described basically as a night-bird.

GM In fact, they were not that incompatible. Mesens was as neat as Magritte. Mesens' nails were as clean, and his face was as well-shaven, his clothes as conventional. The only difference was that Magritte's conventionality was petit-bourgeois and Mesens' was bourgeois, in other words Mesens' suits were of better material, his ties came from better tie places. Although Mesens was a tremendous drinker, he had a conventional side to him, a sort of Belgian bourgeois side. Drink was his form of protest, and the reason for his many explosions. Nor did Magritte not drink. He just drank very modestly, a glass of wine with lunch and dinner. He wasn't a 'drinker'; Mesens was an alcoholic, and indeed drink killed him. After his wife's death, he doubled the amount he was drinking and then trebled it, until eventually he had one breakdown from drink, one D.T. session in a hospital in St John's Wood. When he came out he gradually stepped up his drinking again. The day he collapsed, I believe he drank a bottle of Pernod before lunch. I have postcards from him in which, answering my pleas for him not to drink so much, he claimed that the effects of the drink on him, particularly Pernod, were medically advantageous – from the point of view of killing yourself, yes, but not otherwise. Magritte also, I think, suffered a great deal from his stomach in later years, so that he was probably unable to drink even if he had wanted to, which I don't think he did.

- I believe that Mesens was deeply anti-religious. I heard a story that one day he found himself in hospital, being tended by nuns.

GM He did but he didn't particularly mind that. He commented as usual on the young ones' tits and so on. He was anti-religious, because to be a surrealist one has to be anti-religious and of course his background was Catholic which gives one something to be anti-religious about. One of the reasons why surrealism has more validity on the Continent than here is that Catholicism has more strength than Protestantism when it comes to protesting against it. A protestant blasphemy is never the same as a Catholic one, because it has less to blaspheme against. So Mesens was anti-religious, certainly. He sometimes said that he would like to have retired to a small French country village, where he would have had arguments with the local curé and the schoolmaster. Of course, he didn't believe, and Magritte neither, but Magritte always took a cooler attitude towards the surrealists' tendency to scream and protest. Of course, there is the famous story of 1930 of Georgette with her cross attending a surrealist meeting, and it showed a certain *je m'en fous* on Magritte's part. There is not so much overt blasphemy in Magritte's paintings as there is, for example, in Ernst's, with his 'Good Day, Satan' and the Virgin smacking the infant Christ, although there is a picture of God sitting on a cloud with a railway engine passing underneath, a late picture.[1] His philosophy is expressed very well in that piece printed in the Sylvester catalogue about higher powers and the futility of believing in them. He had a cool attitude to everything, I think, compared with the excitable Parisian surrealists, although he made his protests from time to time.

- Amongst other things, Mesens was a collagiste and musician. Do you think he had anything to do with Magritte's collages of sheet music in 1926?

GM It's very possible. It's very interesting to talk to people unofficially and consider what they say in relation to what they say officially. Mesens always gave his reasons for giving up music as moral. This is of course, in a way, surrealist mystification, and also probably a bow in the direction of Breton, who, being tone deaf, found music unallowable, but many of the surrealists liked music. Magritte for a start was devoted to Brahms very much, did you know that?

- I thought it was Satie.

GM Oh sure he liked Satie, but Satie would be more explicable. However he liked a lot of classical music, and his brother Paul was a musician. He wrote popular music, not particularly popular, but popular in intention!

- He wrote Marie Trombone, *I believe.*

GM Yes, *Marie Trombone* indeed, which has a pretty picture on the cover by Magritte. But Mesens in fact told me that he didn't give up music for moral reasons at all; he gave up music because his father refused to support him at the Conservatoire for further study, and also that he realised that he hadn't got the mathematical intelligence needed for truly important composition. He did write some things; a poem by Philippe Soupault, called *Garage*, had music by Mesens, and Mesens' early music was performed by well-known minor opera singers of the period in recital. But he felt that if he couldn't study more he wouldn't go much further, but he remained devoted to music all his life, and would sometimes play the piano – not too brilliantly, I might say – but with terrific panache. He particularly liked playing things like *The Merry Widow*, and the sentimental music of his youth. He had a sort of tenderness towards what I suppose you would call the life of the *boulevardier*, with girls and champagne, good food and musical comedies. He liked that side of life.

- *Did he keep that up throughout his life?*
GM Not particularly, but he was always a great dandy. He wore quite dandified clothes, he adored gambling too. He would go frequently to the casino, telling me not to tell his wife, and gambled sometimes all the money he had been given for hanging an exhibition in Belgium, but sometimes he would double it. He particularly enjoyed roulette. The element of chance pleased him, and the excitement. He was a *bon viveur*, which Magritte was not. Magritte lived a very austere life. But when they were young and less established, before Magritte married Georgette, he had a studio somewhere in the middle of Brussels. Mesens once told me that Magritte would occasionally put down his brushes and palette, claiming that he had become too randy to continue to paint, and would run 'frantically' to the brothel, so that once Magritte had married Georgette he became more or less faithful. I never heard that he was otherwise. But he was certainly very interested in eroticism, albeit in a rather chilly way, perhaps, because it was never a Dalí-like ecstasy. Eroticism in Magritte is always as chilly as any other subject, but very intense for all that.

- *Eroticism in Magritte's art has not received much attention.*
GM Yes, well, he didn't deny a certain interest in the erotic, but I think he probably didn't do much about it after he was married to Georgette. It was in a way his profoundest joke to live quite so respectably. It was amazing how respectably he lived. A visit to him was like a parody of visiting a petit-bourgeois, with his good manners, his attention, the cleanness of his house, and his treatment of Georgette, which was always formal. As necessary, he paid her those little attentions that the bourgeois can sometimes extend towards his wife. It was almost like a stage play, slightly satirizing the behaviour of a good bourgeois, and yet in his mind he was the opposite. He was totally subversive of bourgeois reality and I think the effect of his paintings was increased by the fact that he played that game for forty years. By playing it he gives his pictures

the conviction that they would not have had if he had been a bearded boisterous fellow, knocking round the cafés. I don't think the pictures would have had those virtues. It was by living in that world, where the commonplace was regarded as the commonplace, and the mad was regarded as the commonplace as well, or the grotesque, that his pictures have an extraordinary conviction beyond any of the rest of the surrealists, for me.

- *You said that your first contact with surrealism was through Herbert Read's book* Surrealism.
GM Of which, I might add, I could understand not a word, but nevertheless which seemed to me the key to a type of 'Alice in Wonderland' state of mind that I was eager to achieve.

- *What could draw you to a philosophy which, unlike Cubism for example, basically left no place for music?*
GM That was Breton who left no place for music. Secondly, I'm not particularly musical. I like jazz, which was always allowed to the surrealists. Many of them were keen jazz fans, because of course they had a sometimes exaggerated respect for the primitive, as they thought, and so jazz they found permissible, probably for the wrong reasons. Many surrealists liked jazz very much. In England, for instance, Simon Watson Taylor had a magnificent collection of 78 rpm jazz records. There was no problem in that, apart from which Mesens adored classical music. So did Magritte and so did many of them. It was Breton's insistence that music was stupid, for which he managed to find a quote in Chirico, because it had no moral content, no surrealist moral content. But Édouard was a great friend of Satie and had many postcards from him in his early days. He remained a friend of Satie and never quarrelled with him.

- *So in this book you were struck by the pictures.*
GM I looked at the pictures, which struck me as both familiar and extraordinary, and I read dutifully the text, but I wasn't really to understand the philosophy behind the text for another ten years. At sixteen, it was just like drinking raw alcohol. It set everything swirling in my head and I began immediately to write surrealist poems. And I realised that surrealism was anti-religious, which was encouraging for me as I was, at a time when it was not usual to admit to it and was vaguely anarchistic, because at that time the links of the Communist Party had broken, although they were interested in Trotsky still. The three things that I found most interesting in my life at that time were jazz, surrealism and anarchism, and none of them cancelled out the others as far as I could see. In England for instance, the surrealists were friendly with the anarchists. The anarchists contributed to surrealist publications at that time, and vice versa.

- *In England there was the* London Bulletin.

GM That was before the war. The last issue was at the beginning of the war, I think. He was always intending to restart it. But Mesens, due to an extraordinary mixture of meticulousness and alcoholism, worked very, very slowly, very meticulously checking everything twenty-five times, going to the same book yet again to check measurements, and being drunk every day by three o'clock, he had to sober up in the night to work, as he worked largely at night. So to edit a magazine was for him, by this time, an immense task. But he did edit some things, *Message from Nowhere*, a few pamphlets during the war and a few afterwards. At the same time, his poems came out here, in the same edition as the poems of Éluard, and eventually his poems came out in full, not here but in Brussels. He got a great deal done, but very slowly. You see, he was a maniac of the bathroom in the mornings. He would never have an appointment before eleven although he got up at seven thirty. So at eleven thirty he would come to the gallery and be brisk and businesslike for an hour, and would then go to the pub, from which he returned at three, say, very drunk but very cheerful, very full of jokes, full of fantasy, delightful. He would stay down in the gallery for half an hour, he would then go upstairs, perhaps have another drink, and come down at about five like a fiend, picking faults with everything, shouting, making me stay after my time to do things. This was just after the war, in 1947, 1948. I'm talking about him as an employer because then I saw him very closely in a certain way and he was a sort of fiend to work for. He combined this fury, if I put a comma in the wrong place in a letter, with a demonic Dadaist fantasy in joking. One never knew which way he was going to turn. But once I left the gallery, I didn't see him too much for about five, six, seven years, even ten. Then I re-entered his life when I left the jazz world with its endless touring, and then I saw him a great deal from the beginning of the sixties until the end of his life. In the last ten years I saw him at least twice a week, and I think at the end when Sybil had died and he was very miserable, I was a comfort to him. Few people would visit him because he was often impossible and I did, every week, every Saturday when I was in London. He quarrelled with a great many people as you can imagine, and when he went to Brussels, he quarrelled with Magritte, I think, too, because Magritte made a slighting remark about his collages to someone who was going to buy one, and he came back and told him. But they made it up. He also quarrelled with Georgette before he died after Magritte's death, and they, in the end, made it up, I think. In London, towards the end, he hung about in his dressing-gown in his flat most of the day and would seldom go out. But when he went abroad, he would be out, neatly dressed, drinking with his chums like a loony, and eventually killing himself. Magritte did none of those things. He was totally constant in his behaviour.

- *When Magritte died you said, 'The stones fell to the ground'. Do you think that the world which he created died with him?*
GM Nobody else can paint another Magritte, and nobody has exactly the sense of the object that he had. What one has seen, of course, done well or badly, as the case may be, is the enormous influence of Magritte in the popular field, such as advertising. Benson and Hedges is perhaps the most obvious, and indeed one of the best. Some of the images in Benson and Hedges are not disgraceful from a Magrittian point of view, except they happen to be advertising cigarettes. Although Magritte was very indignant at being called the father of Pop painting, one sees what people meant by that. Pop painting also painted in the same vaguely realistic negligent manner, but the difference was, of course, that Magritte was aiming at poetry and contra-reality, whereas Pop painting was really saying three cheers for the most shoddy artefacts of our civilization. So, one can understand his rage at being called the father of Pop painting. The language is not dissimilar in certain cases, but the intention was absolutely different.

- *Do you think that his art has made a difference to our culture, what we see around us? You mentioned advertising. Could these things have happened without Magritte?*
GM No. Originally the influence on advertising from the surrealists was that of Dalí. Before the war you saw Dalí's influence and in many musicals of the forties one sees the influence of certain surrealists. I saw the other day an extract from a musical in which the background was a plain pinch from Chirico with arches and towers. And Dalí, both through his own collaborations and because the style was easy to copy, influenced the cinema and advertising a great deal during the thirties and forties. But Magritte did not come into his own until the end of the sixties, I would say, when you suddenly began to notice Magrittian images – the white horse in White Horse whisky looking at itself in the mirror, a wood-cutting firm that sells tools did a series in which everything was of wood – the mouse as well as the cheese – and so on. The thing that happened there was that the huge Magritte exhibition at the Tate in the sixties had a tremendous influence on the art students. Whenever you went to an art school at that time there were people dutifully painting chairs made out of clouds and so on. And these same students went into advertising, in many cases, taking Magritte with them.

- *It's ironic because Magritte started his career as a commercial artist.*
GM Well, he painted a few advertising posters and also roses on wallpaper.

- *In a BBC programme, you said that Magritte was amused by everything. Do you think that his intention was to amuse us?*

GM No, I think to startle us more. There is humour in Magritte, albeit black humour. In my poem I was obviously not saying that the stones literally fell to the ground but that he, by putting up his reality, side by side, sometimes in the same canvas, as in the variations of *La Condition humaine*, by putting up his apparently realistic reality against the real one, called the real one into question. He did, and when he stopped being there, and therefore stopped doing it, in a sense, we have his work now in the past to compare, rather than happening simultaneously alongside. Once things go into the past they become analyzed, they become history. They become values and are perhaps not as effective as when they are actually a part of life, rather than a comment on life in the past.

- *It's easy to take him as a comical figure, a Chaplin.*
GM No, he was too solemn for that in a way. He had a Chaplinesque element but if one had to compare him with a silent film comedian, I would compare him infinitely more closely to Buster Keaton, who remains solemn always and lacks Chaplin's whimsy. There is, after all, a sense of terror in Magritte, which is not present in Chaplin, but which sometimes is present in Keaton. Someone has written that it was Magritte's intention to make a brick wall as terrifying as a lion, which can happen in dreams certainly, to any of us. We are suddenly oppressed by some harmless object in a dream. One can discover it in Alfred Hitchcock, for instance, where circumstance can make an innocent object charged with menace, or terror because of the circumstances in which the object is presented, the bread-knife, for instance, in one of Hitchcock's films. A bread-knife by a loaf of bread is not in itself terrifying, but when you know one of the characters is a murderer, it is. The quality that gives Magritte his strength is his coolness, as opposed to, say Dalí, who was a hot fantasist. Magritte's coolness is what, for me, gives him that edge, the fact that everything is presented poker-faced, without comment, in a straightforward manner. When people do laugh at Magritte, as they sometimes might, when they see an obvious painting of a pipe, with the comment 'This is not a pipe' underneath it, slowly it sinks in that this is a very worrying statement because it is not a pipe. It is a painting of one and so on.

- *Consistent reference is made to Magritte's sober dress and lifestyle, and his insistence on routine and domestic tidiness. Is this, in your view, a deliberate parody of an order which he clearly upsets? Was he conscious of this?*
GM I think he was conscious of it. Mind you, to be conscious of it and to carry it through for so many years is another matter. One wonders in the end if the parody didn't become a reality. I only had one evening with him when he behaved out of character. I went to Brussels with a girlfriend and I asked him and Georgette out for the evening because I wanted to go to a little café

he had frequented in his youth, although in a different place then, but run by the same man, [Geert] van Bruaene, who was a sort of naïve peasant poet and had a café called the Café of the Golden Flower. There is a little book about him. He was a very interesting gnome-like figure. He gave the first exhibition of Ernst's collages in Brussels and he was very friendly with the surrealists. Magritte, against his pattern, came out for the evening and we went there. We drank quite a lot, including Magritte, who had this awful little dog with him, as he always had, a Loulou mark 12, or whatever it was. We had a riotous evening and by the end of the evening Magritte was quite uninhibited and funny because the taxi-man came, a gloomy taxi-man, to take him back to the rue des Mimosas, who said 'Don't let that dog go on the seat with his muddy feet'. It was raining and Magritte said 'Hmmm'. And he walked the dog deliberately up and down the gutter, which was full of muddy water and pointed at the seat. I think he himself sat on the floor of the taxi, which again of course preserves the Magrittian idea of the dog on the seat, the man on the floor, but it was done with a certain venom. He could occasionally relax. On the way to the café there was a little fair in one of the squares and I persuaded him, Georgette, myself and the girl to put our heads through one of those photographer's cut-out stands. I have the photograph of this, showing that there was an extra hole. So one hole is blank.

- *Magritte played with fire and indeed with creation as a whole. Did he want to play God?*

GM I don't think so. I think he was aware that he had understood something nobody else had. I think he had a certain pride in his thought, but I don't think he felt that he could make much effective change in the world, except, perhaps, in the way in which we look at reality. He approaches each painting in the spirit of the object lesson. This is very well carried out by those pictures in which he puts the name of another object under the representation. He felt he might affect our thought and he succeeded, because, however diluted the Benson and Hedges posters may be, nevertheless they introduced to people who may never have seen a Magritte in their lives the spirit of the paradox presented coolly. The pyramids are one of the best ones. These are what you might call exercises in the Magrittian spirit. I suspect that he would have been angry that he should be used as a form of advertisement. At the same time I feel, although they are an advertisement, they nevertheless bring to the attention of the public the paradox which Magritte insisted upon in a non-commercial manner.[2] I went to see Magritte just after the tide had turned, and people were beginning to buy Magrittes in great quantities.

- *In about 1962, I presume.*

GM Yes. I met a bourgeois woman in the rue des Mimosas when I was looking for the house and I said to the woman 'Do you know the house of Mr Magritte?' She said 'Yes, and do you know that his paintings are worth so much a metre, or centimetre?' She spoke before, I suppose, he was considered a figure of weirdness, the artist who looked like everybody else. But, once the auction room had made each picture of his worth so much a square centimetre, she was truly impressed. I told him and he laughed. I said 'Now you've become famous as the man whose pictures are worth so much per square centimetre'.

- *Was Magritte conscious of his fame or did it arrive too late?*
GM Oh no, he knew he was well-known alright, after years of being famous only to a world-wide conspiracy of extremely small dimensions. He then suddenly became somebody in every newspaper, with covers of *Scientific American* using that picture of his called *La Lunette d'approche*, the one with the open window showing it's dark outside, whereas you can see a blue sky on the glass. I think he recognized that he had become famous but I don't think it affected him an iota. In fact, he was more often bored by people wanting to go and see him, because obviously people, especially Americans, who are very earnest in their collection of people, started to try and come to see him every day and he would frequently refuse. But when I went over with Jonathan Miller to make that short film for Monitor, he was affability itself. He took the whole day to do what Jonathan suggested, sit in a chair, move around the room while the camera was stopped and restarted, so that he seemed to appear all over the room. He was fascinated by that and good tempered, although it meant the usual influx of fifty-five BBC technicians with lots of cords and wires and things.

- *I can't imagine that in that meticulously ordered house.*
GM Well, it was there for the day, and my wife was there and Jonathan Miller's wife too, but he didn't mind that. He liked girls, you know, he really liked women, I think. He was always extremely courteous and old-style towards them. And as you know, Suzi Gablik lived with the Magrittes for some time, which is again a rather difficult thing because she is a big, rangy, clumsy girl. Really very nice, but having that American ranginess, which suggests objects falling over, although they probably don't. And she lived with them. I think he probably liked that.

- *If you had to distinguish Magritte from Dalí, how would you do it?*
GM Well, I think Magritte is an infinitely more serious figure. He didn't depend on the inspiration of his madness, which meant that, when Dalí was genuinely probably rather mad between 1931 and, say, 1936, he painted some masterpieces, but at the same time he played the fool. Magritte painted totally consistently his whole life because he didn't depend on madness but on, in a

funny way, logic, albeit that he turned the logic upside down. I think his pictures were considered, whereas Dalí depended on inspiration and Dalí turned into a caricature of himself. Magritte remained constant, and for me the resonance of a great Magritte is deeper, more solid than the resonance of a great Dalí, and there are great Dalís. But they have a sort of flash to them. In the end, even the badly painted Magrittes of the early years, before he could draw very well or paint very well, grow in mystery. And I think Dalí diminishes in mystery. I can see that if you put an early Dalí next to an early Magritte, at the time, there would have been no comparison. One would have thought 'What a dull fellow', compared with this genius of appearance and lunacy. But, in the end, even the dullest Magritte of 1924, 25, 26, 27 carries for me more meaning than the best Dalí of that time.

- *And the Vache period?*

GM I think it's extremely funny, and I don't think it's that bad any more, by the way, because within the context of the work it's so extraordinary and so crackers that I wouldn't mind a Vache one. I wouldn't like a 'Renoir' one much, which was earlier wasn't it? But the Vache ones are in such frantic bad taste, they are painted with such absurd negligence that I wouldn't mind one. I like the one of the rabbit playing the drums, and the man smoking the fifteen pipes. I'm not too fond of the girl with tartan backcloth, licking her shoulder,

- Le Galet, *1948*.

GM Yes, I think if Magritte had painted nothing but Vaches his whole life, I wonder what he would be thought of. But in the context of his whole work – I hated them when I saw them, by the way, they seemed to be a total destruction of everything he stood for, but then he returned after all to his old style – as an isolated joke and as a way of irritating the French for their chauvinism, which is one of the reasons he did them, I think it's a good joke.

14 April 1981, 33 St Lawrence Terrace, London

---

[1] The citation is from Max Ernst's 'Au-delà de la Peinture' in *Cahiers d'art*, 6-7 (1937).

[2] Magritte did, however, prepare advertisements for Belga cigarettes.

LETTER TO FLOUQUET

ILLUSTRATIONS

BIBLIOGRAPHY

INDEX

René Magritte: letter to Pierre-Louis Flouquet, 1921

Cher Pierre,

Je suis 'au travail' depuis mardi, et quoique les dessins que j'ai à faire ne sont pas modernes, la besogne est tout de même intéressante, d'autant plus que dans un an on compte ne faire que des papiers peints modernes. Il y a une technique spéciale à acquérir pour ce métier, de petites choses que l'on ne soupçonne pas, des règles à connaître, et qui sont des lois d'harmonie bien déterminées. Par exemple ce premier dessin que j'ai fait n'est pas bon à cause de deux feuilles qui sont presque horizontales – en supprimer une dira-t-on? mais alors il y a un vide, il faut chercher une autre combinaison. Il faut aussi ne pas avoir de mouvement comme dans un dessin comme ceci :

Il ne faut pas qu'une feuille passe en dessous d'une fleur et cela est très juste puisque dans ce cas il y a deux plans, et que le papier peint étant décoratif les 'deux dimensions' doivent être respectées. Et tout cela en 'style modernisé' et sans fantaisie comme celle-ci : D'ici une quinzaine de jours je serai assez au courant pour toucher trois francs de l'heure – ce qui fera 600 fr. par mois environ – et je crois qu'ils auront bientôt besoin de nouveaux dessinateurs si cela te plaît tu pourrais poser ta candidature?

Entre nous ne parle plus de Georgette dans tes lettres ni de mes appointements car mon père n'a pas besoin de connaître cela, et comme il pourrait lire mes lettres incidemment, épargnons-lui ces connaissances –
A part cela comment ça va ?

à bientôt,
René

PS Je mets ton adresse sur l'enveloppe afin que si elle ne [*sic*] trouve plus à Paris tu la reçoive chez toi au cas où tu serais déjà venu en perin [*sic*, rather than 'pèlerin']

Archives de l'Art Contemporain, Brussels, 36345

Dear Pierre,

I've been 'working' since Tuesday, and even though the drawings I have to do are not modern, the task is nevertheless interesting, all the more so given that in a year's time we expect to make only modern wallpapers. You have to learn a special technique for this job, little things you wouldn't suspect, rules you have to know and which are well-established laws of harmony.

For example, this first drawing of mine is no good because of the two leaves that are nearly horizontal – why not remove one, you may say? But then there is an empty space. Another arrangement is needed. You also need to avoid movement in a drawing, as follows:

A leaf must not pass underneath a flower and rightly so since, if it were to, there would be two planes and so the 'two dimensions' of wallpaper, which is decorative, would not be retained. And all this needs to be done in a 'modernized style' and without excessive adornment, like this:

In a fortnight I'll be sufficiently knowledgeable to earn three francs an hour – which makes about 600 francs a month and I think they'll soon need new design artists. If that appeals to you, you could apply.

Between you and me don't mention Georgette in your letters or how much I'm earning, since my father doesn't need to know these things, and since he could accidentally read my letters, let's spare him from knowing these things –

Apart from that, how are things?

See you soon
René

PS I'm putting your address on the envelope so that, if you are not in Paris, you'll receive it at home in case you've already made the pilgrimage.

Illustrations

Works by René Magritte (1898-1967)

1. Buste en plâtre et fruits, 1917. Private Coll. © 2015 BI, ADAGP, Paris/Scala, Florence. DACS, London 2015
2. La Pipe [Biomorphes avec mots], 1923. Private Coll. Oil on canvas, © 2015. BI, ADAGP, Paris/Scala, Florence. DACS, London 2015
3. La Trahison des images (Ceci n'est pas une pipe), 1929. Los Angeles (CA), Los Angeles County Museum of Art (LACMA). Oil on canvas. Purchased with funds provided by the Mr and Mrs William Preston Harrison Collection (78.7), © 2015. Digital Image Museum Associates/LACMA/Art Resource NY/Scala, Florence. ADAGP, Paris and DACS, London 2015
4. Découverte, 1927. Private Coll. Oil on canvas, © 2015. BI, ADAGP, Paris/ Scala, Florence. DACS, London 2015
5. Harmonie moderne, Alfa Romeo, advertisement from *Englebert Magazine*, n° 59-60, 1924. Brussels, Bibliothèque Royale Albert 1er. Lithography © 2015. BI, DAGP, Paris/Scala, Florence. DACS, London 2015
6. Fleurs devant une fenêtre, 1920. Private Coll. © 2015 BI, ADAGP, Paris/ Scala, Florence. DACS, London 2015
7. La Retraite militaire, 1920. Private Coll. Tempera on paper, © 2015. BI, ADAGP, Paris/Scala, Florence. DACS, London 2015
8. Tête d'homme, 1920. Houston (TX), The Menil Collection. Oil on canvas, © 2015. BI, ADAGP, Paris/Scala, Florence. DACS, London 2015
9. Titania, 1948. Brussels, Musées Royaux des Beaux-Arts. Gouache and watercolour on paper, © 2015. BI, ADAGP, Paris/Scala, Florence. DACS, London 2015
10. Les Droits de l'homme, 1948. Private Coll. Oil on canvas, © 2015. BI, ADAGP, Paris/Scala, Florence. DACS, London 2015
11. L'Arc-en-ciel, 1948. Private Coll. Gouache on paper, © 2015. BI, ADAGP, Paris/Scala, Florence. DACS, London 2015
12. Femme, 1923. Private Collection/The Bridgeman Art Library. Oil on canvas, © 2015. BI, ADAGP, Paris and DACS, London 2015
13. L'Assassin menacé, 1927. New York, Museum of Modern Art (MoMA). Oil on canvas, Kay Sage Tanguy Fund. 247.1966 © 2015. The Museum of Modern Art, New York/Scala, Florence. DACS, London 2015
14. L'Homme du large, 1927. Brussels, Musées Royaux des Beaux-Arts. Oil on canvas, © 2015. BI, ADAGP, Paris/Scala, Florence. DACS, London 2015
15. Les Signes du soir, 1926. Private Collection/ Peter Willi/The Bridgeman Art Library. Oil on canvas, © 2015. BI, ADAGP, Paris. DACS, London 2015
16. Deux Sœurs 1925. Private Coll. Oil and pen and ink on canvas, © 2015. BI, ADAGP, Paris/Scala, Florence. DACS, London 2015
17. Le Mariage de minuit, 1926. Brussels, Musées Royaux des Beaux-Arts. Oil on canvas, © 2015. BI, ADAGP, Paris/Scala, Florence. DACS, London 2015
18. Le Sang du monde, 1926-7. Private Coll. Oil on canvas, © 2015. BI, ADAGP, Paris/Scala, Florence. DACS, London 2015
19. La Fin des contemplations, 1927. Houston (TX), The Menil Collection. Oil on canvas, © 2015. BI, ADAGP, Paris/Scala, Florence. DACS, London 2015
20. La Grande Famille, 1963. Utsunomiya, Utsunomiya Museum of Art. Oil on canvas, © 2015. BI, ADAGP, Paris/Scala, Florence. DACS, London 2015

21. Le Séducteur, 1953. Private Coll. Oil on canvas, © 2015. BI, ADAGP, Paris/Scala, Florence. DACS, London 2015
22. Cinéma bleu, 1925, Private Coll. Oil on canvas, © 2015. BI, ADAGP, Paris/Scala, Florence. DACS, London 2015
23. Couture Norine. Advertisement for the fashion house Norine, 1926. Private Coll. Gouache, watercolour and Indian ink, © 2015. BI, ADAGP, Paris/Scala, Florence. DACS, London 2015
24. La Festa (publicity design for Norine), 1924. Private Coll. Gouache, watercolour and Indian ink on paper, © 2015. BI, ADAGP, Paris/Scala, Florence. DACS, London 2015
25. La Fatigue de vivre, 1927. Private Coll. Oil on canvas, © 2015. BI, ADAGP, Paris/Scala, Florence. DACS, London 2015
26. Le Conquérant, 1925-6. Private Coll. Oil on canvas, © 2015. BI, ADAGP, Paris/Scala, Florence. DACS, London 2015
27. La Fenêtre, 1925. Private Coll. Oil on canvas, © 2015. BI, ADAGP, Paris/Scala, Florence. DACS, London 2015
28. Une Panique au Moyen Âge, 1927. Brussels, Musées Royaux des Beaux-Arts. Oil on canvas, © 2015. BI, ADAGP, Paris/Scala, Florence. DACS, London 2015
29. À la Suite de l'eau, les nuages, 1926. Zurich, Kunsthaus. Oil on canvas, © 2015. BI, ADAGP, Paris/Scala, Florence. DACS, London 2015
30. L'Oasis, 1926. Private Coll. Oil on canvas, © 2015. BI, ADAGP, Paris/Scala, Florence. DACS, London 2015
31. La Raison d'être, 1928. Private Coll. Gouache on paper, © 2015. BI, ADAGP, Paris/Scala, Florence. DACS, London 2015
32. Le Jockey perdu, 1926. Pastel, Indian ink and pencil on paper, © 2015. BI, ADAGP, Paris/Scala, Florence. DACS, London 2015
33. Georgette, 1926. Paris, Musée National d'Art Moderne – Centre Pompidou. Oil on canvas (pencil), © 2015. BI, ADAGP, Paris/Scala, Florence. DACS, London 2015
34. Untitled collage, 1926. Private Coll. Sheet music, photograph, watercolour and pencil on paper, 40 x 55.5 cm. © 2015. BI, ADAGP, Paris/Scala, Florence. DACS, London 2015
35. La Condition humaine, 1933-4. Washington DC, National Gallery of Art. Oil on canvas, © 2015. BI, ADAGP, Paris/Scala, Florence. DACS, London 2015
36. La Lunette d'approche, 1963. Houston (TX), The Menil Collection. Oil on canvas, © 2015. BI, ADAGP, Paris/Scala, Florence. DACS, London 2015
37. Vous ne saurez jamais 1925. Munich, Bayerische Staatsgemäldesammlungen, Sammlung Moderne Kunst in der Pinakothek der Moderne München, on loan from the Theo Wormland Stiftung (inv. L 1950). Watercolour & charcoal on paper, ©2015. BI, ADAGP, Paris. DACS, London 2015
38. Le Prisonnier, 1926. Private Coll. Oil on canvas, © 2015. BI, ADAGP, Paris/Scala, Florence. DACS, London 2015
39. Le Dormeur téméraire, 1927-8. Tate, London. Oil on canvas, © Tate, London 2010. DACS, London 2015
40. Perspective : le balcon de Manet, 1949. Oil on canvas, © 2015. BI, ADAGP, Paris/Scala, Florence. DACS, London 2015
41. Perspective : Madame Récamier de David, 1950. Ottawa, National Gallery of Canada. Oil on canvas, © 2015. BI, ADAGP, Paris/Scala, Florence. DACS, London 2015
42. Le Tombeau des lutteurs, 1960. Private Coll. Oil on canvas, © 2015. BI,

ADAGP, Paris/Scala, Florence. DACS, London 2015
43. La Sortie de l'école, 1927. Private Coll. Oil on canvas, © 2015. BI, ADAGP, Paris/Scala, Florence. DACS, London 2015
44. Les Grands Voyages, 1926. Private Coll. Oil on canvas, © 2015. BI, ADAGP, Paris/Scala, Florence. DACS, London 2015
45. Les Idées de l'acrobate, 1927-8. Munich, Staatsgalerie Moderner Kunst. Oil on canvas, © 2015. BI, ADAGP, Paris/Scala, Florence. DACS, London 2015
46. La Promenade du monstre, 1926-7. Private Coll. Oil on canvas, © 2015. BI, ADAGP, Paris/Scala, Florence. DACS, London 2015
47. Le Repos de l'acrobate, 1928. Private Coll. Oil on canvas, © 2015. BI, ADAGP, Paris/Scala, Florence. DACS, London 2015
48. Les Chasseurs au bord de la nuit, 1928. Private Collection/The Bridgeman Art Library. Oil on canvas, © 2015. BI, ADAGP, Paris. DACS, London 2015
49. Le Village mental, 1926. Private Collection/The Bridgeman Art Library. Oil on canvas, © 2015. BI, ADAGP, Paris. DACS, London 2015
50. Les Complices du magicien, 1926. Private Coll. Oil on canvas, © 2015. BI, ADAGP, Paris/Scala, Florence. DACS, London 2015
51. La Ruse symétrique, 1928. Private Coll. Oil on canvas, © 2015. BI, ADAGP, Paris/Scala, Florence. DACS, London 2015
52. L'Invention de la vie, 1928. Private Coll. Oil on canvas, © 2015. BI, ADAGP, Paris/Scala, Florence. DACS, London 2015
53. La Gravitation universelle, 1943. Private Coll. Oil on canvas, © 2015. BI, ADAGP, Paris/Scala, Florence. DACS, London 2015
54. La Naissance de l'idole, 1926. Montréal, Sobelal Inc. Oil on canvas, © 2015. BI, ADAGP, Paris/Scala, Florence. DACS, London 2015
55. La Traversée difficile, 1926. Private Coll. Oil on canvas, © 2015. BI, ADAGP, Paris/Scala, Florence. DACS, London 2015
56. Le Supplice de la vestale, 1926-7. Private Coll. Oil on canvas, © 2015. BI, ADAGP, Paris/Scala, Florence. DACS, London 2015
57. Dialogue dénoué par le vent, 1928. Private Coll. Oil on canvas, © 2015. BI, ADAGP, Paris/Scala, Florence. DACS, London 2015
58. Le Genre nocturne, 1928. Private Coll. © 2015 White Images/Scala, Florence. DACS, London 2015
59. La Promesse salutaire, 1927. Private Coll. © 2015 BI, ADAGP, Paris/Scala, Florence. DACS, London 2015
60. L'Espion, 1927-8. London, The Mayor Gallery. Oil on canvas, © 2015. BI, ADAGP, Paris/Scala, Florence. DACS, London 2015
61. L'Invention collective, 1935. Private Coll. Oil on canvas, © 2015. BI, ADAGP, Paris/Scala, Florence. DACS, London 2015
62. Entracte, 1927-8. Private Coll. Oil on canvas, © 2015. BI, ADAGP, Paris/Scala, Florence. DACS, London 2015
63. Le Viol, 1934. Houston (TX), The Menil Collection. Oil on canvas, © 2015. BI, ADAGP, Paris/Scala, Florence. DACS, London 2015
64. L'Importance des merveilles, 1927. Private Collection/Giraudon/The Bridgeman Art Library. Oil on canvas, © 2015. BI, ADAGP, Paris. DACS, London 2015
65. Le Monde poétique, 1926. Private Coll. Oil on canvas, © 2015. BI, ADAGP, Paris/Scala, Florence. DACS, London 2015
66. La Grande Nouvelle, 1926. Bogota, Galerie Fernando Quintana. Oil on canvas, © 2015. BI, ADAGP, Paris/Scala, Florence. DACS, London 2015
67. Le Double Secret, 1927. Paris, Musée National d'Art Moderne – Centre

Pompidou. Oil on canvas, © 2015. BI, ADAGP, Paris/Scala, Florence. DACS, London 2015

68. L'Âge des merveilles, 1926. Private Coll. Oil on canvas, © 2015. BI, ADAGP, Paris/Scala, Florence. DACS, London 2015
69. L'Esprit comique, 1927. The Ulla and Heiner Pietzsch Collection, Berlin. Oil on canvas, © 2015. Photo: Jochen Littkemann, Berlin. DACS, London 2015
70. La Parure de l'orage, 1928. Private Coll. Oil on canvas, © 2015. BI, ADAGP, Paris/Scala, Florence. DACS, London 2015
71. L'Âge du feu, 1927. Private Coll. Oil on canvas, © 2015. BI, ADAGP, Paris/Scala, Florence. DACS, London 2015
72. Manuscript letter, *circa* 1927. Collection Mme DeKnop, Brussels. DACS, London 2015
73. La Saison des voyages, 1927. Private Coll. Oil on canvas, © 2015. BI, ADAGP, Paris/Scala, Florence. DACS, London 2015
74. Le Démon de la perversité, 1927. Brussels, Musées Royaux des Beaux-Arts. Oil on canvas, © 2015. BI, ADAGP, Paris/Scala, Florence. DACS, London 2015
75. L'Explication, 1952. Private Coll. Oil on canvas, © 2015. BI, ADAGP, Paris/Scala, Florence. DACS, London 2015
76. Le Bon Sens, 1945-6. Private Coll. Oil on canvas, © 2015. BI, ADAGP, Paris/Scala, Florence. DACS, London 2015
77. L'Empire des lumières II, 1950. New York, Museum of Modern Art (MoMA). Oil on canvas, Gift of D. and J. de Menil. 16.1951 © 2015. Digital image, The Museum of Modern Art, New York/Scala, Florence. ADAGP, Paris. DACS, London 2015
78. Les Promenades d'Euclide, 1955. Minneapolis (MN), Minneapolis Institute of Art, The William Hood Dunwoody Fund. Oil on canvas, © 2015. BI, ADAGP, Paris/Scala, Florence. DACS, London 2015
79. La Culture des idées, 1927-8. Private Coll. Oil on canvas, © 2015. BI, ADAGP, Paris/Scala, Florence. DACS, London 2015
80. Les Marches de l'été, 1938-9. Musée d'Art Moderne de la Ville de Paris, Paris, France/Peter Willi/The Bridgeman Art Library. Oil on canvas, © 2015. BI, ADAGP, Paris. DACS, London 2015
81. Les Valeurs personnelles, 1952. San Francisco (CA), Museum of Modern Art. Oil on canvas, © 2015. BI, ADAGP, Paris/Scala, Florence. DACS, London 2015
82. Les Muscles célestes, 1927. Private Coll. Oil on canvas, © 2015. BI, ADAGP, Paris/Scala, Florence. DACS, London 2015
83. L'Apparition, 1928. Oil on canvas, © 2015. BI, ADAGP, Paris/Scala, Florence. DACS, London 2015
84. L'Usage de la parole I, 1928-9. Private Coll. Oil on canvas, © 2015. BI, ADAGP, Paris/Scala, Florence. DACS, London 2015
85. Les Deux Mystères, 1966. Private Coll. Oil on canvas, © 2015. BI, ADAGP, Paris/Scala, Florence. DACS, London 2015
86. Le Temps menaçant, 1929. Edinburgh, Scottish National Gallery of Modern Art. Oil on canvas, © 2015. BI, ADAGP, Paris/Scala, Florence. DACS, London 2015
87. L'Inondation, 1931. Brussels, Private Coll. Oil on canvas, © 2015. BI, ADAGP, Paris/Scala, Florence. DACS, London 2015
88. La Voix du silence, 1928. Private Coll. Oil on canvas, © 2015. BI, ADAGP, Paris/Scala, Florence. DACS, London 2015
89. Le Musée d'une nuit, 1927. Private Coll. Oil on canvas, © 2015. BI, ADAGP, Paris/Scala, Florence. DACS, London 2015
90. Personnage méditant sur la folie, 1928. Private Coll. Oil on canvas, © 2015.

BI, ADAGP, Paris/Scala, Florence. DACS, London 2015

91. L'Homme au journal, 1927. Oil on canvas, © 2015. BI, ADAGP, Paris/Scala, Florence. DACS, London 2015
92. Le Soupçon mystérieux, 1928. Private Collection/The Bridgeman Art Library. Oil on canvas, © 2015. DACS, London 2015
93. La Lectrice soumise, 1928. Private Coll. Oil on canvas, © 2015. BI, ADAGP, Paris/Scala, Florence. DACS, London 2015
94. La Clef des songes, 1930. Private Coll. Oil on canvas, © 2015. BI, ADAGP, Paris/Scala, Florence. DACS, London 2015
95. La Femme cachée, 1929. Private Coll. Oil on canvas, © 2015. BI, ADAGP, Paris/Scala, Florence. DACS, London 2015
96. Les Affinités électives, 1933. Private Coll. Oil on canvas, © 2015. BI, ADAGP, Paris/Scala, Florence. DACS, London 2015

Other Illustrations

97. *Au Volant. Art et littérature*, 1 (1919)
98. *Le Geste. Critique et action*, 1 (Dec. 1919)
99. Victor Servranckx, *Opus 47. Exaltation du machinisme*, 1923. Musées Royaux des Beaux-Arts de Belgique. Oil on canvas, © 2015. Photo. J. Geleyns / Ro scan. DACS, London 2015
100. *Œsophage*, 1 (Mar. 1925)
101. William Hogarth, *Whoever Makes a Design without the Knowledge of Perspective*, 1754
102. Atelier Robertson, *Le Danseur acrobatique* in *Variétés*, 2ème année, 5 (15 Sept. 1929): unnumbered plate on the fifth of six pages of illustrations inserted between pp. 322 and 323
103. Paul Nougé, *Les Buveurs* from the series *Subversion des images*, 1929-1930, Private Coll. Photograph, © 2015 Dépôt au Musée de la Photographie, Charleroi. DACS, London 2015

Photographs by the Author

104. Georgette Magritte, parlour, rue des Mimosas 97, Brussels, 1981
105. rue des Mimosas 97, Brussels, 1981
106. Georgette Magritte, first floor, rue des Mimosas 97, Brussels, 1981
107. Georgette Magritte, first floor, rue des Mimosas 97, Brussels, 1981
108. Georgette Magritte, parlour, rue des Mimosas 97, Brussels, 1981
109. Bookcase, first floor study, rue des Mimosas 97, Brussels, 1981
110. Parlour, rue des Mimosas 97, Brussels, 1981
111. Irène Hamoir and Louis Scutenaire, rue de la Luserne 20, Brussels, 1981
112. Marcel Mariën, rue Louis Hap 222, Brussels, 1981
113. Marcel Mariën, rue Louis Hap 222, Brussels, 1981
114. George Melly, 33 St Lawrence Terrace, London, 1981
115. rue René Magritte, Brussels, 1981

Bibliography

Primary sources

Archives

Archives de l'Art Contemporain de Belgique, René Magritte, 342.
Archives de l'Art Contemporain de Belgique, René Magritte, 36345.
Archives de l'Art Contemporain de Belgique, René Magritte, 36547.
B.B.C. Talks Department, unpublished transcript, Tape TLN 10 TY 903D.
Bibliothèque royale Albert-1er, René Magritte, letter to Pierre-Louis Flouquet, 1921.
Victoria and Albert Museum Library, 83226.

Private collections

Collection Evelyn DeKnop, Brussels, unpublished manuscript, René Magritte.
Estate of George Melly, unpublished manuscript, René Magritte.
Collection Andrew Murray, Norwich, unpublished manuscript, René Magritte.

Interviews and Private Correspondence

Interview, Georgette Magritte by Silvano Levy, 1981, Brussels.
Interview, Louis Scutenaire and Irène Hamoir by Silvano Levy, 1981, Brussels.
Interview, Marcel Mariën by Silvano Levy, 1981, Brussels.
Interview, Marcel Mariën by Silvano Levy, 1981, Antwerp.
Interview, George Melly by Silvano Levy, 1981, London.
Interview, Conroy Maddox by Silvano Levy, 1981, London.
Correspondence Georgette Magritte and Silvano Levy, 1974-1982.

Secondary sources

Abadie, Daniel (ed.), *Magritte* (Paris, Antwerp: Jeu de Paume, Ludion, 2003).

Ades, Dawn, *Dada and Surrealism Reviewed* (London: Arts Council of Great Britain, 1978).

Alberti, Leon Battista, *On Painting*, trans. John R. Spencer (London: Routledge, 1956).

Alberti, Leon Battista, *On Painting, On Sculpture*, trans. Cecil Grayson (London: Phaidon, 1972).

Alexandrian, Sarane, *Surrealist Art* (London: Thames & Hudson, 1969).

Allmer, Patricia, *René Magritte. Beyond Painting* (Manchester: Manchester University Press, 2009).

Alloway, Lawrence, 'Portrait of the Artist No 125', *Art News and Review*, 5(21) (14 Nov. 1953): 1.

Alquié, Ferdinand, *Philosophie du surréalisme* (Paris: Flammarion, 1955).

Altenloh, C., 'Magritte', *Copères Dinant* (1955): 17-19.

Ampoux, Georges, d', 'Magritte, prince des surréalistes belges', *Phare-Dimanche* (23 Feb. 1958): 1, 9.

Angenot, Marc, 'Objets et machines surréalistes', *Marginales*, 166-167 (Sept.-Oct. 1975): 1-12.

Apollinaire, Guillaume, 'Commencement du cubisme. Réalité, peinture pure', in Robert Delaunay, *Du Cubisme à l'art abstrait, documents inédits publiés par Pierre Francastel, École Pratique des Hautes Études, VIe section* (Paris: S.E.V.P.E.N., 1957).

Apollinaire, Guillaume, *Les Peintres cubistes. Méditations esthétiques* (Geneva: Cailler, 1950).

Aragon, Louis, *Les Collages* (Paris: Hermann, 1965).

Aristotle, *The Metaphysics* (Harmondsworth: Penguin Classics, 2004).

Arnaud, Noël *et al.*, *La Terre n'est pas une vallée de larmes* (Brussels: Didier Devillez, 1996).

Art belge, L', René Magritte (Jan. 1968).

Artley, Alexandra (ed.) *Golden Age of Shop Design: European Shop Interiors 1880-1939* (London: Architectural Press, 1975).

Arwas, Victor, *Art Deco* (London: Academy Editions, 1976).

Aspley, Keith, *Historical Dictionary of Surrealism* (Lanhan: Scarecrow Press, 2010).

Au Volant : Art et littérature, 1-4 (1919).

Baj, Enrico, 'Mesens in Italy', *Transformaction*, 10 (Oct. 1979): 40-41.

Balakian, Anna, *Surrealism: Road to the Absolute* (London: Unwin, 1972).

Barnicoat, John, *A Concise History of Posters* (London: Thames & Hudson, 1979).

Barr, Alfred Hamilton, Jnr. (ed.), *Fantastic Art, Dada, Surrealism* (New York: Arno Press, 1968).

Barrington, John, *Anthropometry and Anatomy* (London: Encyclopaedic Press, 1963).

Barron, Stephanie (ed.), *Magritte and Contemporary Art: The Treachery of Images* (Antwerp, Los Angeles: Ludion, Los Angeles County Museum of Art, 2006).

Barron, Stephanie, 'Enigma: The Problem(s) of René Magritte', in Anon., *Magritte & Contemporary Art: The Treachery of Images* (Los Angeles: Los Angeles County Museum of Art, 2010): 1-11.

Barthes, Roland, 'Eléments de sémiologie', *Communications*, 4 (1964): 91-134.

Barthes, Roland, 'Rhétorique de l'image', *Communications*, 4 (1964): 40-51.

Barthes, Roland, *Système de la mode* (Paris: Le Seuil, 1967).

Battersby, Martin, *The Decorative Twenties* (London: Studio Vista, 1969).

Bayer, Herbert, Gropius, Walter, Gropius, Ise (eds), *Bauhaus 1919-1928* (London: Secker & Warburg, 1979).

Bellmer, Hans, *Petite Anatomie de l'inconscient physique ou l'anatomie de l'image* (Paris: Le Terrain Vague, 1957).

Berger, John, 'A Way to Magritte', *New Society*, 338 (20 Mar. 1969): 450-451.

Berry, William A., *Drawing the Human Form: Methods/Sources/Concepts* (New York: Van Nostrand Reinhold, 1977).

Blavier, André, *Ceci n'est pas une pipe, contribution furtive à l'étude d'un tableau de René Magritte*, (Verviers: La Fondation René Magritte, a.s.b.l., Temps Mêlés, 1973).

Bosmans, André, 'René Magritte ou la connaissance du monde', catalogue of the exhibition *René Magritte*, Musée des Beaux-Arts, Liège (14 Oct.-10 Nov. 1960): n. pag.

Bosschère, Jean, de, 'Notes sur la peinture de Miró', *Variétés*, 3 (15 July 1928): 132-139.

Bosschère, Jean, de, *Essai sur la dialectique du dessin* (Brussels: G. van Oest, 1910).

Bounoure, Vincent, 'Le Thème de la contradiction chez Magritte', *L'Œil*, 206-207 (Feb.-Mar. 1972): 4-11.

Bouret, Jean, 'Magritte l'assembleur des impossibles', *Lettres françaises* (23 Aug. 1967): 28.

Bourgeois, Victor, 'Des Mots', *Au Volant*, 4 (1919): 60-61.

Bousquet, J., 'Et Après', *Variétés*, 9 (15 Jan. 1929): 461-464.

Boydron, Maurice, *L'Étalage* (Paris: Dessein et Tolra, 1975).

Breton, André, 'Devant le Rideau', in catalogue of exhibition *Exposition internationale du surréalisme : le surréalisme en 1947*, Galerie Maeght, Paris (1947).

Breton, André, 'Envergure de René Magritte', in catalogue of exhibition *Magritte*, Arkansas Art Center, Little Rock (15 May-30 June 1964): n. pag.

Breton, André, 'René Magritte', *Studio*, 177(908) (Feb. 1969): 70-71.

Breton, André, *Le Surréalisme et la peinture* (New York: Bretano, 1945).

Breton, André, *Le Surréalisme et la peinture* (Paris: Gallimard, 1965).

Breton, André, *Magritte. Le Sens propre* (Paris: Galerie Alexandre Iolas, 1964).

Breton, André, *Manifestes du surréalisme* (Paris: Gallimard, 1975).

Brockway, F., 'Sidelights on the Magritte Exhibition', *London Bulletin*, 2 (May 1938): 18, 23.

Broodthaers, Marcel, 'Interview imaginaire de René Magritte', *Journal des arts plastiques*, 30 (Jan. 1967): 3-5.

Brunhammer, Yvonne, *The Art Deco Style* (London: Academy Editions, 1983).

Brunhammer, Yvonne, *The Nineteen Twenties Styles* (London: Hamlyn, 1969).

Bussy, Christian, 'Le Surréalisme belge', *Magazine littéraire*, 118 (Nov. 1976): 59-61.

Bussy, Christian, *Anthologie du surréalisme en Belgique* (Paris: Gallimard, 1972).

Butor, Michel, 'Les Mots dans la peinture', in Michel Butor, *Répertoire IV* (Paris: Les Éditions de Minuit, 1974): 31-95.

Butor, Michel, 'Magritte et les mots', *Lettres françaises* (13 Nov. 1968): 7-8.

Calas, Nicholas, 'Letter to the Editor', *Arts Magazine*, 46(7) (May 1972): 24.

Calas, Nicholas, 'Pearls of Magritte', *Arts Magazine*, 46(6) (Apr. 1972): 46-49.

Calas, Nicholas, 'What is the Real Illusion?', *Art News*, 61(4) (Summer 1962): 33-34, 60-61.

Calvocoressi, Richard, *Magritte* (Oxford: Phaidon, 1979).

Cardinal, Roger, Short, Robert, *Surrealism: Permanent Revelation* (London: Studio Vista, 1970).

Carte d'après nature, La, 1-10 (Oct. 1952-Apr. 1956).

Caso, Paul, 'René Magritte : du fils de Fantômas au peintre du merveilleux', *Le Soir*, Brussels (20 Nov. 1966): 10.

Castro, Nestor, *The Handbook of Window Display* (New York: Architectural Press, 1954).

Cavalcanti, Alberto, 'Introducing E.L.T. Mesens', *London Bulletin* (1 Apr. 1938): 19.

Centaure, Le (1926-1930).

Ceuleers, Jan, Sylvester, David, *René Magritte, 135 rue Esseghem, Jette-Bruxelles* (Antwerp: Pandora, 1999).

Char, René, 'La Jeunesse illustrée : Titre d'un tableau de René Magritte', *Cahiers G.L.M.*, 6 (Nov. 1937): 52-53.

Chiavoni, Luca, Ferlisi, Gianfranco, Grassi, Maria Vittoria, *Leon Battista Alberti e il quattrocento: studi in onore di Cecil Grayson e Ernst Gombrich. Atti del convegno internazionale, Mantova, 29-31 ottobre 1998* (Florence: L. S. Olschki, 2001).

Clair, Jean, 'Le Visible et l'imprévisible', in catalogue of the exhibition *Rétrospective Magritte*, Palais des Beaux-Arts, Brussels (27 Oct.-31 Dec. 1978) & Musée National d'Art Moderne, Paris (19 Jan.-9 Apr. 1979): 21-45.

Clark, Kenneth, 'Leon Battista Alberti: On Painting', *Proceedings of the British Academy*, 30 (1944).

Clark, Kenneth, *Looking at Pictures* (London: Murray, 1970).

Clément, Catherine B., 'Lettre à Lacan ou l'oiseau pris', *Magazine littéraire*, 121 (Feb. 1977): 18-20.

Clurman, Irene, *Surrealism and the Painting of Matta and Magritte* (Stanford: Leland Stanford Junior University, 1970).

Colinet, Paul, 'Il y a Quelque Chose', in catalogue of the exhibition *Magritte*, Galerie Dietrich, Brussels (7-18 Apr. 1951): n. pag.

Colinet, Paul, 'Le Domaine enchanté', in catalogue of the exhibition *L'Œuvre de René Magritte*, Casino Communal, Knokke (July-Aug. 1962): 49-50.

Colinet, Paul, 'Pour Se Délivrer Des Explications', in catalogue of the exhibition *René Magritte*, Galleria dell'Obelisco, Rome (19-31 Jan. 1953): n. pag.

Collani, Tania, 'La Génération du sens : une lecture du Catalogue Samuel de Magritte et Nougé', *Synergies Roumanie*, 5 (2010): 233-240.

Colleye, Hubert, 'Magritte', *Métropole* (31 Jan. 1968): 5.

Communications, 4, 15 (1964, 1970).

Connolly, Cyril, 'Surrealism', *Art News Annual*, 21 (Dec. 1951): 133-170.

Correspondance (1924-1926).

Creuz, Serge, 'Journal d'un article pour journal', *Beaux-Arts*, 1166 (6 May 1967): 13-19.

Crispolti, Enrico, 'Brevi Appunti per Magritte', in catalogue of the exhibition *Magritte*, L'Attico, Rome (9-25 Jan. 1963): n. pag.

Crowet, Pierre, 'René Magritte', *Soupirail*, 1 (Feb. 1928): 19-20.

DeKnop, Anne, 'Voir Les Tableaux de René Magritte', in catalogue of the exhibition *Magritte 1898-1967*, Galerie Brachot, Brussels (29 Mar.-26 May 1979): n. pag.

DeKnop-Kornelis, Evelyne, 'Les Samedis de René Magritte ou la linguistique poétique', in catalogue of the exhibition *Magritte 1898-1967*, Galerie Brachot, Brussels (29 Mar.-26 May 1979): n. pag.

Delaunay, Robert, *Du Cubisme à l'art abstrait, documents inédits publiés par Pierre Francastel, École Pratique des Hautes Études, VIe section* (Paris: S.E.V.P.E.N., 1957).

Demarne, Pierre, 'Les Images de Magritte...', in catalogue of the exhibition *L'Œuvre de Magritte*, Casino Communal, Knokke (July-Aug. 1962): 13.

Demarne, Pierre, 'René Magritte', *Rhétorique*, 3 (Sept. 1961): n. pag.

Derrida, Jacques, *La Vérité en peinture* (Paris: Flammarion, 1978).

Distances, 1-3 (Feb.-Apr. 1928).

Documents 34, Intervention surréaliste (1 June 1934).

Dopagne, Jacques, *Magritte* (Paris: Hazan, 1977).

Dotremont, Christian, 'Nos Peintres : René Magritte', *Clarté*, 50 (16-22 Dec. 1945): 4.

Draguet, Michel (ed.), *Magritte tout en papier : collages, dessins, gouaches* (Paris: Fondation Dina Verny-Musée Maillol, Hazan, 2006).

Dypréau, Jean, 'Le Mystère de la réalité', in catalogue of the exhibition *René Magritte. Le Mystère de la réalité*, Museum Boymans-van Beuningen, Rotterdam (4 Aug.-24 Sept. 1967): 9-18.

Englebert Magazine (Jan.-Feb., Mar.-Apr. 1925).

Ernst, Max, 'Au Delà De La Peinture', *Cahiers d'Art*, 11(6-7) (1936): 149-184.

Esprit Nouveau, L', 22 (1924).

Everaert-Desmedt, Nicole (ed.), *Magritte au risque de la sémiotique* (Brussels: Facultés universitaires Saint-Louis Bruxelles, 1999).

Fait Accompli, Le, (1968-1974).

Faure, Élie, 'Preface', catalogue of the exhibition *Exposition internationale d'art moderne*, Bâtiment électoral, Geneva (20 Dec. 1920-25 Jan. 1921): 3-6.

Fazakerley, G. R., *Window Display* (London: English Universities Press, 1957).

Feuille chargée, La, (Mar. 1950).

Fierens, Paul, 'Cocteau et Chirico', *Variétés*, 5 (15 Sept. 1928): 269-270.

Fierens, Paul, *L'Art en Belgique : Du Moyen Âge à nos jours* (Brussels: La Renaissance du Livre, 1939).

Flouquet, Pierre-Louis, 'Servranckx, cet inconnu', *Fantasmagie*, 22 (Mar. 1966): 22-24.

Foucault, Michel, *Ceci n'est pas une pipe* (Montpellier: Fata Morgana, 1973).

Foucault, Michel, *Les Mots et les choses* (Paris: Gallimard, 1966).

Foucault, Michel, *Questa non è una pipa*, trans. Guido Almansi (Milan: Serra e Riva, 1980).

Francastel, Pierre, *Art et technique aux 19ème et 20ème siècle* (Paris: Éditions de Minuit, 1956).

Froment, Jean-Louis, 'Avant-Propos', in catalogue of the exhibition *Magritte*, Centre d'Arts Plastiques Contemporains, Bordeaux (24 May-17 July 1977): n. pag.

Fry, Roger, *Vision and Design* (Harmondsworth: Pelican, 1961).

Gaba, Lester, *The Art of Window Display* (London: Crowell & Studio, 1952).

Gablik, Suzi, 'A Conversation with René Magritte', *Studio International*, 173(887) (Mar. 1967): 128-131.

Gablik, Suzi, 'Le Surréalisme, Magritte et le Pop Art', in catalogue of the exhibition *Magritte*, Centre d'Arts Plastiques Contemporains, Bordeaux (24 May-17 July 1977): n. pag.

Gablik, Suzi, 'Meta-trompe l'œil', *Art News*, 64(1) (Mar. 1965): 46-49.

Gablik, Suzi, 'René Magritte: Mystery Painter', *Harper's Bazaar*, 97(3024) (Nov. 1963): 146-149, 190-191.

Gablik, Suzi, 'To Those who Interpret his Paintings...', in catalogue of the exhibition *The Vision of René Magritte*, Walker Art Center, Minneapolis (16 Sept.-14 Oct. 1962): n. pag.

Gablik, Suzi, *Magritte* (London: Thames & Hudson, 1970).

George, Waldemar, 'Morphologie du Baroque', *Variétés*, 5 (15 Sept. 1929): 341-346.

Geste-Critique et action, Le, 1-2 (Dec. 1919-2 Jan. 1920).

Gimferrer, Pere, *Magritte* (Milan: Rizzoli, 1986).

Gleizes, Albert, *Du Cubisme et les moyens de le comprendre* (Paris: La Cible, 1920).

Gleizes, Albert, Metzinger, Jean, *Du Cubisme* (Paris: Eugène Figuière, 1912).

Goemans, Camille, 'La Jeune Peinture belge', *Bulletin de la vie artistique* (1 Sept. 1926): 266-269.

Goemans, Camille, 'Magritte et ses tableaux parlants', *Beaux-Arts* (11 Feb. 1949): 8.

Goemans, Camille, *Œuvre 1922-57* (Brussels: André de Rache, 1970).

Gohr, Siegfried, *Magritte*, (San Francisco: Museum of Modern Art, 1999).

Gohr, Siegfried, *Magritte: Attempting the Impossible* (Cologne: Dumont Buchverlag Gmbh, 2009).

Gohr, Sigfried, *Magritte*, exhibition catalogue (San Francisco: Museum of Modern Art, 1999).

Gombrich, Ernst Hans, Hochberg, Julian, Black, Max (eds), *Art, Perception and Reality* (London: Hopkins, 1973).

Goodglass, Harold, Blumstein, Sheila (eds), *Psycholinguistics and Aphasia* (Baltimore: John Hopkins University Press, 1973).

Gottlieb, Carla, 'The Pregnant Woman, the Flag and the Eye: Three Motifs in Modern Art', *Journal of Aesthetics and Art Criticism*, 21(2) (1962): 177-187.

Greene, Judith, *Psycholinguistics, Chomsky and Psychology* (Harmondsworth: Penguin, 1977).

Gregory, Richard L., Gombrich, Ernst Hans (eds) *Illusion in Nature and Art* (London: Duckworth, 1973).

Gregory, Richard L., *Seeing Through Illusions* (Oxford: Oxford University Press, 2009).

Guiraud, Pierre. *La Stylistique* (Paris: P.U.F., 1972).

Hale, Robert Beverly, Coyle, Terence, *Anatomy Lessons from the Great Masters* (London: Pitman, 1977).

Hammacher, Abraham, Marie, *Magritte* (New York: Abrams, 1973).

Hawkes, Terence, *Metaphor* (London: Methuen, 1972).

Hawkes, Terence, *Structuralism and Semiotics* (London: Routledge, 2004).

Hayett, William, *Display and Exhibit Handbook* (New York: Reinhold, 1967).

Heath, Adrian, *Abstract Painting: Its Origin and its Meaning* (London: Alex Tiranti, 1953).

Hecke, Paul-Gustave, van, 'La Peinture de René Magritte', in catalogue of the exhibition *René Magritte*, Galerie Le Centaure, Brussels (23 Apr.-3 May 1927): n. pag.

Hecke, Paul-Gustave, van, 'Les Limites de la peinture', *Variétés*, 7 (15 Nov. 1929): 531-533.

Hecke, Paul-Gustave, van, 'René Magritte, peintre de la pensée abstraite', *Sélection* (Mar. 1927): 439-444.

Hecke, Paul-Gustave, van, 'René Magritte', *Le Centaure*, 1(7) (Apr. 1927): 131-133.

Herbst, René, *Devantures, vitrines, installations de magasins à l'Exposition internationale des arts décoratifs, Paris, 1925* (Paris: Moreau, 1925).

Hinde, Robert Aubrey (ed.), *Non-Verbal Communication* (Cambridge: Cambridge University Press, 1972).

Hockett, Charles Francis, 'A Note on Design Features', in Sebeok, Thomas A. (ed.), *Animal Communication* (London: Bloomington, 1968).

Hockett, Charles Francis, 'Linguistic Elements and their Relations', *Language*, 37(1) (Jan.-Mar. 1961): 29-53.

Hockett, Charles Francis, 'Logical Considerations in the Study of Animal Communication', in Lanyon, W. E. & Tavolga, W. N. (eds), *Animal Sounds and Communication* (Washington D. C.: American Institute for Biological Sciences, 1960).

Hockett, Charles Francis, 'The Origin of Speech', *Scientific American*, 203 (1960): 89-96.

Hockett, Charles Francis, *A Course in Modern Linguistics* (New York: Macmillan, 1958).

Hughes, Robert, *Atelier Magritte* (Antwerp: Ludion, 2009).

Jaguer, Édouard, 'L'ABC d'E.L.T. et les collages de Mesens', *Transformaction*, 10 (Oct. 1979): 34-37.

Jakobson, Roman, 'Closing Statement: Linguistics and Poetics', in Sebeok, Thomas A. (ed.), *Style in Language* (Cambridge, Massachussetts: M.I.T.Press, 1960).

Jakobson, Roman, 'Toward a Linguistic Classification of Aphasic Impairments', in Goodglass, Harold, Blumstein, Sheila (eds), *Psycholinguistics and Aphasia* (Baltimore: John Hopkins University Press, 1973).

Jakobson, Roman, Halle, Morris, *Fundamentals of Language* (The Hague: Mouton, 1956).

Jakobson, Roman, *Main Trends in the Science of Language* (London: Allen & Unwin, 1973).

Jakobson, Roman, *Selected Writings* (The Hague: Mouton, 1962).

Jakobson, Roman, *The Framework of Language* (Michigan: University of Michigan/Michigan Slavic, 1980).

Jameson, Fredric, *The Prison-House of Language: A Critical Account of Structuralism and Russian Formalism* (Princeton: Princeton University Press, 1972).

Jean, Marcel, *Histoire de la peinture surréaliste* (Paris: Seuil, 1959).

Jouffroy, Alain, 'La Mort de Magritte', *Les Lettres françaises* (23 Aug. 1967): 28.

Juin, Hubert, 'Images du surréalisme', *Magazine littéraire*, 121 (Feb. 1977): 66-71.

Kandinsky, Wassily, *The Art of Spiritual Harmony* (London: Constable, 1914).

Kaplan, Gilbert E., Baum, Timothy, *The Graphic Work of René Magritte* (New York: II Editions, 1982).

Kornelis, Anne, DeKnop, Evelyne & Char, René, *Magritte. 1898-1967* (Brussels: Galerie Isy Brachot, 1967).

Kubie, Lawrence S., *Neurotic Distortion of the Creative Process* (Kansas: University of Kansas Press, 1958).

Kulvicki, John, *On Images: Their Structure and Content* (Oxford: Oxford University Press, 2006).

La Révolution surréaliste, 1-12 (1924-1929).

Lacoste, Michael Conil, *Kandinsky* (Naefels: Bonfini, 1979).

Laferrière, Daniel, 'Making Room for Semiotics', *Academe* (Nov. 1979): 434-440.

Larkin, David (ed.), *Magritte* (London: Pan/Ballantine, 1972).

Latil, Pierre, de, 'Paul Broca, premier anthropologue français', *Sciences et Avenir*, 402 (Aug. 1980): 92-97.

Lauryssens, Stan, 'Le Modèle du maître', *Panorama*, 32 (6 Aug. 1974): 26-29.

Lebel, Robert, 'Avant Et Après Magritte', *L'Œil*, 159 (Mar. 1968): 28-35.

Lebel, Robert, *Magritte, peintures* (Paris: Hazan, 1969).

Lecomte, Marcel, 'L'Univers des lettres et des mots dans la peinture de René Magritte', *Revue graphique*, 9 (Dec. 1965): 294-295.

Lecomte, Marcel, 'La Cascade', *Rhétorique*, 5 (Apr. 1962): n. pag.

Lecomte, Marcel, 'La Lumière poétique', in catalogue of the exhibition *L'Œuvre de René Magritte*, Casino Communal, Knokke (July-Aug. 1962): 15.

Lecomte, Marcel, 'Les Indices de l'imposture ...', in catalogue of the exhibition *Œuvres récentes de René Magritte*, La Sirène, Brussels (17-28 Oct. 1953): n. pag.

Lecomte, Marcel, 'Quelques Tableaux de Magritte et les textes qu'ils ont suscités', *Bulletin des Musées Royaux des Beaux-Arts de Belgique*, 1-2 (1964): 101-110.

Lecomte, Marcel, 'René Magritte à travers les différents moments de son expérience', in catalogue of the exhibition *Œuvres récentes de René Magritte*, La Sirène, Brussels (17-28 Oct. 1953): n. pag.

Lepschy, Giulio Ciro, *A Survey of Structural Linguistics* (London: Faber, 1972).

Lepschy, Giulio Ciro, *Sulla Linguistica moderna* (Bologna: Il Mulino, 1989).

Levy, Silvano, 'Foucault on Magritte on Resemblance', *Modern Language Review*, 85(1) (Jan. 1990): 50-56.

Levy, Silvano, 'Magritte and the Surrealist Image', *Apollo*, 136(366) (Aug. 1992): 117-119.

Levy, Silvano, 'Magritte and Words', *Journal of European Studies*, 22(4:88) (Dec. 1992): 313-321.

Levy, Silvano, 'Magritte at the Edge of Codes', *Image & Narrative*, 13 (Nov. 2005): n. pag.

Levy, Silvano, 'Magritte, Mesens and Dada', *Aura*, 1 (Jan. 1993): 31-41.

Levy, Silvano, 'Magritte: The Uncanny and the Image', *French Studies Bulletin*, 46 (Spring 1993): 15-17.

Levy, Silvano, 'René Magritte and Window Display', *Artscribe*, 28 (Mar. 1981): 24-28.

Levy, Silvano, 'René Magritte: Representational Iconoclasm', in Silvano Levy (ed.), *Surrealist Visuality* (Keele: Keele University Press, 1996): 15-30.

Levy, Silvano, 'This is a Magritte', *The Times Higher Education Supplement*, 1,028 (17 July 1992): 18.

Levy, Silvano, 'Magritte et le refus de l'authentique', *Cycnos*, 28:1 (July 2012): 53-62.

Libero, Libero, de, 'René Magritte e il miraggio nel deserto', in catalogue of the exhibition *René Magritte*, Galleria dell'Obelisco, Rome (19-31 Jan. 1953): n. pag.

London Bulletin (Apr. 1938-June 1940).

Lyle, John, 'Mesens in England 1946-1971', *Transformaction*, 10 (Oct. 1979): 42-45.

Lyle, John, 'Mesens', *Transformaction*, 10 (Oct. 1979): 1-3.

MacAgy, Douglas, 'About the Art of Magritte', in catalogue of the exhibition *René Magritte in America*, Dallas Museum for Contemporary Arts, Texas (1960): n. pag.

Magazine littéraire, 118 (Nov. 1976).

Magritte, René, 'Deux Entretiens', *Le Fait Accompli*, 108-109 (Mar. 1974): n. pag.

Magritte, René, 'La Leçon de choses', *Rhétorique*, 7 (Oct. 1962): n. pag.

Magritte, René, 'La Proie pour l'ombre', *Le Fait Accompli*, 32 (Feb. 1970): n. pag.

Magritte, René, 'Le Garde-Fou', *Le Fait Accompli*, 76 (Dec. 1972): n. pag.

Magritte, René, 'Les Jambes du ciel', *Le Fait Accompli*, 6 (July 1968): n. pag.

Magritte, René, 'Lettres à Paul Bourgoignie', *Le Fait Accompli*, 49 (Mar. 1971): n. pag.

Magritte, René, 'Lettres à Paul Nougé', *Le Fait Accompli*, 127-129 (Nov. 1974): n. pag.

Magritte, René, 'Magritte contre Delvaux', *Le Fait Accompli*, 101 (Nov. 1973): n. pag.

Magritte, René, 'Nick Carter et cie', *Le Fait Accompli*, 23 (Oct. 1969): n. pag.

Magritte, René, exhibition catalogue *Die Kunst der Konversation* (Düsseldorf: Kunstsammlungen Nordrhein-Westfalen, 1996).

Magritte, René, *Écrits complets*, (Paris: Flammarion, 1979).

Magritte, René, exhibition catalogue *Exposition de peintures et gouaches de René Magritte* (Paris: Galerie Cahiers d'art, 1955).

Magritte, René, exhibition catalogue *Exposition René Magritte* (Liège: Musée des Beaux-Arts, 1960).

Magritte, René, exhibition catalogue *L'Œuvre de René Magritte* (Knokke: Casino Communal, 1962).

Magritte, René, exhibition catalogue *Magritte* (Bordeaux: Centre d'Arts Plastiques Contemporains, 1977).

Magritte, René, exhibition catalogue *Magritte* (Brussels: Palais des Beaux-Arts, 1933).

Magritte, René, exhibition catalogue *Magritte* (Little Rock: Arkansas Art Center, 1964).

Magritte, René, exhibition catalogue *Magritte* (Milan: Galleria Schwarz, 1962).

Magritte, René, exhibition catalogue *Magritte* (Paris: Galerie du Faubourg, 1948).

Magritte, René, exhibition catalogue *Magritte Retrospective Loan Exhibition* (London: Marlborough Gallery, 1973).

Magritte, René, exhibition catalogue *Magritte : Les Images en soi* (Paris: Galerie Iolas, 1967).

Magritte, René, exhibition catalogue *Magritte: Paintings, Drawings, Gouaches* (London: Obelisk Gallery, 1961).

Magritte, René, exhibition catalogue *René Magritte* (Brussels: Palais des Beaux-Arts, 1954)

Magritte, René, exhibition catalogue *René Magritte* (London: Tate Gallery, 1969).

Magritte, René, exhibition catalogue *René Magritte* (New York: Museum of Modern Art, 1965).

Magritte, René, exhibition catalogue *René Magritte* (Verviers: Société Royale des Beaux-Arts, 1947).

Magritte, René, exhibition catalogue *René Magritte in America* (Dallas: Museum for Contemporary Art, 1960).

Magritte, René, exhibition catalogue *René Magritte : Le Mystère de la réalité* (Rotterdam: Museum Boymans-van Beuningen, 1967).

Magritte, René, exhibition catalogue *Rétrospective Magritte* (Paris: Palais des Beaux-Arts, Brussels, Musée National d'Art Moderne, 1979).

Magritte, René, exhibition catalogue *Rétrospective René Magritte* (Ixelles: Musée des Beaux-Arts, 1959).

Magritte, René, exhibition catalogue *The Vision of René Magritte* (Minneapolis: Walker Art Center, 1962).

Magritte, René, *Imagination et imaginaire. Les Lettres à Gualtieri di San Lazzaro* (Milan: Edizioni del Naviglio, 1969).

Magritte, René, *La Destination : lettres à Marcel Mariën 1937-1962, René Magritte* (Brussels: Les Lèvres nues, 1977).

Magritte, René, *Les Couleurs de la nuit* (Brussels: Les Lèvres nues, 1978).

Magritte, René, *Les Mots et les images* (Brussels: Labor, 2000).

Magritte, René, *Lettres à André Bosmans, 1958-1967* (Paris: Seghers, Isy Brachot, 1990).

Magritte, René, *Lettres mêlées (1920-1966)* (Brussels: Les Lèvres nues, 1979).

Magritte, René, exhibition catalogue *René Magritte* (Montreal: Museum of Fine Arts, 1996).

Magritte, René, *Manifestes et autres écrits* (Brussels: Les Lèvres nues, 1972).

Magritte, René, Nougé, Paul, 'Colour-Colours or an Experiment by Roland Penrose', *London Bulletin*, 17 (June 1939): 9-12.

Magritte, René, Nougé, Paul, Gutt, Tom, *Le Catalogue Samuel* (Brussels: Didier Devillez, 1996).

Magritte, René, *Quatre-Vingt-Deux Lettres de René Magritte à Mirabelle Dors et Maurice Rapin, avec des lettres de Noël Arnaud et Georgette Magritte* (Paris: Velizy-Villacoublay, Mirabelle Dors & Maurice Rapin, 1976).

Magritte, René, *Secret Affinities: Words and Images by René Magritte* (Houston: Dominique De Menil, 1976).

Magritte, René, Souris, André, 'Entre Musique et peinture', *Le Fait Accompli*, 67

(June 1972): n. pag.

Magritte, René, Wergifosse, Jacques, 'Le Surréalisme en plein soleil', *Le Fait Accompli*, 111-113 (Apr. 1974): n. pag.

Manvell, Roger, 'Magritte and the Surrealist Image', *Humanist*, 84 (June 1969): 76-179.

Marcadé, Bernard, *Tentative de l'impossible* (Brussels: Labor, Isy Brachot, 1992).

Marcelis, Bernard, 'L'Empire des lumières', *Domus*, 591 (Feb. 1979): 49.

Marcus, Leonard, S., *The American Store Window* (London: Architectural Press, 1978).

Marie, 1-3, final issue (June-July 1926, undated).

Mariën, Marcel (ed.), *L'Activité surréaliste en Belgique (1924-1950)* (Brussels: Lebeer-Hossmann, 1979).

Mariën, Marcel (ed.), *La Terre n'est pas une vallée de larmes* (Brussels: Éditions La Boétie, 1945).

Mariën, Marcel (ed.), *René Magritte, croquer les idées* (Brussels: Les Lèvres nues, 1978).

Mariën, Marcel, 'La Charpente des mirages', *London Bulletin*, 3 (June 1938): 21.

Mariën, Marcel, 'Les Pieds dans les pas', in catalogue of the exhibition *Magritte*, Centre d'Arts Plastiques Contemporains, Bordeaux (24 May-17 July 1977): n. pag.

Mariën, Marcel, *Le Radeau de la mémoire : souvenirs détérminés* (Paris: Le Pré-aux-Clercs, 1983).

Mariën, Marcel, *Les Corrections naturelles* (Brussels: Librairie Sélection, 1947).

Mariën, Marcel, *René Magritte* (Brussels: Les Auteurs Associés, 1943).

Marlier, Georges, 'Du Métier et de l'enseignement artistique', *Le Centaure*, 9-10 (June-July 1930): 180-182.

Martinoir, Brian, de, 'Une Linguistique de l'image', *Atomes*, 24(262) (Feb. 1969): 129-130.

Masheck, Joseph, 'The Imagism of Magritte', *Art Forum* (May 1974): 54-58.

Melville, Robert, 'Inexplicable Genius', *New Statesman*, 21 (Feb. 1969): 268-269.

Menna, Filberto, *La Linea analitica dell'arte moderna* (Turin: Einaudi, 1975).

Mertens, G., 'René Magritte, peintre de l'invisible, retour d'Israël', *Pourquoi Pas?* (26 May 1966): 91-94.

Mesens, Édouard Léon Théodore, 'A Painter's World of Fantasy', *Life* (7 Sept. 1959): 6-7, 9.

Mesens, Édouard Léon Théodore, 'I Was in Marvellous Company', *Transformaction*, 10 (Oct. 1979): 11-16.

Mesens, Édouard Léon Théodore, 'Les Points cardinaux du surréalisme', in catalogue of the exhibition *Magritte, Miró, Tanguy & Ernst*, Zaal C.A.W., Antwerp (15-26 Apr. 1956): n. pag.

Mesens, Édouard Léon Théodore, 'Magritte est donc un peintre surréaliste...', in catalogue of the exhibition *L'Œuvre de René Magritte*, Casino Communal, Knokke (July-Aug. 1962): 12.

Mesens, Édouard Léon Théodore, 'The World of René Magritte', *The Saturday Book*, 19 (1959): 273-283.

Mesens, Édouard Léon Théodore, *Peintres belges contemporains* (Brussels: Éditions Lumière, 1947).

Meuris, Jacques, *Magritte* (Paris: Nouvelles Éditions françaises Casterman, 1988).

Michals, Duane, A Visit with Magritte (Göttingen: Steidl, 2011).

Michaux, Henri, *En Rêvant à Partir de Peintures énigmatiques* (Montpellier: Fata Morgana, 1972).

Mitchell, Alexander Ross Kerr, *Schizophrenia-What it Means* (London: Priory Press, 1972).

Mukařovský, Jan, 'L'Art comme fait sémiologique', *Poétique*, 3 (1970): 387-392.

Mullaly, Terence, 'Clarifying the Work of Magritte', *The Daily Telegraph* (22 Jan. 1979): 9.

Nadeau, Maurice, *L'Histoire du surréalisme* (Paris: Seuil, 1964).

Negri, Antonello, *René Magritte: Il Buon Senso e il senso delle cose* (Milan: Mazzotta, 1984).

Neve, Christopher, 'Holding a Double Mirror to Nature', *Country Life*, 145 (20 Feb. 1969): 404-405.

Newton, E., 'The Self-Sufficient Idea: Magritte and Surrealism', *The Sunday Times* (10 Apr. 1938): 15.

Noël, Bernard, *Magritte* (Paris: Flammarion, 1976).

Norine (Honorine Deschrijuer), 'Les Coulisses de la mode', *Variétés*, 4 (15 Aug. 1928): 219-220.

Nougé, Paul, 'A Cette Peinture...', in catalogue of the exhibition *L'Œuvre de René Magritte*, Casino Communal, Knokke (July-Aug. 1962): 10-11.

Nougé, Paul, 'Pour Illustrer Magritte', *Le Fait Accompli*, 34-35 (Apr. 1970): n. pag.

Nougé, Paul, *Journal (1941-1950)* (Brussels: Les Lèvres nues, 1968).

Nougé, Paul, *L'Histoire de ne pas rire* (Brussels: Les Lèvres nues, 1956).

Nougé, Paul, *La Subversion des images* (Brussels: Les Lèvres nues, 1968).

Nougé, Paul, *René Magritte ou les images défendues* (Brussels: Les Auteurs associés, 1943).

Œsophage, 1 (Mar. 1925).

Ottinger, Didier, *Magritte* (Montreal: The Montreal Museum of Fine Arts, 1996).

Ozenfant, Amédée, Jeanneret, Charles-Édouard, 'Destinée de la peinture', *L'Esprit Nouveau*, 20 (1924): n. pag.

Ozenfant, Amédée, Jeanneret, Charles-Édouard, *Après le Cubisme* (Paris: Éditions des Commentaires, 1918).

Paquet, Marcel, *Photographies de Magritte* (Paris: Contrejour, 1982).

Paquet, Marcel, *René Magritte, la pensée visible* (Cologne: Benedikt Taschen Verlag, 1993).

Passeron, René, *René Magritte* (Paris: Filipacchi, 1972).

Peirce, Charles Sanders, *Collected Papers Vols. 1 & 2* (Cambridge, Massachussetts: Havard University Press, 1960).

Penrose, Roland, Ollinger-Zinque, Gisèle, 'The Belgian Contribution to Surrealism', *Studio International*, 183(937) (Oct. 1971): 150-155.

Pfeiffer, Paul. 'L'Image de Magritte : poésie et peinture', *Journal des poètes* (Jan. 1965): 21.

Piaget, Jean, *Le Structuralisme* (Paris: P.U.F., 1974).

Pierre, José, 'Le Style E.L.T.', *Transformaction*, 10 (Oct. 1979): 30-33.

Pierre, José, *Le Surréalisme* (Lausanne: Rencontre, 1966).

Pierre, José, *Magritte* (Paris: Éditions Aimery Somogy, 1984).

Pleynet, Marcelin, *L'Enseignement de la peinture* (Paris: Seuil, 1971).

Plowman, Allan William, Pearson, Vhairi, *Display Techniques* (London: Blandford, 1966).

Podro, Michael, *Depiction*, (New Haven and London: Yale University Press, 1998).

Pontévia, Jean-Marie, 'La Portée de Magritte : remarques sur la notion d'influence', in catalogue of the exhibition *Magritte*, Centre d'Arts Plastiques Contemporains, Bordeaux (24 May-17 July 1977): n. pag.

Porteus, Hugh G., 'Surrealism', *World Review* (July 1947): 48-54.

Pourquoi Pas? (Nov. 1978).

Ragghianti, Carlo Ludovico, 'Accoucheurs de flammes', *Critica d'arte*, 1(3) (May 1954), 267-273.

Rapin, Maurice, *Aphorismes* (Viry-Châtillon: S.E.D.I.E.P., 1970).

Read, Herbert, *A Concise History of Modern Painting* (London: Thames & Hudson, 1959).

Read, Herbert, *Art Now* (London: Faber, 1933).

Reichardt, Jasia, 'René Magritte', *Apollo*, 75(440) (1961): 115.

Rhétorique, 1-12 (May 1961-Aug. 1964).

Richter, Hans, *Dada: Art and Anti-Art* (London: Thames & Hudson, 1965).

Robbe-Grillet, Alain, *La Belle Captive* (Brussels: Cosmos, 1975).

Roberts-Jones, Philippe, 'Éloge de René Magritte', *Revue de l'Université de Bruxelles* (Feb.-Apr. 1968): 231-236.

Roberts-Jones, Philippe, 'Les Poèmes visibles de René Magritte', *Bulletin des Musées Royaux des Beaux-Arts de Belgique*, 1-2 (1968): 61-90.

Roberts-Jones, Philippe, *Magritte, poète visible* (Brussels: Laconti, 1972).

Robertson, B., 'Good News from Wallonia', *Spectator* (21 Feb. 1969): 247.

Robins, Robert Henry, *General Linguistics: An Introductory Survey* (London: Longman, 1971).

Roegiers, Patrick, *Magritte and Photography* (Antwerp: Ludion, 2005).

Roisin, Jacques, *Ceci n'est pas une biographie de Magritte* (Brussels: Alice Éditions, 1998).

Roque, Georges, 'Magritte et la publicité', in catalogue of the exhibition *Magritte*, Centre d'Arts Plastiques Contemporains, Bordeaux (24 May-17 July 1977): n. pag.

Roque, Georges, *Ceci n'est pas un Magritte* (Paris: Flammarion, 1985).

Rosenberg, Sheldon, Koplin, James H. (eds), *Developments in Applied Psycholinguistic Research* (London: Macmillan, 1968).

Rosenblum, Robert, 'Magritte's Surrealist Grammar', *Art Digest* (15 Mar. 1954): 16, 32.

Rosey, Guy, 'Divagations d'un amant maladroit', in catalogue of the exhibition *Magritte : les images en soi*, Galerie Iolas, Paris (10 Jan. 1967): n. pag.

Rubin, William S., *Dada, Surrealism, and their Heritage*, exhibition catalogue (New York: Museum of Modern Art, 1968).

Samuel, S., Muller, Ch., *La Maison S. Samuel & Cie vous présente quelques modèles pour la saison 1926-1927* (Brussels: Agence Havas, 1926).

Samuel, S., Muller, Ch., *Pour l'Année 1928 la Maison Samuel nous présente quelques manteaux* (Brussels: Bischoftsheim, 1927).

Schliebler, Ralf, *Die Kunsttheorie René Magrittes* (Munich, Vienna: Hanser, 1981).

Schneede, Uwe M., *René Magritte: Leben und Werk* (Cologne: DuMont-Schauberg, 1973).

Schwartz, P. W., 'An Interview with René Magritte', *Studio*, 177(908) (Feb. 1969): 74-75.

Scruton, Roger, *Art and Imagination: A Study in the Philosophy of Mind* (Abingdon: Rougledge & Kegan, 1982).

Scutenaire, Louis, 'Down the Years with René Magritte', in catalogue of the exhibition *Magritte Retrospective Loan Exhibition*, Marlborough Gallery, London (Oct.-Nov. 1973): 11-14.

Scutenaire, Louis, 'Gloser à Propos de l'Exposition parisienne à Paris des œuvres de René Magritte est prématuré. Allons-y donc', *Au Miroir d'Elisabeth* (1948).

Scutenaire, Louis, 'J'ai toujours pensé...', in catalogue of the exhibition *Magritte : les images en soi*, Galerie Iolas, Paris (10 Jan. 1967): n. pag.

Scutenaire, Louis, 'L'Invention de la vie', in catalogue of the exhibition *Rétrospective Magritte*, Palais des Beaux-Arts, Brussels (27 Oct.-31 Dec. 1978) & Musée National d'Art Moderne, Paris (19 Jan.-9 Apr. 1979): 13-20.

Scutenaire, Louis, 'L'Œuvre peinte de René Magritte', *Savoir et Beauté*, 43 (2-3) (1961): 2415-2418.

Scutenaire, Louis, 'L'on ne sait plus trop quel sage de l'Inde...', in catalogue of the exhibition *René Magritte Rétrospective*, Musée des Beaux-Arts, Ixelles (19 Apr.-16 May 1959): 2-4.

Scutenaire, Louis, 'Le Cicerone', *Le Fait Accompli*, 76 (Dec. 1972): n. pag.

Scutenaire, Louis, 'Les Pieds dans le plat', in catalogue of the exhibition *René Magritte Peintures et Gouaches*, Galerie du Faubourg, Paris (11 May-5 June 1948): 3-5.

Scutenaire, Louis, 'Magritte n'a pas eu le désir...', in catalogue of the exhibition *L'Œuvre de René Magritte*, Casino Communal, Knokke (July-Aug. 1962): 9.

Scutenaire, Louis, 'Pour Illustrer Magritte', *Le Fait Accompli*, 24-25 (Aug. 1969): n. pag.

Scutenaire, Louis, 'Ut Pictura Poesis', *Rhétorique*, 6 (July 1962): n. pag.

Scutenaire, Louis, *Avec Magritte* (Brussels: Lebeer-Hossmann, 1977).

Scutenaire, Louis, *La Fidélité des images. René Magritte* (Brussels: Lebeer-Hossmann, 1976).

Scutenaire, Louis, *Les Pieds dans le plat, René Magritte – la période 'vache'* (Marseille, Antwerp: Réunion des Musées Nationaux, Musées de Marseille, Ludion, 1992).

Scutenaire, Louis, *Magritte* (Antwerp: De Sikkel, 1948).

Scutenaire, Louis, *Magritte* (Chicago: William & Noma Copley Foundation, 1958).

Scutenaire, Louis, *Mes Inscriptions 1946-1963* (Brussels: Brachot & Gutt, 1976).

Scutenaire, Louis, *René Magritte* (Brussels: Librairie Sélection, 1947).

Sebeok, Thomas A., *Style in Language* (Cambridge, Massachusetts: M.I.T.Press, 1960).

Shattuck, Roger, 'This is not René Magritte', *Art Forum*, (Sept. 1966): 32-35.

Shattuck, Roger, *The Innocent Eye: On Modern Literature and the Arts* (New York: Farrar Straus Giroux, 1984).

Shelley, R., 'On a Painting, Le Regard Intérieur by René Magritte', *Tiger's Eye*, 1(7) (15 Mar. 1949): 84-85.

Short, Robert, *Dada and Surrealism* (London: Octopus, 1980).

Soby, James Thrall, *René Magritte* (New York: The Museum of Modern Art, 1965).

Sonesson, Göran, *Pictorial Concepts: Inquiries into the Semiotic Heritage and its Relevance for the Analysis of the Visual World* (Lund: Aris/Lund University Press, 1989).

Spector, Jack J., 'Magritte's *La Lampe philosophique*: A Study of Word and Image in Surrealism', *Dada/Surrealism*, 7 (1977).

Spitz, Helen Handler, *Museums of the Mind* (New Haven: Yale University Press, 1994).

Sterckx, Pierre, *René Magritte. L'Empire des images* (Paris: Assouline, 2003).

Stévo, Jean, 'Le Surréalisme et la peinture en Belgique', *L'Art belge* (Jan. 1968).

Sylvester, David, 'Introduction', in catalogue of the exhibition *Magritte*, Tate Gallery, London (14 Feb.-2 Apr. 1969): 5-14.

Sylvester, David, 'Magritte', *The Sunday Times Magazine* (9 Feb. 1969): 24-31.

Sylvester, David, 'Portraits de Magritte', in catalogue of the exhibition *Rétrospective Magritte*, Palais des Beaux-Arts, Brussels (27 Oct.-31 Dec. 1978) & Musée National d'Art Moderne, Paris (19 Jan.-9 Apr. 1979): 47-76.

Sylvester, David, *Magritte* (London: Thames & Hudson, 1992).

Sylvester, David, *Magritte* (New York: Praeger, 1969).

Sylvester, David, *Magritte: The Silence of the World* (Houston: The Menil Foundation and New York: Harry N. Abrams, 1992).

Sylvester, David, *René Magritte: Catalogue Raisonné Volume 1: Oil Paintings 1916-1930* (London: Philip Wilson, 1992).

Sylvester, David, *René Magritte: Catalogue Raisonné Volume 4: Gouaches, Temperas, Watercolours and Papiers Collés 1918-1967* (London: Philip Wilson, 1995).

Sylvester, David, *René Magritte: Catalogue Raisonné Volume 5* (London: Philip Wilson, 1997).

Tate Gallery, *Abstraction: Towards a New Art*, (London: Tate Gallery, 1980).

Thévoz, M., *Le Langage de la rupture* (Paris: P.U.F., 1978).

Thomas, L., 'Un Prince des surréalistes : René Magritte', *Aux Écoutes du Monde* (15 Apr. 1955): 30-31.

Tomassoni, Italo, *Mondrian* (London: Littlehampton, 1970).

Torczyner, Harry, 'The Lucid Magic of René Magritte's Art...', in catalogue of the exhibition *René Magritte in New York*, Landry Galley, New York (17 Oct.-14 Nov. 1961): n. pag.

Torczyner, Harry, 'The Magic of Magritte', *The Art Gallery*, 7(4) (Jan. 1964): 6-11.

Torczyner, Harry, *L'Ami Magritte : correspondance et souvenirs* (Antwerp: Bibliothèque des Amis du Fonds Mercator, 1992).

Torczyner, Harry, *Magritte, le véritable art de peindre* (Paris: Draeger, 1978).

Torczyner, Harry, *Magritte, signes et images* (Paris: Draeger, Le Soleil noir, 1977).

Transformaction, 3-10 (Nov. 1970-Oct. 1979).

Twentieth Century Studies, 15-16 (Dec. 1976).

Tytell, Pamela, 'Lacan et l'anglais tel qu'on le parle', *Magazine littéraire*, 121 (Feb. 1977): 14-18.

Tytell, Pamela, *La Plume sur le divan : psychanalyse et littérature en France* (Paris: Aubier Montaigne, 1982).

Tzara, Tristan, *Œuvres complètes, Tome 1, 1912-1924* (Paris: Flammarion, 1975).

Tzara, Tristan, *Seven Dada Manifestos and Lampisteries* (London: Calder, 1977).

Umland, Anne, D'Alessandro, Stephanie, *Magritte: The Mystery of the Ordinary, 1926-1938* (New York: The Museum of Modern Art, 2013).

Variétés (May 1928-Apr. 1930).

Vasari, Giorgio, *Vasari on Technique: being the introduction to the three arts of design, architecture, sculpture and painting prefixed to the lives of the most excellent painters sculptors and architects* (London: J. M. Dent, 1907).

Verougstraete, Wilhelm, 'Magritte', *Au Large*, 2 (June 1927): 27-8.

Vial, Claude, 'Ceci n'est pas René Magritte', *Femmes d'aujourd'hui*, 1105 (6 July 1966): 22-24.

Vovelle, José, 'Des Magrittiens', in catalogue of the exhibition *Magritte*, Centre d'Arts Plastiques Contemporains, Bordeaux (24 May-17 July 1977): n. pag.

Vovelle, José, 'Magritte à Paris', in catalogue of the exhibition *Magritte*, Centre d'Arts Plastiques Contemporains, Bordeaux (24 May-17 July 1977): n. pag.

Vovelle, José, 'Un Surréaliste belge à Paris : Magritte 1927-1930', *Revue de l'art*, 12 (1971): 55-63.

Vovelle, José, *Le Surréalisme en Belgique* (Brussels: De Rache, 1972).

Waldberg, Patrick, 'René Magritte, l'inspiration et le mystère', *XXe Siècle*, 22 (Dec. 1963): 10-18.

Waldberg, Patrick, *Magritte : Peintures* (Paris: L'Autre Musée, La Différence, 1983).

Waldberg, Patrick, *René Magritte* (Brussels: De Rache, 1965).

Watson-Taylor, Simon, 'André Breton and René Magritte', *Studio*, 177(908) (Feb. 1969): 69-70.

Wergifosse, Jacques, 'La Joie de vivre', in catalogue of the exhibition *René Magritte*, Société Royale des Beaux-Arts, Verviers (19 Jan.-2 Feb. 1947): 1-2.

Wergifosse, Jacques, 'La Partie de plaisir', *Le Fait Accompli*, 99 (Oct. 1973): n. pag.

Wergifosse, Jacques, 'Les Sensations dépaysées', *Le Fait Accompli*, 104 (Jan. 1974): n. pag.

White, John, *The Birth and Rebirth of Pictorial Space* (London: Faber, 1987).

Whitfield, Sarah, *Magritte* (London: Hayward Gallery/The South Bank Centre, 1992).

Whitfield, Sarah, *René Magritte: Catalogue Raisonné Volume 2: Oil Paintings and Objects 1931-1948* (London: Philip Wilson, 1994).

Whitfield, Sarah, *René Magritte: Catalogue Raisonné Volume 3: Oil Paintings, Objects, and Bronzes 1949-1967* (London: Philip Wilson, 1994).

Whitfield, Sarah (ed.), *René Magritte: Newly Discovered Works. Catalogue Raisonné Volume VI: Oil Paintings, Gouaches, Drawings* (Brussels: Mercatorfonds, 2012).

INDEX

Page numbers in *italics* indicate illustrations. References to footnotes are preceded by n.

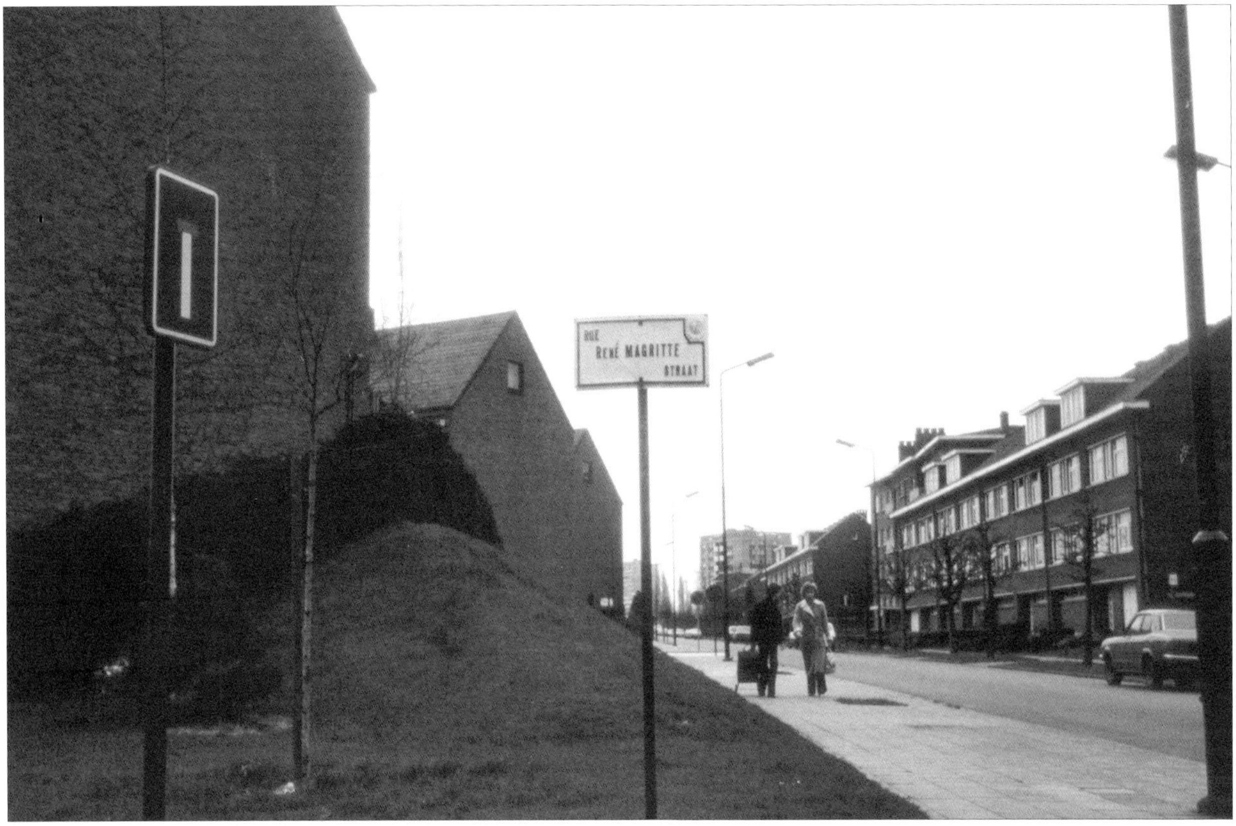
RUE
RENÉ MAGRITTE
STRAAT